PATHOLOGY AND NUTRITION

…A Guide for Professionals

written by…

LILIEANA STADLER MITREA M.D.(EUR), N.D.

COVER ART: Sorin I. Mitrea

COMPUTER DESIGN & GRAPHICS: Sorin I. Mitrea
Cornelia Ureche

LITERARY AGENT & BUSINESS MANAGER: Ernest W. Painter

Printed in Canada,
First Printing: February, 2005
First Revised Edition Printed November, 2005

Produced in co-operation with:
CSNN Publishing, A Division of Canadian School of Natural Nutrition Inc.

Email: lmitrea@healthenhance.ca

ISBN 0 – 9737549-0-7

DISCLAIMER

This book is not intended to take the place of medical advice from a trained medical professional; the author and publisher do not imply or intend that this book should in any way replace the services of a physician. Although it has been written by a trained and qualified professional, it has been prepared as a teaching tool and guide for professionals in, or entering, the complementary medicine modalities, and every prudent precaution should be exercised by such persons when assessing or preparing to provide assistance or guidance in matters of health. All information within this text is provided as reference material for information and not diagnostic or prescriptive; each and every case of illness or disease is to be carefully considered upon all of its merits, particularly the signs and symptoms of the specific individual presenting those signs.

All persons currently, or seeking to become, professionals in this field should always recognize the boundaries of their own capabilities, and never hesitate to seek, or advise the seeking of, further qualified medical advice. Ours is a profession that has no room for ego or error.

PREFACE

...To Mom and Dad with thanks and love!

Here we are again, happily now finishing off the revisions for this, the first revised edition of my very first adventure into professional writing. It has been a memorable journey for me since beginning the writing of my first edition...a time I well remember as full of ideas, inspiration and...fear! But it happened, and I was finished; I even finished it on time thanks to the help of my many friends who assisted me, and my family who supported me; heartfelt thanks again to Cornelia, Crystal, Ernie, Sorin and Sorin Jr. and all my CSNN friends. Sadly enough, I was so wrapped up in the tension and exhilaration of those finishing moments when I was reminded (two minutes to final deadline) that I should be writing a *Preface* in which I might explain the reason for writing this book, and thanking those responsible! Gulp! Well, panic again produced fruit as I rushed to acknowledge the contributions of all those people who had motivated and assisted me in its writing...*except...**Mom and Dad!*** Oops!

So now I take an appropriate, if belated, moment to share with you a sensation which most of you have likely encountered. It is the moment when we are filled with pride in our own achievements, and we mentally wander back through all the struggle and suffering which we endured to bring us to that one particular point on the journey; in fact, we are usually stuck with awe at how we persevered through all that challenge and adversity, and we not-so-humbly murmur that lesser mortals might not have accomplished what we have just mastered. At that moment, we muse, we are not such a 'bad' person after all. But success should always be dressed in modesty, accomplishment with humility, for, in most cases, we have much to thank others for our having arrived at that mighty altar.
In my case, forty-"something" years after arriving on the scene, I cannot help but look back at every one of those years and realize that there were always two people there as well as myself...always supporting, always encouraging, always loving, always motivating and...always sacrificing...*for me!* In this life, we seldom do anything of significance alone, it was not meant to be that way. We were meant to share for others, care for others, and sometimes even provide for others; it is the foundation stone of our profession and it is the foundation stone of our society. I have always been blessed with those two loving and caring parents who, now that I think back and focus upon forty odd years, were always *there*...either physically, or emotionally, and many times financially. What good fortune I have had to have been (still am!) loved and supported by two good people, people who sometimes did not seem to understand when enough had been said, but people who always somehow found time to listen to me long after I, myself, had said far too much.

Thanks, Mom and Dad! Your love has been responsible for this book, just as it was responsible for getting me to where I was competent to write it. You were not missing from my heart when I wrote the first Preface, just missing from my head amongst corrections, revisions, typographical errors and deadlines.

But then, there is a little more truth required to be told here…it was happening at a moment when I was about to go forth for the first time and produce a professional product to be studied by the eyes of many (hopefully) in my classrooms, my patients, and my peers; that was surely no place for ramblings of the heart about one's infancy and childhood memories.

But it was, and I will tell you why.

Our chosen profession in this field of health care is one that must be borne, carried, and expressed…*from the heart!* We must all resist the pressures of modern-day stress for performance, numbers, and quick fixes and choose, instead, to proceed *from the heart.* The path you have chosen, as have I, requires us to be constantly vigilant in our approach to our learning and our practice, to be always open to new ideas, new findings, new approaches, new truths. We must be bold but careful in the ways we choose to assist our fellow man; we must spare no effort to provide a service based upon excellence, a skill based upon knowledge—our society depends upon us, and we can justify no less. We must resist the temptation to memorize results and strive, instead, to master understanding. When errors are made, as they always are, we must step forth and wisely set them right…it is our profession, it is our duty, it is our choice. I encourage you to continue your chosen path with courage and devotion; I challenge you to walk that path with curiosity and wisdom.

Our children will depend upon us for this.

Lilieana

FOREWORD

GENERAL THERAPEUTIC APPROACH

It is important for all of us, as practicing professionals in the complementary alternative modalities, to remember that while we continue to strive to improve our knowledge, our techniques, and our acceptance in the modern-day world of western health and medicine, we must constantly be aware of our role in this industry in that most of us are neither medical doctors nor naturopathic doctors. Our role is to provide competent professional guidance to those who seek our assistance; the more we work at improving our knowledge and our techniques, the more help we will be able to provide unto the community, the more it will accept us, even to embrace us and grant us a position of respect within their health outlook. It is therefore imperative that we all learn to be aware of, and understand, our limitations, and when the involvement of other health professionals should be sought or recommended. There is no dishonor in knowing one's limits as long as one knows their capabilities. Throughout this text you will see that I have carefully attempted to distinguish between gaining additional knowledge versus exceeding beyond the realm of our expertise. It is also a skill to know more than what we outwardly show. With this in mind, I offer you the following general comments.

General therapeutic approach to disease:

As a rule of thumb, every time when you approach therapeutically an imbalance or a disease, please keep in mind that, ideally, you should take into consideration the following:

- Assess the individual, not the imbalance or disease;

- When you design a nutritional protocol, take into consideration all the factors that may have contributed to the apparition of the imbalance/disease, not only the etiologic factors (for example, acne is a skin infection, etiologically speaking, but the condition will be much worse when the client is exposed to stress or when the liver does not function properly);

- Do your best to approach the condition from two points of view: apply the proper protocol for the given condition and support the body at the same time (of course that vitamin C in increased dosage is very beneficial for the immune system, but if your client goes through stress at the same time, you will do well to remember to take care of his/her nervous system as well);

- Always begin with a general cleanse: *liver* (to make sure that toxins are being eliminated from the body), *digestive system* (to ensure proper nutrient digestion and absorption) and *blood* (metabolized toxins are being released in the blood stream);

- If your client is going through stress and/or they are suffering from a chronic disease, keep in mind *Adrenal support*;

• Approach your client from three points of view: *diet* (after all, you are nutritionists… who knows better than you?), *supplementation* and *other approaches* (stress management, exercise, meditation, support groups, walks in the park, etc.);

Try to respect the ***Basic principles*** of nutritional protocols:

1. **Synergy** of nutrients (vitamin C benefits from the presence of bioflavonoids);
2. **Completeness** (apply the correct dosages according to your client's needs);
3. **Biochemical individuality** (diabetes requires a certain nutritional protocol, that may be different from the one you apply for Rheumatoid Arthritis);
4. **Lifestyle dynamics** (you will need more antioxidants if you live in a polluted city as opposed to what you would need if you lived far away, where the air is very clean!);
5. **Precision** (apply the correct dosages taking into consideration toxicity and side effects)
6. **Physiological dynamics** (you will need a certain amount of proteins if you are a body builder that you would not need if you lead a sedentary life).

As for this particular book, allow me to emphasize a few aspects:

- I took the liberty to present a few medical emergencies to you, so you are able to take the necessary precautions, or, if the need arises, to take action; if you ever recognize a medical emergency, do not hesitate and advise your client to seek medical attention immediately;
- The supplements doses presented to you throughout the book are suggested, generally accepted dosages for an adult; they do not apply for children; as mentioned above, assess every client individually and apply your knowledge accordingly;
- The supplement list sometimes contains the words: "*as prescribed*", instead of a dosage; this is due to the great variety of supplements out there, as different companies will suggests different supplements forms with the appropriate dosages;
- You will find, throughout the text, that we follow a pattern: we start with what causes the diseases, then we analyze, when applicable, how does the disease happen, then how does it look like from a clinical point of view (symptoms/signs), and finally, we present the nutrition and holistic approach; for those particular diseases that are not accompanied by a nutritional and holistic protocol, do apply the general supportive measures listed above; even when we can not help a lot, the least we can do is to support the body;
- I have been asked many times by students if we can "cure" a disease; this is a strong word with great implications; my strong belief is in balance; I do know that, when provided with the right food, the right nutritional support and the right frame of mind, a person can be and should be in balance. My aim is always to provide support so the body and the mind can do their magic work. Do not forget that healing comes, ultimately, from within;
- The assessment tables that present the medical assessment in a left column (which assesses the presence of a disease) and the nutrition assessment in a right column (which assesses a possible imbalance) are not to imply that numbers that coincide are, by any means, a comparison between the medical and the nutritional assessment; I merely wished to point out how well we are equipped to prevent the apparition of a disease (so you don't get to go through all those diagnosis procedures in the left column!). These charts are to be read as stand-alone only columns.

Legend of symbols

Diagram

Table

Nutrition and holistic approach

Separates sub-chapters (for example, for the Integumentary system, this symbol will separate the infectious conditions from the allergic conditions; sub-chapters are introduced by the following symbol: ◆)

Separates the general presentation of a system (introduction, important nutrients, assessment), from the pathology of the system; also, for easy identification of subjects, it may separate subdivisions of the same sub-chapter

Signals the end of a chapter

Medical emergency!! Attention!!

TABLE OF CONTENTS

CHAPTER 1

INTRODUCTION TO PATHOLOGY

THE CELL AND THE CELLULAR ENVIRONMENT

Pathology is the study (from the Greek word "*logos*") of suffering (*pathos*). It is actually a science that links the human physiological processes with the clinical practice and with the changes responsible for various diseases that occur at cellular, tissue and organ level.

The science of Pathology is divided into two main categories:

- *General pathology,* which studies the basic, general reactions of cells and tissues to various abnormal stimulations (i.e.: inflammation, cell death, free radical injury, etc.);
- *Special pathology,* which studies the reactions of specialized tissues and organs to various abnormal stimulations (specific disease processes: pneumonia, myocardial infarction, etc.).

A disease process will always be approached from four points of view:

1. **Etiology** (cause) of disease
    - Intrinsic (genetic)
    - Acquired (infectious, nutritional, mechanical, chemical, environmental, etc)
2. **Pathogenesis** (description of the pathological mechanisms responsible for the occurrence of disease)
3. **Morphologic changes** (the structural modifications at cellular, tissue and organ level)
4. **Clinical aspect** (the functional consequences of the structural modifications)

Definitions and terminology:

- **Homeostasis**: a tendency to balance, stability in the physiological processes;
- **Hypertrophy**: enlargement of an organ or organ part due to increase in size of its cells;
- **Atrophy**: decrease in size of cells;
- **Hyperplasia**: increase in cell number;
- **Dysplasia**: abnormal changes in the size and shape of cells;
- **Acute:** severe symptoms and a short course;
- **Chronic**: lasting for a long time (weeks, months);
- **Symptoms**: subjective evidence, as perceived by a person (headache, abdominal pain);
- **Sign**: objective, noticeable and /or measurable evidence pertaining to a person's status (rash, fever);
- **Onset**: beginning, debut;
- **Syndrome:** a set of symptoms occurring together, co-existing;
- **Generalized (systemic):** applied to the whole body;
- **Localized (organic):** applied to a specific organ/part;

- **Prophylaxis**: prevention;
- **Maintenance**: preserving what has been achieved.

Following there is a short list with the most frequently used prefixes and suffixes, their meaning, and some examples. Hopefully, this list will explain some of the medical terminology we encounter as we study medicine. Most of these words come from the Greek language.

Algia: pain (neur*algia*)	**Angi:** vessel (*angio*graphy)
Ankyl: crooked (*ankyl*osis)	**Carcin:** cancer (*carcin*ogen)
Cyan: blue (*cyan*osis)	**Cyt:** cell (*cyto*plasm)
Dys: bad, improper(*dys*biosis)	**Endo:** inside (*endo*crine)
Exo: outside (*exo*crine)	**Gest:** carry (*gest*ational)
-glia: glue(neuro*glia*)	**Gyn:** woman(*gyn*ecology)
Hem: blood (*hem*oglobin)	**Hepat:** liver (*hepat*itis)
Hyper: above, more (*hyper*secretion)	**Hypo:** under, less (*hypo*secretion)
Macro: long, large (*macro*nutrient)	**Mega:** great (*mega*doses)
Micro: small(*micro*nutrient)	**Phleb:** vein (*phleb*itis)
Poly: much, many (*poly*peptides)	**Scler:** hard (*scler*osis)
Soma: body (*soma*tic)	**Stoma:** orifice (colo*stomy*)

Table 1.1- Frequently used prefixes and suffixes

As a general principle, all organs and organ parts injury, manifested by disease, begin with **cellular modifications.**
CELLULAR INJURY: occurs when the limits of adaptation to a stimulus are exceeded or when adaptation is not possible.

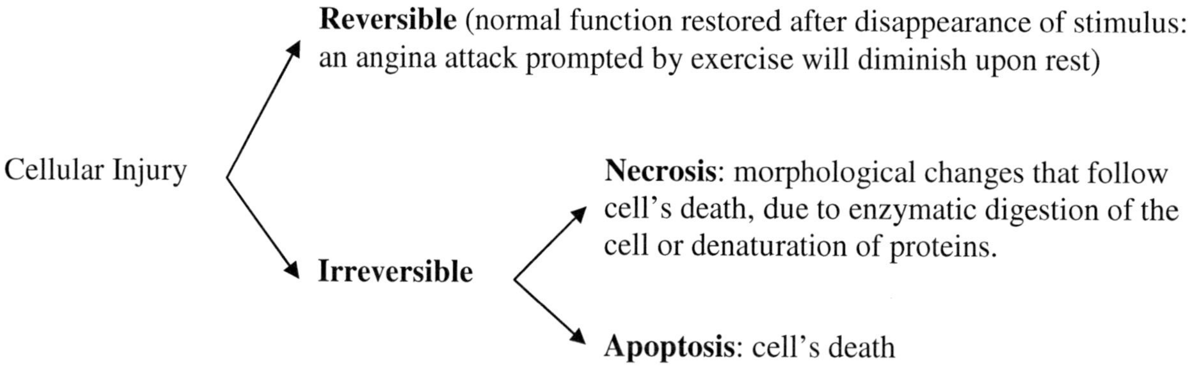

Diagram 1.1- Classification of cellular injury

Causes of Cellular injury:

- **Hypoxia** (lack of oxygen): due to decreased hemoglobin and/or decreased oxygen carrying capacity of cells, poisons, cardio-vascular diseases;

- **Physical agents**: trauma, temperature changes, changes in atmospheric pressure, electrical shock;
- **Nutritional imbalances**: macronutrient and micronutrient deficiencies or excesses (malnutrition, atherosclerosis, diabetes);
- **Chemical agents and drugs**: alcohol, tobacco, drugs, various medications, heavy metals, etc.;
- **Infectious agents**: viruses, bacteria, fungi, parasites, etc.;
- **Immunologic reactions**: such as anaphylactic shock or true allergies;
- **Genetic defects** and/or trends.

Mechanisms of cell injury:

1. **Ischemic** (lack of circulation) and **hypoxic** (lack of oxygen): can cause variable degrees of cellular membrane damage, decrease in ATP production, decreased protein synthesis, cellular swelling;
2. **Free radical damage**: causes lipid peroxidation (oxidation of fats) of plasma membranes and/or oxidation of protein structures;
3. **Chemical injury**: cause membrane damage and formation of free radicals.

When we take a look at the causes of cellular injury, knowing how important it is to keep our body healthy, we can not help but notice that the health and well being of our entire organism depends on the health and well being of our cells.
We can start our journey to health by making sure that we provide proper nutrition at cellular level; all macronutrients (proteins, carbohydrates and quality lipids) are absolutely necessary.
Vitamins and minerals are equally important for various physiological processes and to sustain metabolic and enzymatic reactions.

Important nutrients for the cellular health

Nutrient	Role
Vitamin B_2	➢ Cell respiration and growth
Vitamin B_6	➢ Formation of red blood cells
Vitamin B_{12}	➢ Cell formation
Biotin	➢ Cell growth
Vitamin E	➢ Attacks free radicals in cellular membranes
Vitamin C	➢ Attacks free radicals in body's fluids
Folic acid	➢ Acts in the formation of DNA and RNA
Coenzyme Q10	➢ Increases cellular oxygenation

Table 1.2- Important nutrients for the cellular health

Cells of the same type will form tissues. Tissue health relies on cellular health, but it can also benefit from a few additional measures:

1. **EPITHELIAL TISSUE (EPITHELIUM):** the lining, covering and glandular tissue. *Vitamin A* promotes the integrity and healing of **all** epithelial surfaces

2. **CONNECTIVE TISSUE:** connects body parts and is composed by many types of cells and fibers (collagen fibers health and maintenance depends on the presence of *vitamin C, magnesium and silicon*).

   Bone health will depend on adequate levels of *calcium, phosphorus, vitamin D, proteins,* (for osteocalcin production, which is the calcium binding protein that makes up the bone matrix), and *vitamin C* (needed for collagen fibers formation).

   Blood (the only fluid connective tissue in the body) requires *proteins* (for hemoglobin), *iron, vitamin B_{12}, folic acid* and adequate level of *stomach acid* (in order to be properly absorbed, iron has to be first ionized by the stomach acid).

3. **MUSCLE TISSUE:** specialized to contract and produce movement, requires *calcium, magnesium, sodium, potassium, proteins, carbohydrates and EFA's;*

4. **NERVOUS TISSUE:** conducts impulses from one part of the body to the other and it needs a vast array of macro and micronutrients; among the the most important ones are: *proteins, carbohydrates, EFA's and vitamin B complex.*

THE CELLULAR ENVIRONMENT is composed by fluids, electrolytes, acids and bases

Water: medium in which all other nutrients are found. Our bodies are 60% water.

Functions:

- Main component of body fluids: blood, lymph, digestive juices, urine, sweat;
- Involved in almost every bodily function: circulation, digestion, absorption, etc.;
- Maintains blood volume, transports oxygen, nutrients, waste products;
- Thermo-regulator: prevents overheating (dehydration affects body's normal activities);
- Shock absorbing and joint lubricating properties: water is a major constituent of synovial fluid;
- Homeostasis, enzymatic and neurological functions; vitally important in metabolism;
- Muscular movements depend on water presence;

Water distribution in the body:

Intracellular fluid (ICF): contained inside the cells

Extracellular fluid
ECF (outside of cells)

- Interstitial: outside of the cells, not inside blood vessels.
- Intravascular: inside the blood vessels: the plasma compartment of blood

Diagram 1.2- Water distribution in the body

TBW (total body water): the sum of all fluids in the body. Water moves between the fluid compartments by filtration, osmosis and diffusion.

Alterations in water movement:

EDEMA: accumulation of fluid within the interstitial space, due to an increase in forces favouring fluid movement from the capillaries and lymphatic vessels into the tissue.

PATHOGENESIS:

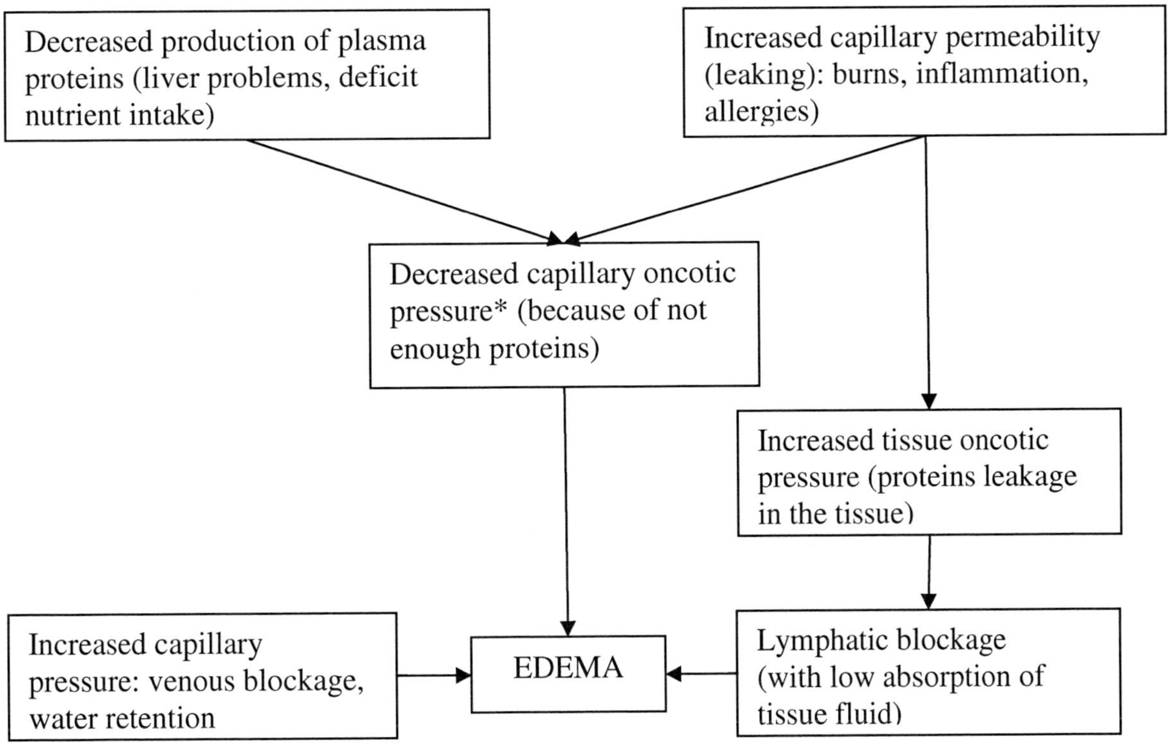

Diagram 1.3- Pathogenesis of edema

*oncotic pressure: due to the presence of colloids (small particles, usually proteins) in a solution.

Clinical manifestations:

1. Localized
   - At the site of trauma (swelling finger)
   - Within a particular organ (pleurisy, ascites)
2. Generalized

> **Note**: Generally, edema associates with weight gain, tight fitting shoes and clothes and limited movement of the affected area.

WATER AND ELECTROLYTE BALANCE

Electrolytes: substances that conduct an electrical current in solution.
Water and sodium balance are closely interrelated.

Water balance: Kidneys absorb more or less water and reclaim ions according to hormonal signals:

- ADH (antidiuretic hormone): responsible for the reabsorption of water at kidney levels when the blood volume is too low.
- Aldosterone: increases reabsorption of sodium at kidney level in response to diminished circulating blood volume; where sodium goes, water will follow.

*more on water balance in the *Endocrine system* and *Cardio-vascular system* chapters

ACID-BASE BALANCE

Our bodies are kept in a continuous balance by homeostatic mechanisms. For us to be healthy, we must be in balance. An important aspect pertains to the acid/base balance of the body, which is illustrated by pH.

pH = concentration of hydrogen ions in the body fluids.
Optimal, neutral (from a chemical point of view) **= 7;** a pH scale ranges from 0 to 14.
Acidic solutions: pH less than 7
Basic/alkaline solutions: pH more than 7

Various body fluids have different pH levels. For example:

- Your gastric juice has a pH of 1.6-1.8,
- The pancreatic juice is alkaline (pH is 7.5-8),

- Saliva is acidic (pH is 5.5-6.9),
- The bile is alkaline (pH is 7.8-8.6) ,
- The urine is acidic (pH is 5.5-6.9) and
- Blood is alkaline (pH is 7.35-7.45)

Please, keep in mind when you look at a fluid's pH that a value below the lowest value of that fluid's pH would have an acidic tendency and, respectively, a value above the highest value of that fluid will have an alkaline tendency. For example, if the blood pH would be 7.34, this means that the blood turned acidic.

REGULATION OF BLOOD pH:

- *Kidney mechanisms*:
  - By secreting (eliminating) bicarbonate ions when pH is basic (alkaline);
  - Reabsorbing bicarbonate ions when pH is low, acidic; (bicarbonate is a base);

  Blood pH: 7.35-7.45
  pH > 7.45: basic, alkaline
  pH <7.35:acidic
- *Blood (chemical) buffers :* tie up excess H ions or bases temporarily; consist of a weak acid and a weak base. When the buffer encounters a strong acid, the weak base part will combine with the strong acid, diminishing the acidity level (an acid will remain acid, as in pH). Consequently, when the buffer encounters a strong base, the weak acid part of the buffer will combine with the strong base, diminishing its alkalinity level.
- *Respiratory Centers:* modify blood pH by retaining CO_2 or by eliminating CO_2 from blood (CO_2 is transported in an acidic form)

It is very important to maintain internal balance (homeostasis). When it comes to acid/base balance, diet is crucial. Our aim should be to alkalinize the body as opposed to acidifying it (it is considered that cancer and chronic diseases are an image of the body's tendency to acidity).
Just as a reminder: fruits and vegetables are alkaline, whereas meats, grains, dairy and refined carbohydrates are acidic. The answer stays in the word: **balance.**

CHAPTER 2

ENVIRONMENTAL DISEASES

Environment means everything that surrounds us, including that which we create or allow existing by way of lifestyle, and is able to influence the manner in which we survive. Consequently, we proceed upon the basis that every disease that is not genetic is likely based upon an environmental factor. On the other hand, it is obvious that genetic diseases, whereas not caused by environmental factors, could be influenced by them (think about genetic errors in metabolism or familial hypercholesterolemia).

We will discuss some genetic diseases in the "Genetic Diseases" chapter; now we will approach the study of how the environment (may it be soil, water, air or food) can be responsible for the development of diseases.

A. AIR POLLUTION RELATED DISEASES

It is said that, from an environment point of view, we are limited in the amount of control we have over our own health. The only aspect we can really control is the food we eat. Otherwise, most environmental factors remain largely beyond our own control, such as the air we breathe. Viruses, bacteria, gases, fumes, and various particles that are present in the air have the potential of harming our respiratory system in various and sometimes, insidious ways. We will not discuss here industrial pollutants; they will be approached with the respiratory system.

A vast array of symptoms may be due to **environmental pollutants,** starting with a dry, persistent cough (a sign of bronchial irritation) and progressing to asthma, emphysema, and, unfortunately, lung cancer. At this time, it is difficult to assess the long-term effects of these pollutants, but there is growing concern that a high amount of respiratory irritants/pollutants may be responsible for various diseases.

Another aspect is the quality of ***indoor air***. Chemicals, asbestos, molds, dust, dust mites, fumes, debris, may all be responsible for future allergic responses, spanning from simple allergic rhinitis to asthma.

One of the worst toxic inhalants is **tobacco**. The tobacco leaf is chemically "enriched" in cigarettes. A smoker will inhale thousands of potentially harmful chemicals. Unfortunately, cigarette smoking has been proven to be responsible for the development of deadly diseases like lung cancer, COPD (Chronic Obstructive Pulmonary Disease), myocardial infarction and atherosclerosis.

B. CHEMICAL AND DRUG-RELATED DISEASES

Chemicals may harm the body in many ways: insidious (by accumulation), accidents, self-administered agents, catastrophes (like industrial spillage). People will experience a vast tableau of symptoms/signs, starting from the very simple (tiredness, insomnia, rashes, etc) and ending with major complications. No body system can escape the effects of chemical injury. In some situations, chemicals may affect one body system more than the others, but it is not unheard of to have the entire body responding negatively, by displaying disease, when exposed to chemicals and/or drugs (for example, recreational drugs effects).

Large attention has been paid lately to **ADR's (Adverse Drug Reactions).** Many are the drugs that can harm us in various ways. In some situations, people may experience various degrees of allergic reactions (from rash to anaphylactic shock). Even worse, most of the commonly used drugs, may they be pharmaceutical agents or not, are accompanied by a vast array of side effects. It is also worth keeping in mind that sometimes, when many chemical agents are used at the same time, we may be experiencing symptoms of side effects of drug interaction.

Among the non-therapeutic agents, attention should be paid to ***alcohol*** intake. Sustained consumption is responsible for liver and nervous system toxicity. Also, the cardio-vascular system and the pancreas may be affected by alcoholism.

The use of ***street drugs*** (cocaine, heroin, marijuana, to name just a few) is responsible for a great variety of disease processes, starting with neurological complications, transmitted infections, behavioral problems and ending up with cardiac arrest.

Heavy metal toxicity is another source of concern, because, in most of the cases, it takes precise diagnosis techniques and findings in order to diagnose with certainty the presence of heavy metals in the human body. Unfortunately, the symptoms of heavy metal toxicity are so extensive (neurological, cardio-vascular, digestive, etc) that it is quite difficult to be precise as to which metal causes each symptoms, especially when there are situations (quite frequent) involving more than one metal. The most frequently accused culprits are lead and mercury. But these two metals are just a few.

Very seldomly one can be assessed on the clinical picture alone. In most cases, the symptoms and signs just suggest that there may be a problem. Extensive investigations (urine testing, blood testing) have to be performed. If heavy metal toxicity is proven, there are quite a few methods of releasing the toxic metals from the body. One involves intravenous therapy (a procedure named Chelation), using chemical agents named EDTA and DMPS. (*See appendix H.)*

The other method employs sustained liver detoxification associated with high doses of vitamin C (which is a weak chelator itself), garlic, cilantro and sea algae, either spirullina or chlorella.

C. PHYSICAL INJURIES

C1. Mechanical force:

Injuries due to mechanical forces can affect the whole body, from lacerations (irregular cuts in the skin layers) and abrasions (which are just scrapes), to contusions (injury caused by a blunt force, causing bleeding but not affecting the continuity of the tissue), to gunshots wounds and massive car accidents. Sometimes only the skin and its underlying tissues are affected, sometimes the injuries caused by mechanical factors are dramatically more severe.

C2. Temperature changes:

Injuries related to *temperature changes* fall into two categories: high heat or hyperthermic and low heat (hypothermic) injuries.

C2a. HYPERTHERMIC INJURIES

1. SYSTEMIC: represented by **Heat stroke**, abnormal increase in body temperature over 40°C, which can occur during febrile events, upon exposure to high temperatures and in exertion conditions (sports players, people who work in heat conditions). Age extremes (very young and very old) and chronically ill people are much more affected. Heat acts by dehydration and by scrambling the protein sequence.

2. LOCALIZED: represented by **Burns**. They are frequently caused by radiation, electricity and chemical exposure and are classified according to the extent of the lesion, in surface and in depth.

***First** degree burns*: are limited to the epidermis, causing redness and discomfort to touch;
***Second** degree burns:* apply to the first two layers (epidermis and dermis) of the skin and manifest themselves with redness, sensitivity, blisters and pain;
***Third** degree burns:* affect all layers of the skin and often the underlying tissues. They are quite serious in nature. The systemic manifestations of burns are quite worrisome: when a high quantity of body fluid is lost, one may go into hypovolemic (low fluid) shock. Also, it is important to remember that burn lesions can also undergo infection.

After first aid and emergency treatments are appropriately applied, **a nutritional approach** can be employed as well, as follows:

- Amino acid complexes, important in tissue healing;
- Vitamins A, B, C, Zinc, and EFA's: all-important in tissue repair and skin health;
- Coenzyme Q10: for circulation improvement and tissue healing.

The following are mostly topical (local) agents:

- Aloe vera speeds up healing and repairs tissues;
- Goldenseal is a natural antiinfectious agent, particularly useful when there is superimposed skin infection;
- Slippery elm helps heal tissues.

C2b .HYPOTHERMIC INJURIES *(Low temperature)* can be **localized** (frostbite) to **systemic** or generalized hypothermia. They are caused by intense exposure to cold and humid conditions or impaired thermoregulation. Among the precipitating factors, a few can be named: substance abuse, especially alcohol, **dehydration,** poor food intake and/or debility. Symptoms can range from shivering, to lethargy, loss of movements and confusion (as low temperatures slow down the metabolic rate). This is usually a medical emergency and has to be handled with care.

C3.Changes in atmospheric pressure

These injuries could be due to:

- *High altitudes,* where the air is rarefied, thin, and gas exchange can be somehow impaired, affecting the cellular metabolism; people may experience dizziness, impaired circulation (because of increased blood viscosity) and, in rare cases, confusion and mental symptoms;
- *Decompression,* encountered in sea divers and underwater workers, can result in bubble gas formation in the blood stream with potential embolism consequences (pulmonary, CNS, inner ear).

C4.Electrical injuries

These injuries, which are caused by the passing of an electrical current throughout the body, may range from no effect or minimal effect on the body, to disruption of nervous transmission and heat production. Lesions could be limited to the skin and its layers or they could be dramatic, resulting in vessel rupture, coagulation and death. Attention should be paid to the fast increasing electro-magnetic stress, which affects our lives in an insidious but constant way: cellular phones, electronic equipment, wires, etc, all release electro-magnetic waves which can disturb the fine homeostatic mechanisms of our bodies.

C5. Radiation related injuries

Radiation is usually encountered in medical settings for diagnosis purposes. Accidental radiation should also be mentioned. Lately, though, the world's population seems to become increasingly worried over the potential carcinogenity of radiation exposure and, also, as to the long term effects of radiation. The direct consequence of radiation exposure is the possibility of mutations, affecting the DNA, with subsequent development of various cancers. The blood elements and lymphatic system are very sensitive to radiation exposure, as are the lungs, the reproductive and the gastro-intestinal systems.

CHAPTER 3

GENETIC (INHERITED) DISORDERS

Introduction:

The nucleus of the cell contains the mechanisms of inheritance: DNA, or deoxyribonucleic acid. While the cell is resting, its genetic material resides inside the nucleus as Chromatin (all DNA molecules and the proteins associated with them). When the cell divides, the genetic material becomes organized in chromosomes. Humans have 23 pairs of chromosomes (one of these pairs is the sex chromosomes pair). Genes are DNA fragments located on chromosomes.

A **mutation** is an inherited alteration of the genetic material (inherited from one's parents and also possibly inherited from an abnormal cell division). Mutations can interfere with protein synthesis at various levels. Substances that can cause mutations are called mutagens. Some examples are: toxins, poisons, drugs, high temperatures, and high level of oxidative stress.

Disorders associated with structural proteins defects:

1. **Marfan syndrome:** disorder of the connective tissue of the body, manifested by changes of the skeletal system, eyes, mitral valve prolapse. It results from mutations in the fibrillin gene (fibrillin is a glycoprotein secreted by fibroblasts and it is part of the extracellular matrix).

2. **Ehlers-Danlos syndromes:** genetic defect in collagen synthesis and structure. Skin is too extensible and the joints are hyper mobile.

Receptor proteins disorders:

1. **Familial hypercholesterolemia:** caused by the mutation of a gene responsible for the encoding of the LDL receptor. Consequently, cholesterol levels will be increased and these individuals are at increased risk for cardio-vascular disorders.

Enzymes defects disorders:

1. **Tay-Sachs disease**: caused by an inability to metabolize gangliosides; this results in motor and mental deterioration, beginning at the age of six months. In most cases, a cherry red spot may appear on the macula of the eye. The disease has a short time span and a negative prognosis. Usually, death occurs at the age of 2 or 3 years.

2. **Niemann-Pick disease**: caused by accumulation of sphingomyelin and cholesterol, manifested by severe neurologic involvement, progressive wasting and death within the first three years of life.

3. **Mucopolysaccharidoses (MPS):** caused by deficit in degradation of mucopolysaccharides (glycosaminoglycans). This is a progressive disorder with multiple organ involvement, characterized by retarded growth, skeletal deformities, and cardio-vascular complications. Death occurs at 6 to 10 years of age.

4. **Glycogen storage disease:** defect in the synthesis or catabolism of glycogen. Three different forms are encountered: hepatic, myopathic and miscellaneous, with various organ system involvements.

5. **Adrenoleukodystrophy (ALD)** is due to lack of an enzyme that breaks down long chain fatty acids. It is recommended to avoid intake of these fatty acids. Lorenzo's oil (erucic acid) has been used for these cases.

6. **Phenylketonuria:** absence of an enzyme that metabolizes phenylalanine; causes mental retardation. Low phenylalanine diet is recommended

Cytogenetic disorders:

1. **Down syndrome**: caused by a chromosomal defect. It is the leading cause of mental retardation. A 90 day study with L-acetylcarnitine (20 mg for every 2 pounds of body weight) resulted in increased visual memory and attention.

Cytogenetic disorders involving sex chromosomes:

1. **Klinefelter syndrome** (male hypogonadism) is a genetic disease involving sex chromosomes. It is the principal cause of male infertility (reduced spermatogenesis associated with morphologic changes in the testes).

2. **Turner syndrome** (female hypogonadism) is another genetic disease involving sex chromosomes. Secondary sex characteristics do not appear at puberty. This syndrome is the main cause of primary amenorrhea.

CHAPTER 4

THE IMMUNE SYSTEM

The study of the immune system is definitely fascinating. After all, this is the system that protects us from external invasion and from culprits that our bodies create. In order to understand how our immune system works, we will begin by reminding you of a few basic concepts.

A. THE LYMPHATIC SYSTEM

Consists of:

- Lymphatic Vessels: which run together with the blood vessels and drain waste leaked from blood capillaries. The fluid contained in the lymphatic vessels is called **Lymph** and it circulates in a one-way fashion only, toward the heart. Eventually, after the lymph goes through a cleaning process, it is being returned to the venous system;

- Lymph nodes: they are clustered along lymphatic vessels and their role is to filter the lymph. As lymph travels through the lymphatic vessels, it will pass through the lymph nodes, which are strategically situated throughout the body, draining precise body territories. When a disease process is under way, the lymph nodes that drain the part of the body that houses the disease will swell up, (lymphadenopathy) informing us that something is going on. The lymph nodes contain two types of cells: Macrophages, which engulf and destroy pathogens, and Lymphocytes, which are cells of the immune system, as we will see later on.

- Other lymphoid organs:
  1. **Thymus:** very active while we are young, is responsible for Lymphocytes T maturation (gaining immunocompetence);
  2. **Spleen:** destroys aged or abnormal red blood cells;
  3. **MALT** (Mucosa Associated Lymphatic Tissue) prevents the invasion of pathogens at respiratory and digestive system level): pharyngeal tonsils, Peyer's patches in the intestines, lymphatic nodules in the respiratory tract.

B. THE BODY'S DEFENSE has three levels:

1. **FIRST LINE OF DEFENSE** consists of anatomic barriers: skin and mucosal membranes, sebaceous glands (sebum has bacteria-killing properties), tears, saliva, hydrochloric acid, vaginal acidity. In order for a pathogen (invader) to gain access inside our body, the first line of defense has to be broken down.

2. **THE SECOND LINE OF DEFENSE** consists of various cells and chemicals that do their best to minimize the effect of pathogen invasion:
   - **Phagocytes** (macrophages and neutrophils) which engulf and destroy pathogens;

- **NK** (Natural Killer) cells, destroy virus infected and malignant cells;

- **Antimicrobial proteins:**

  ▲**Complement** (produced by the liver, involved in the destruction of pathogens by various mechanisms: cell lysis, agglutination, etc.); and

  ▲**Interferon** (group of glycoproteins secreted by virus infected cells; prevent viruses to multiply inside other cells).

- **Fever:** is a protective mechanism that promotes healing by increasing the metabolic rate and by stimulating the liver and spleen to store iron and zinc that bacteria uses for multiplication, thus rendering these nutrients unavailable for bacterial species.

- **Inflammation:** it is a process that occurs in vascularized (rich in blood vessels) tissues. It prevents the spread of injury, disposes of pathogens and promotes resolution and healing. It is a non-specific response, because it manifests in the same way, regardless of the type of pathogen that enters the body. The inflammatory process starts with cell injury:

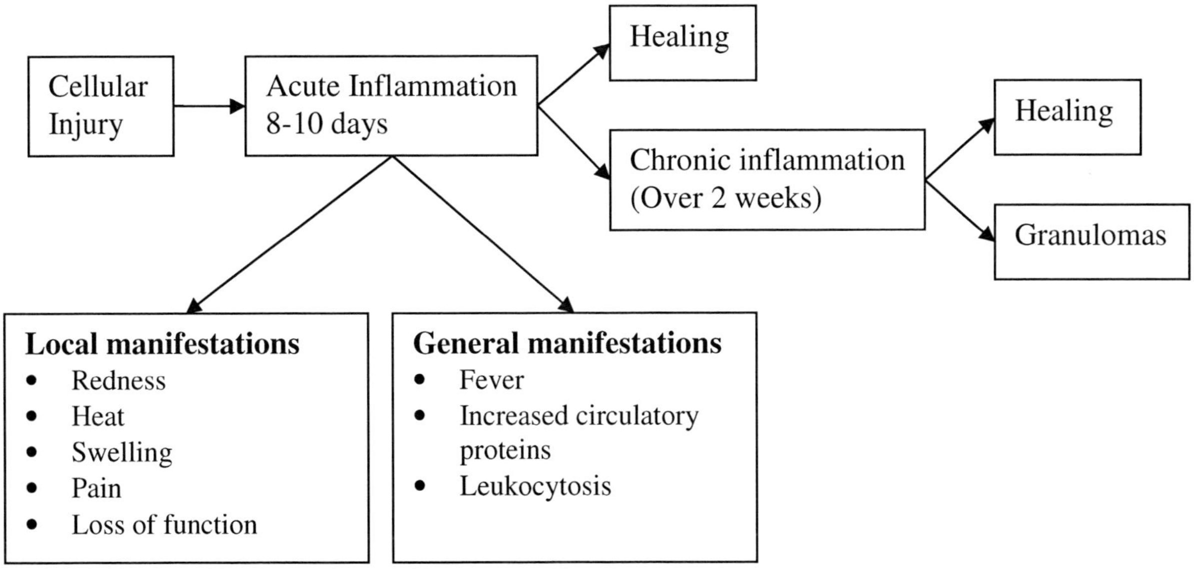

Diagram 4.1: The Inflammatory Process

When the cellular environment sustains an injury, various chemicals are released (kinines, serotonin, histamine), resulting in **vasodilation,** (which in turn is responsible for the *heat* and the *redness* at injury level) and in **increased capillary permeability**, which allows intravascular fluid to flow in the interstitial space and create *edema* (swelling).

The last described process is called exudation, and the inflammatory fluid is an exudate. When the exudate is rich in destroyed cells and cellular debris, it is called **pus**.

The swelling will press on the local nerve endings and the end result is *pain*. On top of the four main signs of inflammation: *redness, heat, swelling and pain*, another factor that is being mentioned is *loss of function.*

Very soon, hungry neutrophils will come into the area and start engulfing and destroying pathogens. These cells can last only for a short length of time, as they are **acute phase fighters.**

Sometimes after a few hours, neutrophils will be replaced by monocytes, which, in tissues, turn into hungry **macrophages.**

Macrophages are very strong phagocytic cells. Their intracellular environment is rich in lysosomes, organelles containing enzymes capable of destroying pathogens. As the invaders are being destroyed, the macrophage will carry small particles of the pathogen on their surface and it will present them to the lymphocytes, for recognition; (becoming **Antigen-presenting cells)**

One of the most important roles of inflammation is to **prevent the spread of injury.** This is accomplished thanks to the presence of **clotting proteins** and **fibrin nets**, which wall off the area. Local heat will allow for increased metabolic rate and will set the parameters for healing.

Normally, after a maximum of 8-10 days, the healing should occur. Repair mechanisms are set in place and body functions will be restored to normal.
Sometimes, though, the virulence of the infectious agents and/or the host's weak terrain may postpone the healing and **chronic inflammation** develops.

Chronic inflammation is characterized by the presence of inflammatory markers, tissue destruction and attempts to healing, which happen at the same time.
Such inflammation can happen under certain conditions:

- *Persistent infections*, by various microorganisms;
- *Prolonged exposure* to internal (plasma lipid components) or external (non-degradable materials, like particles of coal) toxic substances.

Chronic inflammation may be followed by healing or by **granulomas** formation (local area of chronic inflammation, characterized by the presence of modified macrophages). It is characteristic in diseases like tuberculosis, sarcoidosis, and leprosy.

Suppuration (pus formation) is a form of inflammation characterized by presence of pus exudate (dead neutrophils, cells and edema fluid). Certain bacteria always produce pus (pyogenic bacteria). Some forms of suppuration are:

A. Abscess: localized pus collection caused by suppuration in a tissue or organ;
B. Ulcer: localized loss of tissue, produced by the sloughing off of inflammatory tissue.

The body can repair by **regeneration**, which means repair of the tissue by the same type of cells, or by **fibrosis** (scar formation). The inflammation process is very closely linked with the repair mechanisms.

3. THE THIRD LINE OF DEFENSE is your immune system, which is very specific and always acts against a particular culprit (pathogen).

Your immune system works in two ways: by activity of the cells of the immune system (lymphocytes and macrophages) and by involvement of various chemicals (complement) and antibodies production. If we are resistant to disease, it is said that we achieved **immunity.**

The immune system will respond to a threat by eliciting an **immune response**, which is highly *specific* (developed against a particular pathogen, and only one at a time), *generalized* (once you develop immunity, it protects your whole body against the particular pathogen, not only the organ system that was sick), and thirdly, it *"remembers"* the pathogen, so the next encounter with the same pathogen will not catch us unprepared against it.

Let us move one step forward and define two very important elements of the immune system:

- **Antigens**: large molecules that your body does not recognize as belonging to it (nonself) and consequently, it will consider them "foreign" and start a defense against them. Not only microorganisms are considered antigens, but any large molecule (proteins, carbohydrates,) that does not fit the physiological model of the human body.

- **Antibodies** (immunoglobulins/Ig): plasma proteins that can fight against a particular antigen. On top of the antibodies that are created against a particular pathogen, your body has a few classes of immunoglobulins designed to offer general protection:

Classes of antibodies (Immunoglobulins)	Location and function
IgA	Mucus, saliva, tears, gut and mother's milk, bathe the body's surface and prevent pathogen entry
IgG	Plasma. Can cross placenta
IgE	Involved in allergies and reactions to parasites

Table 4.1- Classes of antibodies

To do its work, the immune system enlists the help of two types of cells:

Lymphocytes
- **T**: mature in Thymus and destroy intracellular pathogens
- **B**: mature in Bone marrow and are responsible for antibodies production

Summary:

Once a foreign agent gets access inside our bodies (for example, the flu virus), it will have to break through the first line of defense in order to harm us.

As soon as the first line of defense is broken, cells and chemicals will step in, eliciting an **inflammatory response**. During inflammation, macrophages turn into *antigen presenting cells* and they will carry their burden, for recognition, to Lymphocytes.

If the culprit is new to our bodies, lymphocytes B will create **specific antibodies** against it and it will store them for future use. At this time, lymphocytes T and other cells and chemicals will destroy the flu virus.

Let us just say, for the sake of the argument that next year **the same strain** of flu virus decides to visit us again. It will still have to break through the first line of defense (which, in this case would be the respiratory mucosa), and then it will elicit inflammation again (in this case, runny nose, fever, etc).

Following inflammation, macrophages will turn again into *antigen presenting cells* and they will carry this flu virus to the lymphocytes. The lymphocytes B will take a look, and then realize that there are antibodies already stored against this virus.

Upon release, the antibodies will destroy the antigen in many possible ways (in some cases, it will dig holes in its membrane, in other cases, it will make it clump, in other cases the complement will step in and take care of the bug. And this will be the end of this strain of flu virus…this time!

PATHOLOGY OF THE IMMUNE SYSYEM

CAUSES OF IMPAIRED IMMUNE SYSTEM:

1. **Stress** impairs the immune system in two ways:

    - by weakening the adrenal glands, which in turn will be able to deal with stress less and less, creating a vicious cycle;

    - by slowing down or shutting down the digestion , which opens the door for disturbances at digestive system levels, resulting in maldigestion (improper digestion) with subsequent malnutrition.

2. **Improper nutrition**: lack of nutrients will allow for malfunctioning of the immune system, because the building blocks necessary for creating immune system cells are missing;

3. **Malabsorption and maldigestion,** which are consequences of digestive system imbalances (leaky gut, dysbiosis, candidiasis, hypochlorhydria); if the digestive system is excessively permeable or/and if the transit is too slow or affected by disease processes, then large, abnormal molecules resulted from improper digestion will be allowed to be absorbed from the gut into the circulation; the immune system will attack and try to destroy them, becoming weaker and weaker as the abnormal molecules continue to be released into the circulation (more information on the digestive system in the *Digestive system* chapter)

4. **Improper liver function**:

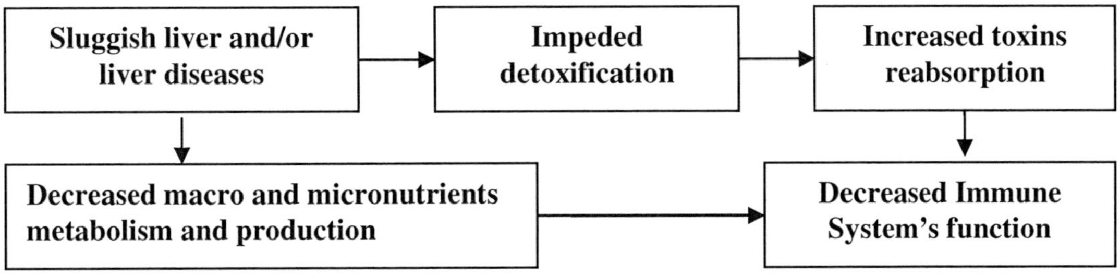

Diagram 4.2-The relationship between improper liver function and immune system pathologies

5. **Chronic diseases**, due to the impact on the adrenal glands by the stress levels;

6. **Drugs**: (antibiotics, steroids drugs) by different mechanisms: some affect the digestive system's functions, some depress the function of the elements of the immune system;

7. **Toxins, pollutants, infections**: release "foreign" molecules in the human body, which the immune system has to attack and destroy.

SIGNS OF IMPAIRED IMMUNE SYSTEM:

- Fatigue;
- Repeated infections;
- Allergic reactions, autoimmune diseases;
- Slow wound healing.

SUPPORTING THE IMMUNE SYSTEM:

A. Lifestyle:

- Decrease/avoid smoking;
- Decrease/avoid alcohol consumption(decreases white blood cells mobilization to areas where they are needed);
- Decrease/avoid sugar intake(decreases the destroying power of phagocytes);
- Decrease fat intake (too much fat will impede white blood cells' movement to areas where they are needed);
- Good sleep;
- Regular meals;
- Proper body weight;
- Regular exercise;
- Adequate water intake.

B. Nutrition

B1. IMMUNE SYSTEM BUILDERS: build the elements of the immune system

- **Proteins:**
  1. Decrease occurrence of bacterial and parasitic infections;
  2. Stimulate macrophage activity;
  3. Support cell-mediated immune response;
  4. Antibodies (immunoglobulins) are proteins.
- **Vitamins:**
  1. Vitamin A: antioxidant, necessary for normal T cell metabolism, required specifically for IgA production; strengthens mucous membranes;
  2. Vitamin B_6: required for conjugation in the Liver (breaking toxins);
  3. Vitamin B_{12} and folic acid: T-cell and B-cell production;
  4. Vitamin E**:** antioxidant, normal immunoglobulines production;
  5. Vitamin C: antioxidant, effect stronger in the presence of bioflavonoids; collagen production; normal adrenal function; normal killing activity of macrophages.
- **Minerals:**
  1. Zinc: reproduction of DNA, increased cell-mediated immune response, increases NK cells activity, increases macrophages activity; part of most of the enzymatic processes in the body;
  2. Iron: involved in normal cell-mediated immune response, antibodies production;
  3. Copper: needed for macrophage/monocyte function;
  4. Selenium: antioxidant properties, part of an enzyme (*gluthatione peroxidase*) that helps eliminate free radicals; involved in cell-mediated immune response and macrophages activity.
- **Fatty Acids:**
  1. Stabilization of cell membranes;
  2. Antibodies production;
  3. Anti-inflammatory properties;

B2. IMMUNE SYSTEM BOOSTERS: boost the existing immune system

- Antioxidants: protect the immune system from the effects of excess free radical damage;
- Echinacea: activates complement activity; stimulates antibodies production, increases phagocytosis, has anti-tumour effects, encourages suppuration; do not use it for more than 5-7 days, because it may depress the immune system upon prolonged usage;
- Astragalus**:** enhances phagocytosis and interferon production; promotes T-cell maturation and increases IgA levels; contains glyconutrients and Quercetin;
- Ligusticum and Reishi: mushrooms that boost a compromised immune system;
- Garlic: natural antibiotic, antibacterial, antiviral; involved in liver detoxification;
- Exercise.

DISORDERS OF IMMUNITY

1. HYPERSENSITIVITY REACTIONS can manifest as multiple disease processes, spanning from the classic allergy and ending up with the anaphylactic shock. They can affect practically every organ system in various ways. When we react to an antigen by having an allergic reaction, the antigen is called an **allergen**. We are exposed to two allergen categories:

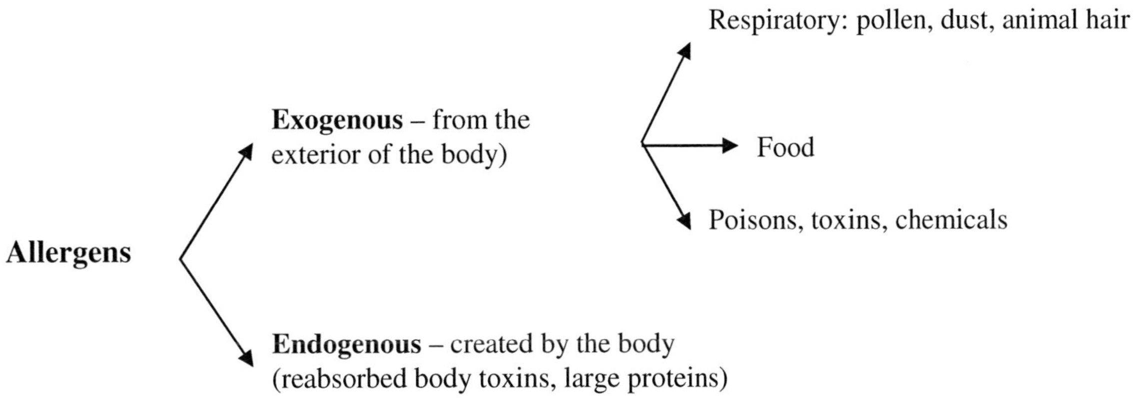

Diagram 4.3-Allergens

Allergies are states of altered reactivity of the immune system.
When it comes to the mechanism of action, there are four main types of allergic reactions

Types of allergic reaction	**Type 1: Immediate hypersensitivity; atopic or anaphylactic**	**Type 2: Cytotoxic antibody**	**Type 3: Immune complexes**	**Type 4: Delayed hypersensitivity**
Antibodies involved	IgE	IgG	IgG	T-cells
Mode of action	IgE attach to mast cells promoting release of histamine ,resulting in vasodilation, bronchoconstriction;	IgG react to surface antigens of whole cells, exposing them to phagocytosis or lysis (breaking down);	IgG reacts with soluble antigens, forming **Immune complexes**, that cause complement fixation;	T-cells react to an allergen and cells are damaged in the process
Examples	Hives, allergic rhinitis,allergic asthma, anaphylactic shock	Autoimmune, haemolytic anaemia, graft rejections, drug reactions	SLE, food allergies, rheumatoid arthritis	Contact dermatitis

Table 4.2- Allergic reactions

Nutrition and holistic approach for allergies:

- Identify the presence of allergic terrain (food allergies, environmental allergies) and make sure that you do your best to avoid the substances and the environmental factors to which you are reacting;
- Employ all lifestyle measures as described above, under *Supporting the Immune System;*
- Good vitamin-mineral formula with added antioxidants;
- Do be careful with use of immune system boosters (they may increase the reactivity of the immune system);
- It is very important to address the health of the liver and the digestive system status, as directed by the client's condition (liver detoxification and support, slow digestion, treatment of hypochlorhydria, leaky gut, candidiasis, etc.);
- Support the health of the adrenal glands, as they are involved in the stress response

2. AUTOIMMUNE DISORDERS: are caused by immune reactions against self (when your immune system identifies structures and molecules belonging to it-*self*- as *nonself*)**;**

Autoimmune diseases can affect
- *Single organs or cell type:* Hashimoto thyroiditis, multiple sclerosis
- *Systemic:* SLE (lupus), Rheumatoid arthritis

Following you will find a few examples of autoimmune diseases. More will be discussed when we study the organ systems of the body:

- SCLERODERMA: antibodies against skin and connective tissue: subcutaneous sclerosis with deformity, multiple organ involvement;

- OTHER EXAMPLES: multiple sclerosis, rheumathoid arthritis, Grave's disease, myasthenia gravis, etc.

Nutrition and holistic approach: do follow the same advice as for the hypersensitivity reactions, but do not forget to take into consideration the particular organ system that is affected. Again, as with the allergies, you can slowly build an immune system, but do not boost it, as it already is in a state of over reactivity.

CHAPTER 5

INFECTIONS AND INFECTIOUS DISEASES

Infection means invasion and multiplication of microorganisms in body tissues.

Factors that influence infection:

- Mechanism of action (i.e:toxin release, using cell's own metabolism as viruses do, etc);
- Infectivity: ability of pathogen to invade and multiplicate in the host's tissues;
- Pathogenity: ability of a pathogen to produce a disease;
- Virulence: potency of a pathogen;
- Immunogenity: ability of a pathogen to induce an immune response;
- Toxigenity: ability of a pathogen to elicit toxic reactions.

Bacteriemia (septicemia): proliferation of microorganisms in blood.

INFECTIOUS DISEASES (See Appendices A-1, A-2, & A-3);

Infectious agents:

- **Viruses**: intracellular pathogens; they damage the cells by entering the cell and replicating at the host's expense (over 400 known virus species);
- **Bacteria:** has a cell wall; they damage the host cell either by adherence to the cell or by releasing toxins (staphylococcus, streptococcus, salmonella, shigella);
- Mycoplasma, Rickettsia, Chlamydia classes: similar to bacteria, sensible to antibiotics;
- **Fungi**: produce spores or budding yeast cells (hyphae);
- **Protozoa;** single cell organisms that have motility (Entamoeba, Giardia);
- **Helmints / worms;**

How microorganisms cause disease:

- They can come in contact or enter host cells and directly cause cell death;
- May release toxins that kill cells at distance, or enzymes that degrade tissue components or damage blood vessels;
- Induce host cellular responses that may damage the cell.

Infection Stages:

- <u>INCUBATION</u>: the time between exposure to pathogen and onset of symptoms; highly contagious; duration depends on the type of microorganism involved and the host resistance; you don't feel a thing…yet;
- <u>PRODROM:</u> very early signs of disease, non specific symptoms (for example fever, chills, fatigue, when you get the flu);

- FASTIGIUM: acute stage of disease, manifestation of characteristic symptoms (sneezing, running nose, cough);
- CONVALESCENCE: recovery period, symptoms subside.

Classification of Infections:

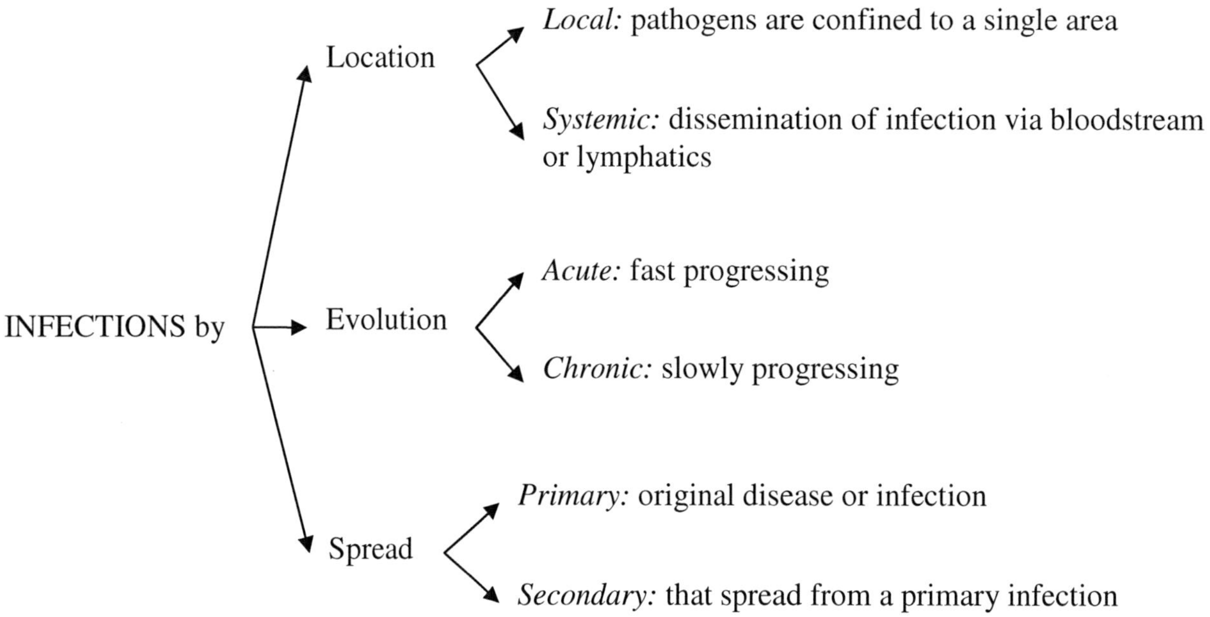

Diagram 5.1-Classification of infections

SPECTRUM OF INFLAMMATORY RESPONSES TO INFECTION:

- Suppurative inflammation: formation of pus (abscess);
- Granulomas: local area of chronic inflammation, characterized by the presence of modified macrophages;
- Necrosis: severe tissue damage following toxin release;
- Chronic inflammation and scarring.

Sources of infection: living or non-living material that a pathogen uses to develop on (your hands, the counter top, etc).
Carrier: an infected individual who does not display symptoms but is capable of transmitting the disease.
Vector: a carrier of pathogenic organisms from one host to another (like the mosquito which can transmit malaria).

Disease transmission:
- **Direct contact**: person to person;
- **Indirect contact:** via air (airborne), contaminated food or water (fecal-oral), non sterile equipment;
- **Animal and insects bites.**

NUTRITIONAL AND HOLISTIC APPROACH TO INFECTIONS:

- Immune system support (as listed under the Immune system chapter);
- If your client is taking antibiotics, a good probiotic supplement (taken away from antibiotic time), will decrease the possibility of developing dysbiosis;

- Antimicrobial herbs:
    - ☐ Cinnamon: Antiseptic, antifungal;
    - ☐ Myrrh: Antibacterial, antiseptic, antifungal;
    - ☐ St. John's Wort: Antidepressant, antiviral;
    - ☐ Oregon grape: Antibacterial, antiparasitic, antiseptic;
    - ☐ Oregano: Antioxidant, antimutagenic, antifungal, antibacterial;
    - ☐ Tea tree: Antibacterial, antifungal, antiseptic;
    - ☐ Pau D'arco: Antimicrobial, antifungal, antimalarial, anti-inflammatory;
    - ☐ Goldenseal: Antimicrobial, antipyretic, antihelminthic; is endangered - source out a sustainably harvested source
    - ☐ Garlic: natural antibiotic. -raw

- Antiparasitic herbs:
    - ♦ Wormwood: antihelminthic;
    - ♦ Pumpkin: Antihelminthic, reduces prostate enlargement;
    - ♦ Black walnut: antihelminthic.

*For comprehensive information on Infectious diseases, *see appendix A*.

CHAPTER 6

NEOPLASIA

Definitions:

Neoplasia:	The formation of a neoplasm;
Neoplasm:	Tumour, growth that depends on the host for their nutrition and vascularization;
Carcinogenesis:	Cancer formation;
Cancer:	Common term for all malignant tumours;
Angiogenesis:	Development of new blood vessels that support the tumour's growth;
Oncology:	The study of tumours and neoplasms;
Metastasis:	Transfer of disease from one part of the body to another not connected to it;
Mutation:	A permanent transmissible alteration of genetic materials;
Mutagenes:	Substances that cause mutations;
Oncogenes:	Cancer-causing genes.

Table 6.1- Neoplasia: definitions

Tumors
- → **Benign** growth formed by cells that are similar to the original cell
- → **Malignant:** growth formed by cells different from the original cell

Diagram 6.1-Classification of tumours

Physiologically, your immune system is well equipped to take care of abnormal cells that are born frequently (by using self defense mechanisms like *tumour necrotizing factor*, *natural killer cells*, and *lymphocytes)*. But certain circumstances allow tumours to form by uncontrolled cellular proliferation (multiplication).

Uncontrolled cell proliferation is the result of the following:

- Stimulation of a gene that causes hyperactivity (**oncogene**);
- Inhibition of a gene that causes inactivity **(tumor suppressor gene).**

CANCER

PATHOGENESIS

1. **Free radical damage:**
   <u>*Free radical*</u>: an unstable molecule with an odd number of electrons, often a form of oxygen, that reacts with other molecules in a destructive way, by stealing electrons. By attacking the DNA, free radicals may cause mutations. Toxins, poisons, medication, chemicals, excess heat, and excess oxidation are all sources of free radical damage;
2. **Weak immune system**: is not able to deal with the development of abnormal cells. Even on a non-specific level, we have natural killer cells that can fight with and destroy abnormal cells;
3. **Malnutrition:** is responsible for the weakening of the immune system by not providing the "building blocks" for the cells of the immune system;

> **Note:** Diet can act as cancer promoting and as cancer inhibiting!

4. **Genetical factors**: by transmitting of oncogenes;
5. **Tumour viruses**: can release oncogenes; (some examples of such viruses are: Human T cell leukemia-lymphoma virus, Human papilloma virus); they act by <u>insertional</u> <u>mutagenesis</u> (insertion of the virus genes into the host's genetic material);
6. **Radiation**
   - → Ultraviolet light exposure: risk factor for skin cancer
   - → Ionizing radiation: inhibits cell division
7. **Increased stress levels and personal attitude:** responsible for a weak immune system and a weak adrenal gland.

Carcinogenesis: process of tumor development.

Stages of carcinogenesis:

1. **Initiaton stage**: irreversible changes in DNA, after exposure to a carcinogen;

2. **Promotion stage**: initiated cells become cancerous.

<u>Initiators and promoters:</u>

- Hormones, drugs, environmental agents,
- Personal behaviour
  - → *Smoking:* causes cancer of lungs, bladder, oral cavity, esophagus, kidneys
  - → *Diet:* increased fat, artificial additives/preservatives
  - → *Environment*: air pollution, occupational exposure (asbestos)

Diagram 6.2-Initiators and promoters of carcinogenesis

3. Progression stage: altered cells become more and more biologically defective

Clinical manifestations
- *General:* pain, cachexia (profound general ill health), anemia, leucopenia, and infection
- *Local:* depending on the affected organ

Diagram 6.3- Cancer: clinical manifestations

Spread of tumours (Metastasis*):
- Direct invasion
- Metastasis of distant organs by lymphatic and veins
- Metastasis by implantation

Diagram 6.4- Metastasis

*Metastasis has been related to disrupted cellular intercommunication

RECOMMENDATIONS FOR CANCER PREVENTION

- Avoid body's stressors: smoking, alcohol, coffee, additives, chemicals, drugs, milk products (galactose has been linked to increased risk of ovarian cancer), increased sugar and refined carbohydrates;
- Increase water intake;
- Increase fiber intake;
- Increase exercise or Do exercise!
- Avoid obesity.

Eat a healthy, wholesome diet, rich in fruits and vegetables, grains, legumes, quality meats (if you are an omnivorous), choose organic when possible (for details regarding the activity of various foods, see below under "THERAPEUTIC NUTRITIONAL APPROACH FOR CANCER"):

- Live a healthy lifestyle and maintain a positive mental attitude; according to personality trends, people may behave differently when facing various stress situations; ideally, in order to counteract the effects of stress, do employ a variety of helpful measures: walks, hobbies, meditation, clubs, etc. Also, don't forget vitamin R (rest) and vitamin H (happiness).

THERAPEUTIC NUTRITIONAL APPROACH FOR CANCER:

There are many approaches that claim to be helpful as a cancer "cure". Whereas it is not impossible to achieve great success, please keep in mind that the information listed below serves as a guideline so you, as a practitioner, will be able to develop the appropriate protocol, according to the individual case.

1. DIET

- **Short cleansing fasts** (juice fasts, water fasts); do use plenty of carrot and beet juice, as it is very beneficial for the liver;
- **Liver detoxification protocols**: lemon water in the morning, fresh fruits and vegetables, dandelion root products; proceed with care and adapt to the body's response, as a toxic body will be more than likely to exhibit "side effects of detoxification" (headache, nausea, intense tiredness);
- **Undereating** (a significant amount of energy is required for digestion and it will be directed away from the healing process);do not starve; just do not overeat; nourish your body!
- **EFA**: increase of TNF (tumour necrotizing factor) and removal of fat soluble pesticide;
- **Vegetables**: increase the cytotoxic (cell killing) activity of NK (Natural Killer) cells

    - Sulphur-containing foods: onions, garlic, leeks, chives: contain allyl sulfides that inhibit carcinogenesis;
    - Carotenoids and bioflavonoids: inhibit tumour enlargement and decrease DNA damage;
    - Cruciferous vegetables: (broccoli, cauliflower, cabbage, Brussels sprouts) contain *glucarate*, which inhibits the effects of carcinogens on the body, *glucoraphanin*, a substance that protects the cell against the effects of free radical damage, and *indoles,* chemicals that reduce the effects of surplus estrogen (vegetarian women excrete two times as much estrogen through their feces than the omnivorous women);
    - Mushrooms (reishi, shiitake, maitake*):* contain *beta-glucan* (a polysaccharide), which stimulates the immune system;
    - Soy: decreases carcinogenesis, inhibit angiogenesis, increases cancer cell apoptosis (death);
    - Flaxseed*s* (source of dietary lignans) reduces cell proliferation and nuclear aberrations in breast cells;
    - Legumes*:* decrease cancer growth;
    - Tomatoes: contain lycopene, which prevent formation of nitrosamines in gut.

- **Yogurt and other fermented cultures***:* increase of interferon production and NK cells; blocks production of carcinogenic compounds in colon.

2. SUPPLEMENTS:

- **Niacin***:* promotes the repair and proper DNA replication;
- **Antioxidants:** protect against and repair free radical damage (vitamins C, E, A);

- **Vitamin A:** increases the efficacy of the immune system;
- **Beta carotenes**: block the initiation of cancer by binding with free radicals;
- **Vitamin K**: seems to act by diminishing the ATP production of the cancer cell;
- **Vitamin C**: helps prevent tumour growth, antioxidant;
- **Bioflavonoids:** prevent cancer prone substances from attaching to cells;
- **Vitamin B complex:** vital in the energy producing process of every cell;
- **Selenium:** can repair DNA damage, stimulates NK cell activity and helps reduce tumour size;
- **Zinc**: increases the number of T cells and improves phagocytosis;
- **Molybdenum:** seems to be effective against stomach cancer;
- **Magnesium**: needed in glutathione (very powerful antioxidant produced by the liver) metabolism;
- **Coenzyme Q10**: increases oxygen uptake in the cell (cancer cells do not thrive in a well oxygenated body);
- **Alpha lipoic acid:**(produced in liver) prevents cellular damage, reduces the effect of environmental toxins, antioxidant, promotes glutathione production;
- **Melatonin**: (levels decrease with age, increase with meditation and bananas consumption), decreases the numbers of estrogen receptors, normalizes cell division and decreases tumour growth;
- **NAC (N-acetyl cysteine):** helps liver detoxification and helps with glutathione production;
- **Grapeseed extract:** contains bioflavonoids that act as potent free radical scavengers, helps slowing down the rate of DNA mutation and slows down the aging process;
- **Glutathione**: strong antioxidant that helps the liver detoxify.

3. OTHER MEASURES:

- **Stress management**, visualization, meditation, support groups;
- **Lavender oil:** massaged in breast, encourages apoptosis (cellurar death) in breast cancer cells;
- **Green Tea:** contains polyphenols, which are strong antioxidants;
- **Ginseng:** helps body cope with stress and replenishes vital energy;
- **Oregano**: antimutagenic;
- **MCP (modified citrus pectin):** decreases stickiness of cancer cells (cancer cells have specific carbohydrate –binding protein molecules on their surface, named *galectins*, which allow for increased cellular adhesion; MCT blocks galectins);
- **Curcumin:** causes cancer cells apoptosis;
- **Shark cartilage:** inhibits angiogenesis.

Notes on chemotherapy and radiation therapies

- Supplements that <u>*can*</u> be taken with chemotherapy/radiation: all but the antioxidants;
- Supplements that <u>*may interact*</u> with chemotherapy/radiation: vitamins C and E.

Helpful supplements for clients who are going through radiation and /or chemotherapy:

- **Vitamin A** (can be administered in local preparations, as the mucus membranes become very frail under chemotherapy): improves tissue tolerance;
- **Alpha lipoic acid**: decreases susceptibility to radiation, decreases toxic side effects of chemotherapy;
- **NAC (N-acetyl cysteine)**: protects against side effects of chemotherapy;
- **Astragalus:** can counteract tiredness and lack of appetite in clients undergoing chemotherapy and /or radiation;

CHAPTER 7

NUTRITIONAL DISEASES

**diseases caused by nutrient deficiency or nutrient excess;*

Nutrient: a nutritious substance used by the body for growth, maintenance and /or repair.

The terminologies utilized to describe deficient nutrients are**:**

- **Under nutrition** (not enough nutrients);
- **Malnutrition** (which means improper nutrition, not necessarily applied to all macro and micronutrients, but to one or a few, for example, protein malnutrition).

Protein Energy Malnutrition means lack of proteins and/or calories, very frequently encountered in Third World countries. It is not limited to the above-mentioned aspects, as quite frequently there is some vitamin deficiency as well.

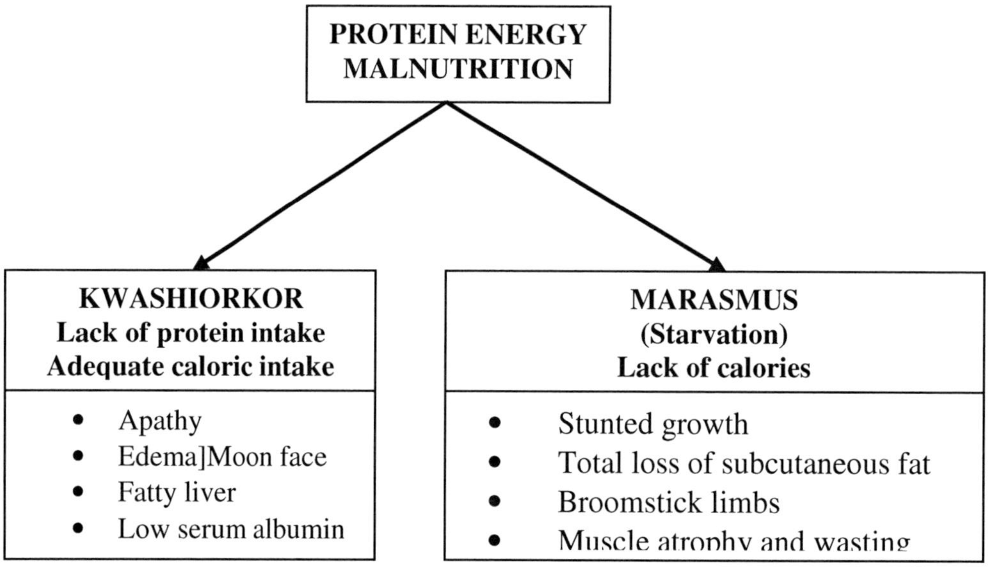

Diagram 7.1- Protein-Energy malnutrition

Vitamin pathologies: (**here**, we are describing <u>disease</u> processes, not only imbalances; this is why you will not see all known vitamin deficiencies and excesses**). Also,** the therapeutic aspect will not be particularly discussed here, as it is obvious that a deficiency disease would be corrected by the supplementation of the deficient nutrient and the excess situation would be corrected by the stopping of ingestion of the excessive nutrient.

◆FAT SOLUBLE VITAMINS

VITAMIN A

A. DEFICIENCY

- One of the most prevalent deficiency conditions worldwide;
- Carotenoids are converted to vitamin A in the intestines.

Pathogenesis:

- Low vitamin A intake;
- Deficient absorption and/or storage;
- Protein or zinc deficiency can reduce the amounts of vitamin A released from the liver (where most of the vitamin A is stored);
- Thyroxin and vitamin E deficiency can impede vitamin A's metabolism by diminishing the conversion of carotenes to retinal.

Consequences of deficiency:

- Impaired vision, particularly in dim light; long term deficiencies may lead to xerophtalmia (dryness and thickening of conjunctiva and cornea);
- Impaired immune system function: low protective function of mucosal membranes and decreased number of lymphocytes T;
- Stunted growth and bone development; enamel-forming cells also require vitamin A;
- Impaired reproductive function, as vitamin A is involved in steroid hormones synthesis.

B. TOXICITY

Toxicity
→ **Acute:** increased intracranial pressure and vomiting in children
→ **Chronic:** irritability, headache, liver damage

Diagram 7.2- Vitamin A toxicity

VITAMIN D

A. DEFICIENCY

Whereas Rickets and Osteomalacia are frequently encountered worldwide, in developed countries they are not consequences of impaired intake, but rather of absorption and/or metabolism problems;

- The organs involved in vitamin D metabolism are: the skin, liver, kidneys and the intestines;
- Vitamin D is stored in the liver, bone, brain and skin. Cortisone interferes with vitamin D absorption.

Sources of Vitamin D

→ **Endogenous:** conversion of a precursor (7-dehydrocholesterol) to Vitamin D_3, in the skin, by UV light

→ **Exogenous:** from dietary sources that contain Ergosterol, which is converted to Vitamin D_2 in the body

Diagram 7.3- Vitamin D sources

Vitamins D_2 and D_3 have the same function in the body and are therefore named by a common denominator: vitamin D.

Pathogenesis:

- Inadequate exposure to UV light;
- Lack of intake;
- Malabsorption, due to diseases that affect the intestines and fat absorption problems;
- Diseases of the organs involved in vitamin D metabolism: liver, kidneys.

Consequences of deficiency:

- Rickets in children;
- Osteomalacia in adults.

B. TOXICITY

- Initially, anorexia, nausea, vomiting, then polyuria, polydipsia;
- Impaired renal function;
- Hypercalcemia.

VITAMIN E

A. DEFICIENCY

- Tocopherols are oily liquids;
  - Transported in the body by fats (chylomicrons, LDL's);
  - Stored in the adipose tissue, liver and muscle;
- Some vitamin E is stored in the adrenal glands;
  - Dietary deficiency is very rare;
- Diets rich in polyunsaturated fatty acids require increased intake of vitamin E and other antioxidants;
- Iron binds with vitamin E and may impede its absorption
  - Large doses may impede vitamin K's absorption and result in prolonged bleeding time.

Pathogenesis:
- Disorders of the fat metabolism, which will impede the vitamin E transport;
- Diseases of liver, pancreas and gall bladder, which will interfere with fat absorption;
- Small intestine disorders, which will interfere with fat absorption.

Consequences of deficiency:
- Central Nervous System changes: spinocerebellar degeneration;
- Liver degeneration;
- Impaired reproductive function;
- Skeletal muscle changes: dystrophies.

B. TOXICITY

Occasionally, muscle weakness, nausea, diarrhea

VITAMIN K

A. DEFICIENCY

- Stored in the liver; absorbed in the upper Gastro-intestinal tract; requires bile salts for absorption;
- Needed for synthesis of osteocalcin, the calcium-binding protein found in bones;
- Involved in the synthesis of a protein secreted by the kidney, that inhibits calcium oxalate kidney stones formation;
- Involved in synthesis of two proteins (C and S), very important in the coagulation process;
- Acidophilus may interfere with vitamin K synthesis.

Sources of Vitamin K

→ **Green leafy vegetables:** Vitamin K (phytonodione) accumulates in the chlorophyll forming parts of leaves

→ **Bacteria in the Large intestine:** synthesizes vitamin K_2 (menaquinone)

Diagram 7.4-Vitamin K sources

Pathogenesis:
- Fat malabsorption (liver, gallbladder, pancreatic conditions);
- Use of antibiotics, which seems to impair vitamin K recycling;
- Use of anticoagulants, which interfere with vitamin K synthesis.

Consequences of deficiency:

- Hemorrhagic disease of the newborn, in infancy;
- Bleeding disorders;
- Secondary: osteoporosis.

B. TOXICITY

- Menadione (precursor) can cause hemolytic anemia and hyperbilirubinemia

◆ WATER SOLUBLE VITAMINS

VITAMIN B_1 (Thiamin)

A. DEFICIENCY:

- Black tea, which contains an antithiamine factor, coffee and chlorinated water may destroy vitamin B_1;
- Stored in very low quantities in the skeletal muscle, heart, liver, kidneys and brain;
- Absorbed at duodenal level;
- Allicin, in onions and garlic facilitates the absorption of thiamin;
- Vitally important for cellular respiration and for all macronutrients metabolism;
- Acts on the nerve cells membrane to facilitate sodium transport and nerve transmission, mostly in peripheral nerves;
- Deficiency frequent in alcoholics.

Pathogenesis:

- Low dietary intake;
- Malabsorption.

Consequences of deficiency:

- Cardio-vascular syndrome ("Wet beriberi"): edema, heart failure
- Polyneuropathy ("Dry beriberi")
- Wernicke-Korsakoff syndrome, affecting the central nervous system (encephalopathy and psychosis)

B. TOXICITY

- Well-tolerated vitamin, no known toxic effects.

VITAMIN B_2 (Riboflavin)

DEFICIENCY:
Not specific, but associated with cheilosis, burning eyes, glossitis

VITAMIN B_3 (Niacin)

A. DEFICIENCY

- Niacin has cholesterol-lowering properties and it is responsible for the flushing effect;
- Niacinamide is used for arthritis; it may cause glucose intolerance;
- Niacin may increase uric acid levels;
- Absorbed at small intestine level;
- Can be synthesized from tryptophan in the presence of vitamins B_1, B_2 and B_6;
- Lime makes the type of niacin found in corn more absorbable;
- Vitally important in countless metabolic pathways, Krebs cycle being just an example.

Pathogenesis:
- Lack of intake;
- Malabsorption;
- High corn intake;
- Alcoholism.

Consequences of deficiency: The 4 D's (Pellagra)
- *Dermatitis*: exacerbated by sun exposure;
- *Diarrhea:* caused by inflammation of the gastro-intestinal tract;
- *Dementia*: irritability, headaches, followed by mental confusion and depression;
- *Death.*

B. TOXICITY

- Flushing, itching, liver damage;
- Nausea is the first sign of toxicity with both niacin and niacinamide

VITAMIN B_6 (Pyridoxine)

A. DEFICIENCY

- Rare, results from malabsorption, alcoholism, BCP (Birth Control Pills) use;
- Seborrheic dermatitis, glossitis, cheilosis, peripheral neuropathy.

B. TOXICITY

- Mega doses result in peripheral neuropathy.

VITAMIN C (Ascorbic acid)

A. DEFICIENCY

- Humans and mammals can not synthesize vitamin C, so the only source is the diet;
- True deficiency would manifest after 30-40 days, if no vitamin C is provided;
- Very important as an antioxidant, for collagen production and for norepinephrine synthesis;
- Can increase uric acid excretion;
- Very high dosages in sensitive individuals or in cases with renal conditions may increase the oxalic acid precipitation, resulting in kidney stone formation;

Consequences of deficiency:

- **Scurvy:** restlessness, fatigue, weakness, muscle cramps, joint pain, rashes, easy bleeding and bruising.

NUTRITIONAL EXCESS

OBESITY:

**The excessive accumulation of body fat.*

Obesity used to be defined as a body weight grater than 30% above ideal body weight as presented in weight/height tables. Presently, it is defined as BMI (Body Mass Index = weight in kilograms, divided by the square of the height in meters).

It is quite difficult to objectively assess the degree of obesity. Many measurement approaches have been employed:

- BMI (Body Mass Index): takes into consideration the relationship between height and weight, applied to gender and age, but it does not consider the fat distribution (it seems that abdominal fat deposits are more related to increased health risks);
- Skin fold measurements;
- Waist-hip ratio;
- Body fat scales (which can assess the amount of body fat).

Fat distribution

- **Gynoid** (female pattern)**:** gluteal region and upper part of legs
- **Android** (male pattern): abdominal deposits

Diagram 7.5-Fat distribution

Types of Obesity

- **Hyperplastic:** an increase number of fat cells throughout the body. It depends of the diet of the mother while the person was still in the uterus and on the diet during early infancy. Less related to serious health consequences.
- **Hypertrophic:** increased size of each individual fat cell. Linked to serious health consequences

Diagram 7.6- Types of obesity

Etiology:

1. **PSYCHOLOGICAL FACTORS:** states that obese individuals are barely sensitive to internal signals for hunger, but very sensitive to external signals (sight, smell, taste);

2. **PHYSIOLOGICAL FACTORS:** states that obese individuals are very sensitive to internal signals for hunger and satiety. In many cases, we think that obesity is just of matter of the imbalance between the quantity and quality of food ingested and the lack of exercise. Whereas the instant mentioned etiology is valid, there are other factors to be taken into consideration:

   - **Low brain serotonin**: can increase the appetite dramatically, because the brain thinks that the body is starving. This seems to be the case of craving for carbohydrates, and, in a lesser extent, for fats. This individuals would benefit from ingestion of tryptophan rich foods;

   - **The Set-Point theory** states that the body is trying to maintain a certain body weight according to the signals from fat cells: when the fat cells lose some of their content, powerful signals will be sent to the brain and the appetite will increase accordingly, manifested by a strong desire to eat. It seems that this body reaction is very much dependent on decreased insulin sensitivity (the larger the fat cell, the lower the number for insulin receptors). The insulin insensitivity consequences are not only impaired blood sugar transport and control, but the burning of fat deposits for energy will also be impeded;

- **Decreased heat production** (heat production is a result of food burning). It seems that obese individuals have a minimal increase in heat production after eating, which means that food energy is stored as opposed to being burned. This theory also relates to insulin insensitivity .It seems that obese individuals have a slower reacting sympathetic nervous system (which controls the metabolism, among other functions).

Consequences of obesity:

- *Insulin resistance,* because increased in size fat cells have a lower number of insulin receptors;
- *Diabetes mellitus type 2;*
- *Hypertension;*
- *Coronary artery disease;*
- *Atherosclerosis;*
- *Gallstones;*
- *Osteoarthritis;*
- *Cancer.*

Nutrition and holistic approach:

1. Proper diet: low in refined carbohydrates and saturated fat; rich in fiber, fruits, vegetables, grains;
2. Liver and digestive system cleansing programs;
3. Adrenal support;
4. Stress management, emphasis on a positive mental attitude;
5. Adequate exercise (depending on lifestyle and physiological/pathological demands);
6. Supplementation:
    - Quality multivitamin/multimineral formula;
    - Vitamin B complex: 50 mg/day;
    - Coenzyme Q10: 100-300 mg/day.

CHAPTER 8

THE DIGESTIVE SYSTEM

We eat in order to get nourished (and because we like it!), to build internal structures, to maintain what we have already built up and to repair what we damaged. Unfortunately, most of the people you know will use their digestive system as a means for disease and sufferance. We eat a nice – non-fat, of course- piece of chicken breast, which should provide us with quite a good amount of proteins (which would be enough to build elements of the immune system-remember, antibodies are proteins-, and to repair a skeletal muscle which we overworked, etc.).

But if we fry that piece of chicken, then we add many sauces rich in additives, not to mention the fact that the chicken has been fed chemically enriched food, then we end up setting the basis for atherosclerosis (from the trans fatty acids released by frying) and for free radical damage (from the additives and chemicals).And this was just one common example.

In the following chapter, we will describe the most important mechanisms of digestive system diseases and in which way they greatly affect the whole body's health.

IMPORTANT NUTRIENTS FOR THE DIGESTIVE SYSTEM

NUTRIENT	ROLE
Vitamin A	Mucus membranes protection; helpful in healing ulcers;
Vitamin B complex	Helps maintain healthy muscle tone in the gastro-intestinal tract;
Vitamins B_1, B_3 and B_6	Hydrochloric acid production;
Vitamin B_2	Along with vitamin A supports mucus membranes;
Vitamin B_3	Involved in bile secretion;
Vitamin B_5	Helps fat conversion into energy;
Biotin	Helps with fatty acids synthesis;
Choline	Helps gallbladder regulation and liver function;
Inositol	Involved in fat and cholesterol metabolism;
PABA	Maintains healthy intestinal flora;
Vitamin C	Collagen formation and antioxidant;
Bioflavonoids	Stimulate bile production;
Calcium	Helps lower cholesterol levels;
Chromium	Important in fat and cholesterol synthesis;
Magnesium	Relaxes smooth muscle tonus;

NUTRIENT	ROLE
Zinc	Increases vitamin A absorption, therefore protecting mucus membranes;
Methionine	Important in detoxification;
Cysteine	Important in detoxification;
Glutamine	Helps heal mucus membranes;
Glutathione	Strong antioxidant; important in detoxification;
Taurine	Bile component.

Table 8.1-Important nutrients for the digestive system

Common signs/symptoms:

- Upper GI (Gastro-intestinal) tract: comprised of mouth, pharynx, esophagus, stomach; gas (belching/eructation), heartburn, hiccup, stomach pain, upper abdomen distension, bleeding (looks like coffee grounds), vomiting, nausea;
- Lower GI tract: small intestine and large intestine: abdominal pain of various locations, distension (increase in size due to gas accumulation), gas (wind/flatulence), stool abnormalities (diarrhea, constipation), presence of blood and/or mucus in stools, bleeding (looks like black stools);
- Others: jaundice.

ASSESSMENT

MEDICAL	NUTRITIONAL
1. Clinical aspect, based on the signs/symptoms mentioned above; 2. Physical examination: assesses size of organs, pain distribution, abnormal findings (blood, etc.); 3. Laboratory analysis: of pancreatic enzymes, liver enzymes, lipid levels, etc. 4. Barium swallow: by ingesting a contrast substance, upon performing an x-ray, the elements of the GI system are clearly seen (ulcers, hiatus hernia, gastric reflux, tumors, etc.); 5. Gastric analysis: to assess levels of hydrochloric acid; performed by introducing a nasogastric tube into the stomach followed by hydrochloric acid aspiration;	1. Liver function status, as an overloaded liver will allow toxins to circulate, overburdening all systems and also, a sluggish liver will not be able to process nutrients properly, which will affect the repair and maintenance mechanisms necessary for the health of the digestive system; 2. Digestive system status, as problems of the digestive system will lead to malnutrition, and consequently to difficulties in repairing and maintaining the structures of the digestive system; 3. Diet analysis, as intake of certain substances may impede on the health of the digestive system (excessive use of sugar can contribute to bacterial overgrowth);

MEDICAL	NUTRITIONAL
6. Endoscopy: visualization of the gastric mucosa through a device named endoscope; 7. Colonoscopy/anoscopy/ sigmoidoscopy: allows visualization of the lower GI tract; 8. Laparascopy: surgical opening of the abdomen and visualization of its structures;	4. Hydrochloric acid level assessment, as imbalances may lead into various digestive system problems; 5. Candida/Dysbiosis/Parasitosis questionnaires as any of the above mentioned conditions may impede on the nutritional status of the body, by creating maldigestion/malnutrition.

Table 8.2-Digestive system assessment

*All the Assessment charts are to be read as **stand-alone only** columns. See *General Therapeutic Approach.*

BASIC MECHANISMS OF THE DIGESTIVE SYSTEM PATHOLOGY

The following synopsis will describe the where, the how and the why digestive system disease happens and why the digestive system is so closely linked to all the other body systems, influencing their performance. We will begin by describing "The Life of a nutrient".

Nutrient means, by various definitions, a nutritive substance, something that is there to nourish, support growth, to maintain what has been achieved so far and to repair when the body needs "fixing".

JUST A REMINDER:

PROTEINS are broken down into amino acids, which are absorbed at small intestine level, then travel to the liver where they are being processed and dispatched within the body according to the body's needs: they will turn into vitally important immunoglobulins, enzymes, hormones, protein carriers...

CARBOHYDRATES are broken down into monosaccharides, which, after absorption at small intestine level, travel to the liver as well; liver will process them then send glucose molecule wherever they are needed: immediate source of energy, brain fuel, glycogen reserves...

LIPIDS are broken down into fatty acids, absorbed at small intestine level, then travel to the liver where processing takes place; they will eventually form the fat deposits, the myelin sheath, the lipoproteins, the cholesterol...

Basic Mechanisms of the Digestive System's Pathology

Now that we know in which way all the body systems are depending on the nutrient intake, absorption and on the digestive system's health, we shall next proceed to describe what happens at every level of the digestive system.

MOUTH:

- Tooth decay or dental problems;
- Tongue pathologies (like pain from glossitis, which is an inflammation of the tongue mucosa; vitamin B_{12} deficiency may lead to glossitis);
- Bucal mucosa (the mucosa that lines up the inside of the cheeks, the roof and the bottom of the mouth) infections or pathologies (tumors, etc.);

These aspects may impede on the proper chewing of food or on the food intake itself (if it hurts too much, people will avoid eating), which results into larger food particles than normal being swallowed and reaching the stomach at a certain size; this will put a strain on the stomach, as it has to break down the food further and also on the pancreas, as it will be called in to release more and more pancreatic juice components.

*Note: pharynx is just a passageway, but its local pathologies (like pharyngitis or tumors) may impede on the digestion if the person can not eat too much or if they have difficulty swallowing.

1. **ESOPHAGUS**: is lined by a very fine mucosa, very sensitive to pH changes;
   - Tumors, infections;
   - Esophagitis, from acid reflux (this aspect will influence the digestive process the most). A person with GERD (Gastro-esophageal reflux disease) will be exposed to acid released through

the cardia sphincter upwards, onto the esophageal mucosa, which is not able to physiologically deal with increased acidity (it simply burns!). The body will react by exhibiting heartburn and vomiting. In time, one of the unfortunate consequences of GERD could be esophageal cancer, due to cellular modifications of the esophageal mucosa by the stomach acid.

2. **STOMACH**
   - Hyperchlorhydria (increased stomach acid) will eventually result in GERD, affecting the esophagus health;
   - Hypochlorhydria (low stomach acid) will result in improper protein digestion, as we need hydrochloric acid to stimulate the transformation of **pepsinogen** (secreted by cells of the stomach mucosa) into **pepsin,** which is ultimately responsible for protein digestion; improper protein digestion will result in the release of longer aminoacids chains (usually called macromolecules) towards the small intestine. When macronutrients are not properly digested, the process is called **maldigestion**.

As they reach the small intestine level, because of their size, the macromolecules will not be able to be absorbed into the blood stream through the physiologic absorption process, so they will have a tendency to elicit a **local low inflammatory** process; in time, this will lead to enlargement of the spaces between the small intestine's cells and a condition named **Leaky Gut** will be created.

It should be mentioned that incomplete protein digestion allows for a process called **putrefaction** (breakdown of proteins by bacteria), which increases the likelihood of allergic reactions because of the toxic byproducts that putrefaction entails.
Leaky Gut will allow these macromolecules and practically everything else (toxins, for example) to leave the intestinal lumen into the blood circulation.

This process will have two consequences:

- Liver overload, as the liver will have to deal with the circulating toxins;
- Immune System overload, as the cells of the immune system will try to get rid of "abnormal" structures; in time, this opens the door to development of allergies and even autoimmune disease.

3. **SMALL AND LARGE INTESTINE:** being the site for food absorption, the small intestine's health is of vital importance. Some medical conditions that impede on the normal physiology of the intestines are:

- Functional intestinal disorders, like Irritable Bowel Syndrome;
- Inflammations (like Inflammatory Bowel Disease, Celiac Disease);
- Tumors (from polyps to cancer);
- Dysbiosis (abnormal intestinal flora);
- Candida, parasites;
- Leaky Gut;
- Constipation

All of the above may pose quite a burden on the small intestine. If disease processes affect the small intestine, it is to be anticipated that the absorption process will be impeded, a situation called **malabsorption**.
Malabsorption has dramatic consequences: **ALL body's systems will suffer from lack of nutrients:**

- The immune system will not be able to create immunoglobulins;
- The endocrine glands will not have enough ingredients to produce their hormones;
- The pancreas will not have the basic substances to produce pancreatic juice , which will impede on digestion even further;
- The liver will not have the nutrient base for its own functioning, nor for bile secretion, which will impede the fat digestion;
- There will not be enough nutrients to repair the gut wall (sick with leaky gut or inflammation), which will lead to further malnutrition.

The large intestine is very important for our health, as water and electrolytes are absorbed at this level and as the large intestine is responsible for the elimination process. Slow transit time (normal transit time is 18-28 hours) impedes greatly on our health. Constipation burdens the body because toxins, which should be eliminated in a timely fashion, will be reabsorbed into the blood stream (remember, the large intestine is the storage place for waste, but only for a limited time) and overloading of the liver and the immune system may result.

4. LIVER AND GALL BLADDER

Liver is making the bile, which the gall bladder stores. The bile is extremely important in lipid digestion and also in keeping the small intestine free of microorganisms.
Liver overload is caused by circulating toxins of various sources:

- Reabsorption from the intestines;
- High chemical intake, as in additives, alcohol, coffee;
- High chemical exposure, as in environmental and occupational toxicity;
- Use of drugs or medication;
- Stress;
- A diet rich in stressors, like saturated fat and sugar will result **firstly**, in allowing toxins, which should normally be detoxified, to travel freely throughout the body and attack various organ systems (for example, the nervous system is particularly susceptible to mercury and alcohol), and **secondly,** in improper and insufficient nutrient metabolism, which will affect the health of every organ and organ system by nutrient depletion.

5. PANCREAS

The pancreas is responsible for secreting (producing) the alkaline pancreatic juice, which contains enzymes able to digest each of the macronutrients.

- **Lipases** are to help in the digestion of fats;
- **Amylases** are to digest carbohydrates;
- **Proteases** are very important, as they break down proteins into aminoacids, therefore minimizing the risk for putrefaction (a process that occurs in the small intestine as a result of incomplete protein digestion), which releases toxic substances. Also, proteases are very important as they keep the intestines clean and free from parasites.

An overloaded and/or malnourished pancreas will have **diminished pancreatic juice output**. This will result in:

- Maldigestion of practically every macronutrient (carbohydrates, proteins or fats);
- Maldigestion leads to further malnutrition and also creates the premises for the development of leaky gut and dysbiosis;
- Leaky gut will allow for further liver overload and immune system overload by allowing large molecules and toxins to exit the small intestine lumen into the blood.

PATHOLOGY OF THE DIGESTIVE TRACT

♦DISEASES OF THE ORAL CAVITY

PERIODONTAL DISEASE

**disease of the gums (gingivitis) and of the teeth elements (odontitis)*

1. Gingivitis: gums inflammation (redness, swelling, bleeding);
2. Periodontitis: (redness, swelling, loose teeth, infections).

Etiology:

- Faulty dental work;
- Faulty dental hygiene;
- Low immune system status;
- Smoking;
- Increased refined carbohydrate intake.

Nutrition and holistic approach:

- Immune system building and support;
- Germanium containing foods, which increase tissue oxygenation;

Supplements:

- Vitamin C and bioflavonoids, 2-4 g/day, or up to bowel tolerance, as it increases the local defense and improves the collagen matrix;
- Vitamin E, 400 IU/day, as it acts as a local antioxidant;
- Beta-carotenes, 250000 IU/day, as they seem to be more protective than vitamin A against the side effects of the periodontal disease;
- Zinc, 30-45 mg/day, as it increases the local antioxidant activity and it inhibits the dental plaque's growth;

Other measures:

- Mouthwashes with folic acid and zinc;
- Mouth rinses with bilberry, grape seed extract, chamomile;
- Bloodroot mouthwash and/or toothpaste, as it protects against plaque formation.

♦ESOPHAGEAL DISORDERS

A. DYSPHAGIA

**difficulty in swallowing; sensation of "food sticking" after swallowing.*

Types of dysphagia:

- Oropharyngeal: difficulty in initiating swallowing (inability to transfer food from mouth to esophagus; due to neurological factors (nerve dysfunctions, MS) or muscular (muscular dystrophy, pharyngeal diverticulum (a local pouch or sac);
- Esophageal: due to mechanical obstruction (tumor) or neurological causes (palsy, CNS lesions).

Treatment approach will vary according with the cause.

B. GASTROESOPHAGEAL REFLUX DISEASE (GERD)

**reflux of stomach content severe enough to produce symptoms and/or complications*

Etiology:

- Low esophageal sphincter pathology (decreased tonus, inappropriate relaxation);
- Delayed gastric emptying (because of improper digestion);
- Obesity (because of the upward pressure on the cardia sphincter);
- Stress (which increases stomach acid secretion);
- Drugs/medications (NSAID), which increase the stomach acid;
- Smoking.

Pathogenesis: acid regurgitation leads to esophageal inflammation, ulceration and bleeding, followed by muscle spasm and/or stricture (narrowing), which poses a risk of metaplasia/cancerous modifications.

Clinical presentation:

- Heartburn;
- Acid regurgitation;
- Non-specific chest pain;
- Dysphagia (difficulty swallowing);
- Symptoms aggravated by position (lying down), increased intraabdominal pressure (which increases the upward pressure against the cardia sphincter), stress, spicy food, medication.

Diagnosis:

- Clinical aspect;
- 24 hrs pH monitoring;
- Barium swallow;
- Endoscopy.

Nutrition and holistic approach:

- Avoid intake of spicy foods and or medication that can increase the stomach acid secretion;
- Avoid stress or take measures to manage stressful situations differently;
- Avoid situations that result in increased intraabdominal pressure (like obesity or indigestion, which is associated with increased gas release, which leads into abdominal distension);
- Sleep with the head of the bed elevated;
- Food combining works very well, as it decreases the workload of the stomach and diminishes the risk of indigestion;
- At the first sign of heartburn, drink one or two large glasses of water, as it dilutes the acid;
- Increase intake of celery, as it greatly diminishes the discomfort due to heartburn.

Supplements:

- Vitamin A, beta carotenes and zinc, as they have healing properties for the mucosa membranes;
- Vitamin C and bioflavonoids, 1-2 g/day, as antioxidants and for collagen formation;
- Glutamine, as prescribed, for its healing properties;
- Flax seed oil, one tablespoon/day, for anti-inflammatory and healing properties;
- Digestive enzymes, as prescribed, to ensure proper digestion;
- Probiotics, when indigestion is the cause.

Others:

- Demulcents (soothing agents) will coat the inner wall of the digestive tract and have a protective and healing effect: aloe vera juice, licorice, slippery elm and marshmallow;
- Do not use peppermint tea (which is largely used for indigestion), as it increases the laxity of the esophageal sphincter, allowing acid to pass;
- Chamomile and fennel tea may be helpful.

C. ESOPHAGITIS

**inflammation of the esophageal mucosa*

Etiology:

- GERD;
- Ingestion of caustic substances;
- Excessive vomiting (like in bulimia).

Clinical aspect:

- Heartburn
- Vomiting

Complications: risk of strictures or metaplasia
Treatment will apply to the cause.

D. HIATUS HERNIA

**outpouch of a portion of the stomach through the esophageal opening, above the diaphragm, into the esophagus*

Etiology:

- Unknown; in some cases, it could be present at birth;
- Weakened tissue, by the factors that have been described under GERD etiology.

Clinical aspect:

- Severe heartburn that worsens upon lying down or straining;
- Belching, acid taste, possible difficulty swallowing.

For **nutrition and holistic approach**, please cross-reference GERD's treatment.

♦ STOMACH DISORDERS

A. HYPERCHLORHYDRIA (high stomach acid)

Etiology:

- High stress, which in certain individuals elicits vagal nerve stimulation with subsequent release of hydrochloric acid;

- Spicy foods, coffee, smoking and alcohol may irritate the stomach mucosa and increase hydrochloric acid secretion;
- Use of medication like NSAID (non steroidal anti-inflammatory drugs) irritate the gastric mucosa;
- Infection with Helicobacter Pylori, which causes irritation, also; the presence of this microorganism is measured by identifying the antibodies against H. pylori in blood or saliva or by culture of the endoscopy sample;
- Other organs disease: some pancreatic tumors (Zollinger Ellison) stimulate the gastric mucosa to produce more hydrochloric acid.

Clinical aspect:

- Heartburn and belching;
- Upper abdomen discomfort.

Nutrition and holistic approach comprises mostly prevention and approach according to etiologic factors. The infectious theory and its therapeutic approach will be discussed under *Gastric ulcer.*

B. HYPOCHLORHYDRIA (low stomach acid)

Achlorhydria: complete lack of stomach acid

Etiology:

- Aging (secretion of hydrochloric acid decreases with age);
- Some authors quote infectious etiology: Helicobacter pylori (see under PUD below);
- Low immune system status: which allows H. pylori to grow;
- Malnutrition, due to all causes listed under Basic mechanisms, causes lack of the building blocks necessary to create hydrochloric acid;
- Very large protein meals, that will eventually exhaust the hydrochloric acid power of secretion;
- Stress, which shuts down the digestion process, resulting in maldigestion and eventually, malabsorption.

Clinical aspect:

- It is closely related with Dyspepsia, which will be discussed shortly;
- Bloating, fullness after meals, belching;
- Abdominal distension and discomfort;
- Possible sensation of mild, diffuse heartburn, because the stomach is trying to release hydrochloric acid for digestion; its secretion is not sufficient, therefore maldigestion of proteins will develop; as the body is trying to digest, putrefaction and gas release are common results; the gas will expand the size of the abdomen and it will push upwards against the cardia sphincter; small amount of gastric content mixed with a small quantity of hydrochloric acid may escape, giving the sensation of heartburn.

Diagnosis and assessment:

> **Note**: it is very important to be able to differentiate between too much and not sufficient stomach acid. Both of them have consequences on your health, as listed above. The problem is that if we give hydrochloric acid supplementation to a person with already excessively high levels, but with a low pain threshold (some people perceive pain much differently than the others), the risk of complications will be much increased, exposing the person to the likelihood of developing esophageal cancer later on in life:

- **Acid self test**: if you experience any of the symptoms listed above under hypochlorhydria, you can take a tablespoon of apple cider vinegar with your meals (my advice is to dilute it, as it may irritate the gastric mucosa in some cases); if the symptoms improve, it could be that you do lack hydrochloric acid to some extent and you may benefit from supplementation;

- **Hydrochloric acid supplementation test** is somehow more precise, as it suggests the intake of gradually increasing number of hydrochloric acid capsules until the symptoms subside or there is warmth/burning in the stomach; in time, as the client is feeling better, the number of necessary pills will decrease; check the insert of the hydrochloric capsules package for using instructions;

- **Heidelberg test (gastric analysis)** is much more precise than any of the others and it will give you the correct interpretation of hydrochloric acid levels.

Nutrition and holistic approach: will very much depend on the cause of the condition, when identified. The approach for hypochlorhydria merges with the approach for dyspepsia, outlined below.

C. DYSPEPSIA (Indigestion)

**general term that depicts discomfort of the upper gastro-intestinal tract , but not limited to this location*

Etiology:

- Increased food intake, which sets a burden on the digestion and it may slow it down, resulting in dysbiosis and malabsorption;
- Intake of spicy, rich and fatty foods, as they overload the digestive processes;
- Hypochlorhydria, as it allows for insufficient protein digestion;
- Excessive smoking , coffee and alcohol intake, as it imbalances the release of digestive secretions (for example, hydrochloric acid excess);
- Stress, as it slows down the digestion;
- Low pancreatic function, either from malnutrition or from overburden, as it impedes on the normal digestion process by decreased pancreatic juice release;
- Diseases of the gastro-intestinal tract (ulcer, gallstones), as they will impede on the digestion; mechanisms will be explained with the specified diseases;
- Food intolerances.

Clinical aspect:

- Abdominal pain and distension;
- Possible heartburn;
- Nausea associated or not with feelings of vomiting;
- Gastro-intestinal gas, either belching or flatulence;
- Sensation of "heaviness" of the upper abdomen, usually.

Nutrition and holistic approach:

- Identify sources of discomfort and eliminate them from the diet or lifestyle;
- Identify food sensitivities/intolerances and address appropriately;
- Gentle but sustained liver detoxification and support, as all products of incomplete or improper digestion will eventually overload the liver;
- Digestive system status assessment: hydrochloric acid level, dysbiosis, etc

Food therapy:

- Employ a diet rich in wholesome, natural foods; increase fiber and fish intake;
- Food combining works very well, as it decreases the digestion overload;
- Increase intake of fresh papaya and pineapple, for their enzymatic content (bromelain and papain).

Supplements:

- If hypochlorhydria is present, either apple cider vinegar in water or hydrochloric acid supplementation may be required;
- For hyperchlorhydria, employ the measures listed above;
- Digestive enzymes, taken as prescribed (there are many discussions pertaining to digestive enzymes; some authors recommend the vegetarian form only, whereas others suggest the intake of pancreas extract (pancreatin); you will apply your protocol according to the client's status and beliefs; it does seem that the comprehensive formula, which comprises vegetarian and animal sources works quite well, but I have accomplished good and stable results on the vegetarian source alone-bromelain and papain);
- Probiotics, as prescribed, as it will ensure a balanced intestinal flora with improved digestive capability; written information varies greatly when it comes to dosage; we do recommend at least 2-4 billions of germs/day.

Other measures:

- Fennel, chamomile, anise, ginger, peppermint (except in cases with GERD) and lemon balm work very well;
- Aloe vera, slippery elm and marshmallow root are demulcents/soothing agents.

D. GASTRITIS

**inflammation of the stomach lining, due to repetitive irritation*

Etiology and clinical aspect: gastritis is a cross between hyperchlorhydria and dyspepsia. All etiological factors expressed under the above-mentioned conditions apply to Gastritis.

Types of Gastritis:

1. Acute: causes apply to drugs, especially NSAID (non-steroidal anti-inflammatory drugs), alcohol and acute stress;
2. Chronic: chronic use of antiinflammatories, smoking, coffee, stressful dietary habits, chronic stress.

Complications:

1. Atrophy: the stomach mucosa (lining) becomes thinner and all secretions may be diminished (acid, pepsin intrinsic factor);
2. Metaplasia (cancerous transformation of cells).

Treatment is a cross between hyperchlorhydria and dyspepsia.

E. PEPTIC ULCER DISEASE (PUD)

**erosion of tissue of the stomach/duodenal lining; it is the result of the imbalance between the protective mucosal factors and the aggressors (as listed under etiology)*

Etiology:

- H. Pylori; low stomach acid may allow for bacterial overgrowth; as the bacteria multiplies, it increases the stomach acidity, allowing for sustained irritation and ulcer formation; both hyper and hypochlorhydria may be etiologic factors for ulcer;
- NSAIDS and aspirin intake.

Associated etiologic factors:

- Smoking: increases risk of ulcer and the risk of complications (bleeding, metaplasia);
- Diet: causes dyspepsia and continuous irritation;
- Stress, which may cause ulcer in two ways: one, by vagal nerve stimulation and increased acidic secretion, secondly, by the body's response to chronic stress, which is shutting down the digestion; the last occurrence will allow for low gastric acid output and improper protein digestion, with all consequences listed under Hypochlorhydria;
- Food allergies, because of the local irritation they may produce.

Clinical presentation:

FEATURE	DUODENAL ULCER* (first few centimeters of duodenum)	GASTRIC ULCER
Acid levels	Hyperchlorhydria predisposes to duodenal ulcer	Hypochlorhydria and hyperchlorhydria
Chronic gastritis	Rare	Very common
Pain character	Gnawing, burning, hunger	
Pain after meal	1.5-3 hrs later	½ hr later
Food intake effect on pain	Relieves	No major effect
Genetics	Major link	Minor link
H. Pylori	75%	90%+

FEATURE	DUODENAL ULCER* (first few centimeters of duodenum)	GASTRIC ULCER
Male: female	3:1	2:1
Relationship to coffee, NSAIDS, tobacco	Weak	Strong

Table 8.3- Clinical presentation of PUD

*Pain awakening the client at night is due to duodenal ulcer

Complications:

- Bleeding: shows up either as upper or/and lower GI bleeding; can be associated with anemia;
- Perforation: is an ACUTE situation, as the stomach wall perforates and releases secretions in the abdominal cavity;
- Penetration: the lesion may penetrate the nearby organs.

Diagnosis:

- Medical history;
- Clinical presentation;
- H. Pylori presence;
- Endoscopy;
- Upper GI series.

Medical treatment: will employ antacids, antibiotics (for H. pylori control), and H2 blockers (which diminish the acidic secretion); surgery is performed usually in cases with complications.

Nutrition and holistic approach:

- Identify the etiologic factors and avoid them;
- Change eating habits (eating on the run, in stressful conditions);
- Avoid fatty foods, excessive sugar, alcohol, smoking, vinegar, coffee or tea, as they may increase the stomach acidity.

<u>Food therapy:</u>

- Cabbage and carrot juice are soothing (glutamine contained in the cabbage juice has healing properties);
- Celery juice may be added, as it helps with hyperacidity;

<u>Supplements:</u>

- Vitamin A, 5000 IU/day, as it increases the strength of the mucosa lining;
- Vitamin C and bioflavonoids, 1-1.5 g/day;
- Vitamin E, 400 IU/day;
- Zinc, 30 mg/day; the last three supplements have a healing effect on the mucosa;
- Evening Primrose Oil, 500 mg three times a day, as it is anti-inflammatory and has healing effects;

- DGL (deglyrrhizinated licorice), as prescribed, as it seems to have very good results in healing ulcers; also, some authors suggest that the licorice's antimicrobial properties play an important role against H. pylori; (DGL can be given to cases with high blood pressure, as it does not have water retaining properties);
- Glutamine, as prescribed, for its healing effects on the GI mucosa.

Other measures:
- Chamomile (unless allergic to the ragweed family, which chamomile is a member of), comfrey (which repairs tissues), aloe and slippery elm(which are demulcents) are very helpful;
- Licorice tea has healing and antimicrobial properties;
- Essential oils of chamomile, geranium and marjoram could be massaged into the abdomen.

♦DISEASES OF THE PANCREAS

PANCREATITIS

**inflammation of the pancreas*

	Acute pancreatitis	Chronic pancreatitis
Causes	• Gallstones (by lodging into the duct that goes to the pancreas and pancreatic enzymes will back up); • Alcohol, tumours, • Infections; • Autoimmune (lupus); • Post surgery; • Post-traumatic; • Emboli; • Toxins/drugs.	Nearly always alcoholic
Presentation	Abdominal pain, nausea, vomiting, abdominal distension, fever, jaundice, shock;	Recurrent attacks of abdominal pain, malabsorption, calcifications, jaundice, weight loss, GI bleeding.
Investigations*	Increased pancreatic enzymes, (amylase, lipase), increased WBC.	Hyperglycemia, increased pancreatic amylase.
Course and complications	Usually benign course, occasionally severe leading to shock, renal and pulmonary insufficiency, pancreatic abscess, death.	May manifest with occasional flare-ups

Table 8.4- Presentation of pancreatitis

*assess both endocrine and exocrine functions

Note: acute form is a **MEDICAL EMERGENCY;** we will approach here the chronic form; treatment may prove somehow difficult, as the nutrients will not be properly absorbed

Nutrition and holistic approach:

- Eliminate alcohol intake, also avoid fatty meals, excessive protein intake, spicy foods;
- Slow liver cleanse and support, according to the cause of the condition;
- The diet should be very clean and wholesome, rich in vegetables, nuts, fruits;
- Take all measures to avoid blood sugar irregularities, as outlined in the *Endocrine system* chapter;

Food therapy:

- Black radish, carrot and beet juices are healing;
- Use pineapple and papaya to supply digestive enzymes.

Supplements:

- Digestive enzymes, as prescribed;
- Multivitamin and mineral formula;
- Probiotics, as prescribed, to ensure intestinal health;
- Vitamin B complex, 50-100 mg/day, as antistress and supportive;
- Some authors suggest Pancreatic glandular; use as prescribed.

Other measures:

- Dandelion root helps the health of liver and pancreas;
- Yellow dock has good effects in pancreatitis;
- Licorice root is soothing.

♦BOWEL MOVEMENT IRREGULARITIES

Notes on normal stool:

- Transit time of food: 18-28 hours;
- Colon elimination time: 6-18 hours;
- Number of stools: at least one a day (the naturopathic profession emphasizes that we should have a bowel movement after every main meal!);
- Aspect: well formed, floating halfway through the water's depth;
- Color: depends on the diet, but usually brown.

A. DIARRHEA

**frequent evacuation of watery stools*; it is usually a sign of other problems in the body;
It develops when increased mucus and fluids are released (see etiology below) and not enough water is absorbed in the large intestine; the excessive water is due to the fact that the body is trying to" flush out" toxins, irritation and disease.

Pathogenesis:

1. Increased fluid accumulation in the GI tract;
2. Increased intestinal movement (the intestines are trying to eliminate the excessive fluid).

Etiology:

- Infectious; various microorganisms may be responsible for diarrhea
- Increased intake of unripe fruits or vegetables;
- Mixing too many food categories.

When diarrhea lasts for only a day or two, we do not need to be concerned. Prolonged diarrhea needs to be properly investigated, as it may be a sign of a disease:

- Parasitosis;
- Dysbiosis;
- Irritable Bowel Syndrome;
- Inflammatory Bowel Disease;
- Celiac disease;
- Colon cancer, and
- Pancreatitis.

Clinical aspect:

- Increased frequency of watery stools;
- Fever; suggests infection;
- Increased intestinal movement, which may result in cramping and discomfort;
- In some cases, symptoms like urging or tenesmus (ineffectual straining when having a bowel movement) may be present;
- Gurgling (in medical terms, borborygmus), which is a rumbling noise caused by the passing of intestinal gas;
- Flatulence, nausea.

Complications of diarrhea: dehydration

Nutrition and holistic approach will be applied to the etiology. Here we will present the general approach to a simple diarrhea episode:

- Drink plenty of fluids to avoid dehydration; use clear broth, diluted juices and tea freely;
- Do not eat solid foods for a few days, as it gives the intestines a chance to heal;
- Solid foods are introduced slowly: soups, cooked fruits, rice puree;
- Avoid milk, fat, sugar and excessive meat;

Food therapy:

- Banana and apple juice are helpful; you can mix with carrot juice;
- Blueberry and black currant juices help with diarrhea;

Other measures:

- Chamomile and peppermint may relieve diarrhea and are antispasmodics;
- Raspberry leaf is astringent (takes away the excess fluid); agrimony and bilberry are useful, also;
- Ginger is a wonderful GI remedy;
- Fennel relieves gas.

Supplements: after the attack

- Multivitamin and mineral formula for replacement;
- Vitamin A, 5000 IU/day, vitamin C,1-2 g/day, zinc,30 mg/day, to heal the digestive tract mucosa;
- Probiotics, as prescribed, to replenish the friendly flora;
- Increase intake of green supplements, as prescribed.

B. CONSTIPATION

**difficulty and/or infrequent passing of stool or incomplete evacuation;* it is usually harmless, unless it is an indication of an underlying disorder.

Etiology:

- Insufficient fiber in the diet, which slows down the transit time;
- Increased immobility, which affects the muscular tonus;
- Rectum pathologies (hemorrhoids, anal fissure), which increase the likelihood of constipation because of the pain that the passing of stool elicits);
- Hypothyroidism, which decreases the body's metabolic rate;
- Inadequate fluid intake;
- Medication/supplementation: iron tablets, laxatives, antibiotics, Tylenol, cough medicine;
- Stress: which slows down the digestive processes;
- Diet: too much protein, too much fat (creates maldigestion), too much sugar (slows down peristalsis);
- Nutrient deficiencies: magnesium, vitamin B complex;
- Intestinal parasites;
- Slow functioning liver, as it affects the bile secretion and release.

Constipation could be also associated with irritable bowel syndrome, nervous system diseases (multiple sclerosis), and cancer.

Clinical picture:

- Slow transit time;
- Stool may be in small quantities, hard, non-continuous, difficult to eliminate;
- Pain or discomfort present on defecation (elimination of feces);
- Bloating, gas;
- Possible nausea.

Nutrition and holistic approach: applies to common causes of constipation;

*constipation associated with chronic or acute diseases will be approached with the disease in cause

- Identify and approach etiologic factors;
- Increase water and fiber intake; increase exercise; increases intake of EFA containing foods;
- Avoid dietary stressors, as mentioned under *Etiology;*

Food therapy:

- Bran is good source of fiber;

- Sauerkraut activates intestinal movement (contains choline);
- Papaya stimulates bowel activity;
- Prunes and figs have a laxative effect; gooseberries have the same effect;

Supplements:

- Fiber supplements of your liking, as prescribed (do increase the water intake when they are taken; they should not replace the dietary fiber);
- Probiotics, as prescribed, to ensure intestinal health;
- Flax seed oil, 1-2 tablespoons/day.

Other measures:

- Senna leaves, rhubarb root, and cascara are powerful laxatives; use with caution;
- Helpful herbs: chamomile, aloe vera, slippery elm, marshmallow, licorice;
- Plantain leaves are helpful; psyllium (Plantago psyllium) belongs to the plantain family;
- Essential oils of rosemary and fennel in carrier oil (plain oil) can be massaged into the abdomen.

♦MALABSORPTION SYNDROMES

CELIAC DISEASE (SPRUE)

**chronic intestinal malabsorption syndrome caused by gluten intolerance*

The reaction is to the gliadin fraction of gluten; gluten is mostly found in wheat, rye, barley and oats; the end results are malabsorption and malnutrition. Affects children and adults and it can appear at any age; strong genetic component is involved.

Pathogenesis: intestinal villi with damage and destruction, due to the local inflammation that the gluten allergy elicits.

Clinical aspect:

- Diarrhea, as the body is trying to eliminate the offending culprit residing in the intestines;
- Weight loss, due to malnutrition;
- Nutritional deficiencies, due to maldigestion and malabsorption;
- Food allergies, due to the inflammatory reaction at intestinal level, which resembles leaky gut and it allows undigested food particles and/or large molecules to travel outside of the intestines and into the blood stream, where they put a strain on the immune system by overloading it;
- Nausea, bloating, large, pale, foul smelling stools, fatigue.

In children:

- Impaired growth, due to maldigestion and malabsorption;
- Vomiting;
- Weight fluctuations, poor appetite;
- Allergic reactions (see explanation above, under *Food allergies*).

Consequences:
- Bone disease, due to lack of nutrients that support the bone health;
- PNS and CNS impairment, due to various malnutrition syndromes;
- Internal bleeding, due to the inflammatory reaction that the allergy elicits
- Pancreatic insufficiency (see above, under *Pancreas*).

Nutrition and holistic approach:
- Completely eliminate any gluten containing foods; read labels carefully, as gluten may be in trace (small) quantities in many food products (alcoholic beverages may contain gluten as well);
- Identify and approach any food allergies, as their presence will overload both the digestive system and the immune system;
- Employ a clean, wholesome, natural diet;
- Eat plenty of fruits and vegetables, as they are rich in nutrients and plant enzymes
- Increase intake of EFA.

Supplements:
- Multivitamin and mineral formula, as directed, as the nutrient deficiencies are frequent in these cases (this author suggests liquid or powder forms, as the absorption surface increases)
- Digestive enzymes, as prescribed, to support a slow functioning pancreas;
- Flax seed oil, one tablespoon/day;
- Vitamin C with bioflavonoids, 1-2 g/day, for its immune system support qualities;
- Vitamin A, 5000 IU/day, to improve health of the intestinal mucosa;
- Vitamin B complex, 50-100 mg/day, as it is very important in the energy pathway;
- Probiotics, as prescribed, to ensure intestinal health.

Other measures:
- Chamomile (avoid if allergy present), peppermint, fennel, slippery elm, marshmallow root, licorice; they are all helpful in various combinations;
- For gas relief, see below, under *Gas*.

♦FUNCTIONAL BOWEL DISORDERS
**disorders of the bowel not associated with structural abnormalities*

A. IRRITABLE BOWEL SYNDROME (IBS) (SPASTIC COLON)
**motility (the ability to move spontaneously) disorder of the GI tract with no evidence of accompanying structural defect;* the normal and regular movement of the GI tract becomes uncoordinated and irregular.

Etiology:
- Stress, as it slows down the digestion;
- Intestinal parasitosis or fungal infections;

- Dysbiosis, as it increases the burden on the bowel;
- Food allergies, as it creates the premises for local inflammation and leaky gut;
- Dietary factors: increased fat and refined sugar intake, less fiber.

Clinical aspect:
- Abdominal pain and distension that is relieved by defecation;
- Pain will bring in another bowel movement;
- Diarrhea or constipation (usually IBS is associated with constipation);
- Hypersecretion of the colonic mucus;
- Dyspeptic symptoms (flatulence, nausea, anorexia);
- Anxiety/depression.

Clinical aspects that **should not** be present: weight loss, nocturnal defecation, blood or pus in stool, fever, anemia, abnormal radiological findings (all these point to diseases other than IBS).

Diagnosis:
- Clinical features;
- Physical exam (should be unremarkable);
- Laboratory and radiological findings (should be negative);

Diagnosis of IBS is ***by exclusion*** of other conditions, as IBS symptoms may mimic many digestive tract disorders: cancer, inflammatory bowel disease, malabsorption disease, etc.

Nutrition and holistic approach:

This may not prove to be an easy approach. Some of the cases with IBS respond well to raw fruits and vegetables, whereas some will become sicker, for example. You will have to approach a case like this slowly and you will have to monitor it closely, as reactions to food may change frequently:
- Eliminate intake of high fat and sugars (decreases intestinal motility), as they pose a overload on the digestion;
- High protein intake may result in hypochlorhydria;
- Avoid spicy food, alcohol, smoking, coffee, as they interfere with the digestive process;
- Identify and approach food allergies;
- When a flare-up develops, go on a bland diet until it remits;
- Avoid intake of gas forming foods: legumes, cabbage;
- Digestive system and liver status assessment;
- Increase intake of pure water and fiber (try to avoid wheat bran, as it may seem to promote allergic reactions);
- Increase intake of papaya and pineapple, for their digestive enzymes content;
- Increase intake of magnesium rich foods, as magnesium relaxes the muscular tonus of the intestines.

Supplements:
- Multivitamin and mineral formula, as prescribed, as nutritional deficiencies are frequently encountered with this condition;

- Probiotics, as prescribed, to ensure intestinal health;
- Digestive enzymes, as prescribed, to ensure proper digestion;
- Magnesium, 400-600 mg/day, as it relaxes the smooth muscle of the intestine;
- Vitamin A , 5000 IU/day, for its gut healing properties;
- Glutamine, as prescribed, for its gut healing properties.

Other measures:

- Enteric Coated Volatile Oils (peppermint is widely used), as prescribed; exhibit relaxing properties on the muscular wall;
- For gas presence, see below, under *Gas;*
- Chamomile, fennel, slippery elm, licorice, marshmallow root, aloe vera, lemon balm, are all very helpful;
- Lemon balm, passion flora and valerian are calming and soothing;
- Essential oils of chamomile and lavender massaged into the abdomen help with relieve the cramps;
- Mild exercise program, according to the severity of the condition;
- Stress management: meditation, visualization, support groups, walks in the parks, aromatherapy bath.

B. GAS

Types:

1. **Upper GI tract gas** (eructation or belching) is due to:
   a. Swallowing high quantities of air when we eat (aerophagy);
   b. Indigestion, hypochlorhydria.
2. **Lower GI tract gas** (flatulence); the particular unpleasant smell is due to a gas called hydrogen sulfide. Gas is formed as a result of action of gut bacteria on carbohydrates and proteins in the digested food;
   - Irritable bowel syndrome;
   - Gut dysbiosis;
   - High intake of gas forming foods;
   - Parasitosis, etc.

Nutrition and holistic approach: will apply to the cause

- Very useful herbs: peppermint, fennel, anise, dill, cinnamon, chamomile, ginger.

♦INFLAMMATORY BOWEL DISEASE (IBD)

**chronic inflammation at different sites of the intestines*; it is comprised by two conditions: CROHN'S DISEASE and ULCERATIVE COLITIS

Etiology:

- Genetic aspect; only in theory so far;
- Autoimmune involvement, also in theory;

- Food allergies and sensitivities, which counts mostly as a risk factor, as their presence creates local inflammation;
- Infectious etiology: by various viruses, fungi and parasites; no specific causal agent discovered so far;
- Dietary factors: mostly involving the so-called "western diet", which, again, seems to be more of a risk factor.

CROHN'S **inflammatory reaction throughout the entire thickness of bowel wall* • **Involves any part of the GI tract**	**ULCERATIVE COLITIS** **non specific inflammatory response limited to lining of colon* • **Always involves rectum** • **Low mucin production (leads to decreased protective capacity)**
• Intermittent accesses of diarrhea; • Low-grade fever; • Lower abdominal pain, especially on the right side; • Anorexia (appetite loss); • Weight loss, flatulence.	• Bloody diarrhea, sometimes with mucus and pus; • Cramps in lower abdomen; • Fever, weight loss. • Rectal exam: anal fissures, hemorrhoids, abscesses;
• Recurs after surgery	• Cured after surgery
• Granuloma (inflammatory local lesions) present;	• Granuloma absent, diffuse inflammation;
• X-Ray shows abnormality of small intestine, with asymmetrical distribution of lesions.	• Diagnosis by X-Ray, which shows characteristic patterns.

Table 8.5-Presentation of IBD

Complications:

- Serious vitamin and mineral deficiencies, as digestion and absorption are greatly impaired;
- Malnutrition/malabsorption;
- Dysbiosis;
- Retardation of growth;
- Urinary calculi(from disorders of metabolism);
- Cholelithiasis;
- Articular disorders;
- Cancer, obstruction, perforation, anemia.

Medical treatment will focus on a combination of antiinflamatories, corticosteroids, antibiotics, spasmolytics, etc. Surgery is also an option.

Nutrition and holistic approach:

Tread very carefully, as these clients are in a lot of pain and distress. Often enough they respect all the dietary advice and all the supplements protocol, but they may still encounter the occasional flare-up.

Patience is very important, as is the careful therapeutic approach. Do not employ drastic measures, even when they seem justified, as the health status may deteriorate.

- Identify and approach food allergies and sensitivities and dysbiosis;
- Slow, mild liver detoxification and support, as they will have an overburdened liver from the stress and the toxic level that their body is exposed to (improper digestion will allow for toxins to accumulate in the gut and be transported from there);
- Gentle immune system building (their immune system status is quite low, from malnutrition and from the increased intestinal permeability, which is a consequence of maldigestion); do not employ immune system boosting, as IBD may carry some autoimmune trends, and boosting will accentuate them;
- Eliminate all food stressors: saturated fat, sugar, spicy foods, "chemically enriched" food, alcohol, coffee, pop, smoking;
- Increase intake of fruits and vegetables (in any form that is acceptable to the body), sources of EFA, water intake and fiber intake;
- Depending on the status of the case, food intake may have to be pureed or juiced, as to decrease the load on the digestive system;
- Grains, yogurt, kefir, complex carbohydrates are all good choices.

<u>Supplements:</u>

- These cases usually follow the "*elemental diet*", which provides all necessary nutrients and the aminoacids in free forms (their most pure form, need no digestion for absorption);
- Green food supplements, as prescribed (be careful as they may exhibit increased gaseousness);
- Probiotics, at least 5-6 billions germs/day;
- Flax seed oil, 1-2 tablespoons/day or Evening Primrose Oil, 500 mg three times/day;
- A multivitamin and mineral formula, in a liquid or powder form;
- Digestive enzymes (most sources recommend Pancreatin), as prescribed;
- Vitamin A, 5000 IU/day, to increase the strength of intestinal mucosa;
- Vitamin C, 2-4 g/day, or up to bowel tolerance, vitamin E,400 IU/day, for their antioxidant properties;
- Calcium and magnesium, 800-1000 mg/day to 400-500 mg/day, for their relaxing properties;
- Vitamin B complex, 50-100 mg/day, as it is anti stress and is important for the energy pathway.

<u>Other measures:</u>

- A highly recommended formula is "*Robert's formula*", which consists of a combination of demulcents, anti-inflammatory and antibacterial herbs; take as prescribed;
- Chamomile and peppermint may help in relieving the gas and distension;
- Hops and lemon balm are calming and soothing;
- Slippery elm and licorice are demulcents;
- Essential oils of lavender and chamomile are soothing when massaged into the abdomen.

♦ DIVERTICULITIS

**inflammation secondary to infection of diverticula* (the pouch fills with matter);
*Diverticulum/diverticula: abnormal sac or pouch protruding from the wall of a hollow organ;
*Diverticulosis: presence of diverticulum.

Etiology:

- Aging, which results in weakened tissue;
- Low intestinal transit;
- Decreased fiber diet;
- Increased fat and refined carbohydrates in diet;
- Adjacent (close by) infection;
- Dysbiosis, indigestion
- Food allergies.

Clinical presentation:

- Low left side abdominal pain and tenderness, palpable mass;
- Constipation or frequent defecation common;
- Low grade fever, leukocytosis (increased WBC, sign of an infection).

Complications: abscess formation, peritonitis, perforation, fistula.

Nutrition and holistic approach:

- Identify and approach etiologic factors;
- Gentle liver detoxification and support;
- Immune system boosting, as we are dealing with an infection;
- Avoid saturated fat, sugar;
- Increase intake of fruits and vegetables, EFA and water.

Supplements:

- Green food supplements, as prescribed;
- Probiotics, as prescribed;
- Vitamin A, 5000 IU/day;
- Vitamin C, 1-3 g/day;
- Vitamin B complex, 50-100 mg/day;
- Vitamin E, 400 IU/day;
- Flax seed oil, one tablespoon/day;

*for explanation of mechanisms of action of supplements, see under IBD

Other measures:

- Chamomile is soothing;
- Yucca and feverfew are anti-inflammatory;
- Echinacea (taken for a maximum of 5-7 days at a time) boosts the immune system.

♦DYSBIOSIS

**altered balance of gut microbial flora*

Our gut is populated with over four pounds of microorganisms, comprising over 400 species! Some of them are helpful, friendly and live in harmony with us (*friendly bacteria*, ***symbionts***) and some of them would do anything to bring us harm (***pathogens***). The microbial flora is in a continuous fight for space and nutrients. If the friendly bacteria prevail (which depends on what we eat, how we eat it and how well we digest it), then we ensure a healthy digestion, healthy liver (by not overloading it and providing its nutrients), healthy blood and healthy immune system. If, on the other hand, we allow the unfriendly bacteria to multiply, then the reverse will happen.

Etiology:

- Use of antibiotics (which kill anything that is alive, including your friendly bugs), corticosteroids, anti-inflammatory medication;
- Excessive use of chlorinated water and all other chemicals that we ingest;
- Large, bulky meals, as they will overload the digestive processes;
- High intake of refined sugar, which affects the intestinal motility, on one hand, not allowing for proper peristalsis, and secondly by destroying the mucosal defense (it affects the IgA mostly);
- Excessive use of saturated fat, alcohol, coffee, anti nutrients;
- Poor food digestion (not enough stomach acid, insufficient bile release, etc.);
- Slow transit time, which allows waste to stay longer in the gut, allowing for further degradation of food particles by microbes, and for increased toxin absorption;
- Ileocecal valve syndrome, which means a slow functioning valve, will allow for slower transit time; constipation and straining may be responsible for the malfunctioning of the ileocecal valve;
- Stress, which slows down digestion.

PATHOGENESIS:

The digestive process is of great importance here. If the digestion proceeds smoothly (if you provide the body with the right nutrient balance and if you have enough stomach acid, bile and pancreatic juice to digest the food), then you will end up with building blocks (aminoacids, fatty acids and monosugars) that are easily absorbed through the mucosa of your intestine and they will nourish you.

Any anti-nutrients (like refined sugar and additives or other chemicals) will greatly overload the digestive process, because they are not absorbed as nutrients, of course, but they create the conditions for a porous gut just by mere presence. A leaky gut will allow toxins to travel into the blood stream with all the health consequences we talked about already, under *Basic mechanisms.*

If the food intake is unbalanced (too much of a macronutrient or the other, too little fiber, too many additives, too much processed food), then the digestive process will be impeded, digestion will be incomplete, and the pathogenic bacteria in your gut will be more than happy to finish the work for you. Well-fed bacteria will multiply quickly, diminishing the surviving chances of the friendly type.
Some bacteria will digest carbohydrates, and the end result will be release of excessive gas and abdominal distension. Some other bacteria will act upon undigested proteins, by putrefaction, creating chemical substances called *vasoactive amines,* which act on the intestinal blood vessels (one of the

actions is constriction) and the end result will be abdominal pain, increased intestinal permeability (leaky gut) and abnormal gut peristalsis.

THE INTESTINAL MICROFLORA

a) The Friendly Bacteria
The main population of friendly bacteria is being composed by the Lactobacillus family (acidophilus, bifidus, bulgaris, casei) and streptococcus lactis. Here is a short list with all benefits of our friendly bacteria.

- Re-implants friendly bacteria in colon, by multiplication;
- Improves immunity, by releasing chemicals able to enhance the mucosal defense and by inhibiting the growth of pathogenic bacteria;
- Produces its own antibiotics;
- Lessens cancer risk;
- Synthesizes B vitamins and vitamin K;
- Digests fats into fatty acids;
- Ensure bowel health and proper digestion;
- Helps deactivating toxins.

When your friendly bacteria diminish in strength and in number, the **clinical aspect** is:

- Abdominal pain, distension, bloating;
- Gas release, gurgling sounds;
- Possible nausea and /or alteration of bowel movements;
- Signs of liver overload (see Liver chapter);
- Signs of the immune system overload;
- Depressed IgA;
- Fatigue;
- Food allergy;
- Foul smelling stool;
- Headache, hives;
- Increased intestinal permeability, indigestion, IBS;
- Malabsorption, weight loss.

b) The Yeast
*in normal, healthy condition, the yeast does not interfere with our health. This is why it is not classified as being harmful. The problems arise when the friendly bacteria diminish and the yeast has enough space and nutrients to grow. The health condition that the yeast overgrowth creates will be approached below, under Candidiasis.

c) The Pathogens/parasites
These microbes are harmful. They populate the gut and are in a continuous search for food and space, and they accomplish their goals by living off their host. Parasites will be described below, under Parasitosis.

PREVENTION OF DYSBIOSIS:

- Eat as healthy as possible, balanced meals as in composition and size;
- Drink plenty of pure water, to flush out toxins;
- Increase intake of dietary fiber, to ensure optimal transit time;
- Avoid exposure to ingested additives and/or chemicals;
- Identify and approach low stomach acid, low pancreatic juice output and low bile output;
- Identify and approach a poorly functioning liver.

Nutrition and holistic approach for dysbiosis:

- Identify and approach accordingly the etiologic factors;
- Employ the general measures described above, under prevention;
- The diet should be as healthy as possible, eliminating any possible allergens;
- **Probiotics supplementation:** these are friendly bacteria in supplement form; they may come as capsules, or powders, or yogurts. Usually, the dosage is expressed in number of germs per unit. The unit varies from one company to another (a unit could be a teaspoon of yogurt or two capsules, etc). Generally, it has been suggested that the number of microorganisms per unit should be in the range of billions. As in dosage, the opinions vary. In dysbiosis cases, according to the gravity of the case, you will adjust the dosage accordingly. In serious cases with utter discomfort and multiple body systems involvement, 8 to 12 billions germs a day is an acceptable dosage. For milder cases and maintenance, 3 to 6 billions germs a day should suffice. Again, work closely with your client. Their body will let you know how well the case progresses.
- If gas is present, employ the measures underlined above, under Gas;
- Cleanses, as to allow the body a chance to properly filter, detoxify, transport and nutrient absorption (these cleanses are not limited only to Dysbiosis protocol; they can be used at any times when you assess a client and you decide that a particular organ system needs a cleanse).

1. **Liver cleanse**, absolutely necessary, as the liver will have to detoxify all toxic products from the intestines; see liver cleanse in the Liver chapter;
2. **Colon cleanse**, which is very important as a sluggish colon will allow for increased transit time and toxic accumulation;

   2a. Increased water and fiber intake, either dietary fiber or fiber supplements (in which case, be sure and increase water intake by at least 0.5 times);
   2b. Healthy diet; low saturated fat and sugar;
   2c. Some authors suggest a fast for colon cleansing; it very much depends upon your clients (if they work, if they are hypoglycemic, etc.); remember, all protocols, even fasting protocols should be individualized; you may employ various types of fasts: water fasts, juice fasts, etc.;
   2d. Aloe vera juice, ½ cup two or three times a day, as it has healing effects;
   2e. Probiotics, as prescribed;
   2f. Wheatgrass juice;
   2g. Some authors recommend brown rice diets; I have had very good results with it, but be aware that not everybody can stomach it;
   2h. Herbs: garlic, burdock, licorice (do not use in cases with hypertension; use DGL instead), senna, fennel, marshmallow.

3. **Blood cleanse**, as the blood is the medium that transports everything throughout your body, may it be nutrients or waste; another aspect that you may wish to keep in mind is that when bacteria dies, there is a phenomenon that is called " the dying off", which means increased toxins release; these toxins will be transported to the liver for detoxification via the blood
   3a. Ideally, fasts should be employed, but again, adapt to your client; if a fast is not doable, then make sure that all dietary stressors are eliminated, along with smoking and alcohol intake; the diet should be as healthy as possible, comprised of macro and micronutrients and increased intake of water; increased intake of fruits and vegetables;
   3b. Chlorophyll, as it is a blood cleanser;
   3c. Herbal teas: dandelion, licorice, yellow dock ("the purifier of the body"), burdock, red clover and chamomile;
   3d. Blood cleansing juices: lemon, carrot, leafy greens and beets.

A. YEAST OVERGROWTH/ CANDIDIASIS

**overgrowth of the yeast Candida albicans*; this yeast normally lives in our gut and vaginal tract, along with the friendly bacteria; its excessive growth results in multiple systems involvement

Etiology:

- Altered bowel flora, due to antibiotic use;
- Decreased digestive secretions;
- High intake of sugar/dairy;
- Impaired immunity;
- Impaired liver function.

Clinical aspect:

Major symptoms:

- Fatigue, feeling of "being drained";
- Poor memory, feeling "spacey";
- Depression;
- Numbness, tingling, muscle aches and weakness
- Abdominal pain and bloating, altered bowel movements;
- Vaginal infections;
- Visual disturbances.

Minor/other symptoms and consequences:

- Irritability, mood swings;
- Headache, dizziness;
- Skin rashes;
- Allergies, multiple chemical sensitivities;
- Increased sensitivity for smells;
- Sugar cravings (candida will digest carbohydrates easily, hence the abdominal gas and discomfort associated with candidiasis).

Notes on Candida:

- It has been suggested that practically, Candida may mimic many disease processes, because it has many variations from its normal form, which allow it to" fool" your immune system;
- Candida secretes estrogen-like molecules, which can add to the estrogen burden;
- Intolerances to cheese, wine and perfumes are quoted as being part of the Candida picture;
- It seems that Candida is able to cross placenta;
- It seems that Candida toxic by-products and cells are able to be absorbed into the circulation through a leaky gut and travel throughout the body, affecting various organ systems.

Diagnosis:

- Clinical picture;
- Candida questionnaires, which are suggestive or not of the presence of the yeast and also assess the degree of infestation;
- Some doctors employ stool analysis, vaginal swabs and/or antibodies measurement; these tests will be positive when Candida infestation is quite serious; we hope to be able to identify the imbalance before it turns into a disease.

Medical treatment will employ the use of antifungal preparations.

Nutrition and holistic approach:

- Identify and approach the etiologic factors;
- Proceed into a liver and colon cleanse, but very carefully, as the dying off phenomenon of Candida may accentuate the clinical picture;
- Eliminate refined and simple sugars, diary, all food allergens, foods with high yeast/mold content (breads, alcohol, cheese, dried fruits, etc.);
- Increase fiber and water intake;
- Improve elimination.

*I personally suggest the dietary aspects first; only in that Candida will start dying; the general supplements (see below) could be used at the same time with the diet; the anti-candida agents will be used after 7-10 days, as they will result in an intense die off phenomenon, which is very uncomfortable for your clients; we know that the anti-candida diet is very restrictive; make sure that your clients will eat sufficiently, though; hypoglycemia accidents and intense fatigue are not unheard of and you should make sure that they are avoided; some authors suggest complete elimination of fruits; whereas I agree with the principle, sometimes it is difficult to be applied; at least suggest that only fruits on the low glycemic index side are consumed, and in small quantities.

<u>Supplements:</u>

- Multivitamin and mineral formula;
- Flax seed oil, one or two tablespoons/day;
- Vitamin C and bioflavonoids 1-2 g/day and vitamin E , 400 IU/day, for their antioxidant effect;

- Garlic, as prescribed, or consume liberally;
- Probiotics, 3-8 billions germs/day.

Anti- candida agents:
- Caprylic acid ,1-1.5 g/day or as prescribed;
- Berberine (plant substance with antibiotic properties) containing plants-Goldenseal, Barberry, Oregon Grape.

B. INTESTINAL PARASITOSIS

**overgrowth of intestinal parasites*

Parasites: organisms that derive food, nutrition and shelter by living in or on another organism and do not contribute beneficially to that organism.

Types of parasites:
1. Protozoa (organisms made of one cell only): Ameba, Giardia, Trichomonas;
2. Helminths (worms): Roundworm (ascaris), pinworm, hookworm, tapeworm, etc.

Pathogenesis: parasites can harm us in two ways:
- Impeding digestion, by consuming our food and eliminating toxins;
- Damage to the intestinal lining, on which they attach.

***Testing for parasites*:**
1. Purged stool test (needs to be repeated, as parasites need to go through a certain life cycle, from eggs to larvae, to parasite, to eggs again; only certain development stages could be identified on testing, this is why we may need to repeat these tests on a periodical basis);
2. Rectal swab;
3. Blood test
4. Sputum test (phlegm);
5. Urine test.

How parasites gain access to the human body:
- Ingestion, by food or water intake;
- Skin contact;
- Transplacentar;
- Sexual activity;
- Injection of infective material (for example, a mosquito that bites you may carry malaria);
- Inhalation (of infected dust).

Consequences of parasitic infestation:
- Malabsorption;
- Immune system overload and suppression;
- Liver overload.

Clinical aspect:
- Abdominal cramps and distension; gas;

- Anemia, as parasites action may result in occult (not seen) bleeding and/or in rectal bleeding;
- Stool abnormalities, as in frequency and consistency;
- Fatigue, dizziness, “brain fog”;
- Rectal pruritus (itching);
- Increased tendency to allergies;
- Skin rashes;
- Increased appetite with increased weight loss.

Nutrition and holistic approach:

- Assess digestive system status, as abnormalities (low gastric acid, low pancreatic juice output, dysbiosis), may create the conditions for parasitic growth and multiplication;
- As you apply your treatment, please employ liver and colon cleanse;
- Increase water and fiber intake;
- Increase antioxidant and beta carotene rich foods, as protective measures;

Food therapy

- Cabbage does not allow parasitic growth;
- Eat garlic and pumpkin seeds between meals, as they are strong anti-parasitic agents;
- Increase papaya intake, as it contains digestive enzymes that may contribute to destroying of parasites.

Supplements:

- Probiotics, as prescribed;
- Garlic, as prescribed;
- Grapefruit seed extract, as prescribed;
- Digestive enzymes, as prescribed.

Other:

- Herbs are very useful and they should be used for at least 30 days, as the parasites go through life cycles:walnut, black walnut, cloves, tansy, wormwood.

♦ANO-RECTAL DISORDERS

A. HEMORRHOIDS

**enlarged anal veins that lost their elasticity.*

Etiology:

- Genetic weakness of veins;
- Excessive pressure on the veins due to straining during defecation, pregnancy, heavy lifting, obesity, standing or sitting for long periods of time;
- Lack of exercise;

- Liver damage;
- Lack of dietary fiber;
- Constipation.

Types:
- Internal hemorrhoids: non visible from the outside;
- External hemorrhoids: protruding through the anus.

Cinical aspect:
- Bright red bleeding;
- Pain, mostly on defecation;
- Itching and discomfort around the anus;
- Lumps may appear outside the anus.

Nutrition and holistic approach:
- Identify etiologic factors and approach them;
- Gentle liver detoxification and support;
- Increase fiber, water and EFA intake;
- Increase fruit and vegetables intake; increased intake of bioflavonoids rich foods, as they strengthen the vascular wall; increase intake of beta carotene rich foods, as they protect the intestinal/colon lining.

Supplements:
- Vitamin C, 2-3 g/day, for collagen formation and support;
- Bioflavonoid complex (especially Rutin and Hesperidin) to improve vascular fragility;
- Flax seed oil, one tablespoon/day, as an anti-inflammatory and emollient agent;
- Vitamin E, 400 IU/day, for its antioxidant properties;
- Vitamin A, 5000 IU/day, for mucosa protection;
- Probiotics, as prescribed, to ensure intestinal health.

Other measures:

- Witch hazel is very helpful, as it is an stringent (decreases size of tissues); it can be used in a topical (local) cream or in a sitz bath (make a tea and pour it in a bowl, then sit in it);
- Cocoa butter applied topically may help;
- Calendula, plantain, slippery elm make good local treatments in sitz bath or compresses; they can be taken internally, as well;
- Aloe vera gel and calendula cream, applied topically are quite soothing.

♦DIGESTIVE SYSTEM TUMORS

*will be described as in etiology and clinical aspect; nutrition and holistic approach always follows the principles explained under Neoplasia (with the exception of polyposis, described below)

A. ESOPHAGEAL CANCER

**cancer of the esophagus*

Etiology:

- Chronic hyperacidity conditions like chronic esophagitis or hiatus hernia;
- Smoking;
- Exposure to environmental chemicals;
- High intake of spicy food and alcohol.

Clinical aspect:

- Dysphagia (difficulty swallowing), begins with difficulty swallowing solid food and progressing into difficulty swallowing liquids, as the tumor grows and occupies the esophageal lumen;
- Pain that radiates in the back;
- Weight loss, malaise (a state of feeling very badly);
- If the tumor compresses on the larynx, there may be hoarseness.

Diagnosis: by clinical aspect, X-ray and CT scan

B. GASTRIC CANCER

**cancer of stomach*

Risk factors:

- Smoking, alcohol, food additives;
- H. Pylori infection;
- Chronic gastritis.

Clinical presentation:

- Suspect when ulcer fails to heal;
- Late onset (start, beginning) of symptoms;
- Postprandial (after meals) abdominal fullness, weight loss, anorexia, dysphagia;
- Non characteristic abdominal pain;
- Epigastric mass, in the later stages.

Diagnosis:

- Clinical aspect;
- Physical examination;
- Upper GI series;
- CT scan;
- Biopsy.

C. COLORECTAL POLYPS

**benign tumors protruding from the mucous lining of the colon;* they usually grow in groups

Etiology:

- Injury or irritation to the mucosa of the intestinal tract;
- Genetic factors;
- Dietary aspect: diet low in fiber, high in refined sugar and saturated fat.

Clinical aspect:

- Mostly asymptomatic;
- Rectal bleeding, change in bowel habits.

*they are considered pre-malignant

Nutrition approach:

- Identify and correct etiologic factors, if possible;
- Vitamin C with bioflavonoids, 1-2 g/day;
- Vitamin A, 5000 IU/day;
- Flax seed oil, one tablespoon/day;
- Probiotics, as prescribed;
- Vitamin E, 400 IU/day.

D. COLORECTAL CARCINOMA

**cancer located at the last portion of the colon and rectum*

Risk factors:

- Familial polyposis;
- Previous colon cancer;
- IBD;
- Diet (increased fat, decreased fiber);
- Increased exposure to smoking, free radical damage;
- Sluggish liver;
- Low immune system status.

Clinical presentation:

	Right colon	**Left colon**	**Rectum**
Pathology	Large polypoid (looks like a polyp) lesions that tend to bleed without being noticed;	Annular (like a coin) lesions leading to obstruction;	Ulcerating lesion
Symptoms	Weight loss, weakness, sided abdominal pain especially on the right side;	Alternation of diarrhea/constipation, abdominal pain, "pencil stool"(long and very thin)	Obstruction, tenesmus (spastic sensation at rectum level);
Signs	Palpable mass in the lower right part of the abdomen, anemia	Bleeding	Palpable mass on rectal exam, rectal bleeding

Table 8.6- Colon cancer

Spread:

- Direct extension;
- Lymphatic nodes;
- Hematogenous (via the blood).

Diagnosis:

- Sigmoidoscopy;
- Colonoscopy;
- Hemoccult (analysis of blood presence);
- Digital rectal exam.

FOR ALL CANCERS, EMPLOY THE MEASURES OUTLINED IN THE NEOPLASIA CHAPTER

CHAPTER 9

THE LIVER AND THE BILIARY TRACT

For an alternative medicine practitioner, the Liver seems to be the center of our undivided attention. And no wonder…

The liver detoxifies the smoke from your cigarettes and the smoke from your next door neighbour's cigarettes, the Pina colada we had yesterday on the beach, the Tylenol we took for a headache, the hair colour shampoo, the make-up, the dishwasher detergent, the soap, the toothpaste. And if all of these would not be enough, the Liver has to process every class of nutrients as well; and make new lipoproteins; and produce some more bile; and produce some more coagulation factors; and some more glutathione.
The air we breath impacts on the liver; so does you getting upset with your boss, bus driver or mother in law. Plus, the liver can regenerate if damaged.

It is no wonder that the Liver should be the center of our undivided attention, as we will see in the following chapter.

IMPORTANT NUTRIENTS FOR THE LIVER

Nutrient	Role
Vitamin B_3	Involved in bile synthesis
Choline	Gall bladder regulation
Vitamin C	Cofactor in bile acids synthesis
Inositol	Helps remove fats from liver
Bioflavonoids	Stimulate bile production
Carnitine	Indicated in fatty liver
Cysteine	Precursor for glutathione
Glutathione	Strong antioxidant
Taurine Glycine	Bile acids production
Copper Magnesium Zinc Vitamin C	Support phase I liver detoxification
Vitamin B complex Zinc Magnesium Sulfur Germanium	Support phase II liver detoxification

Nutrient	Role
Choline	Promote bile flow
Methionine	
Vitamin B6	
Vitamin B12	
Folic acid	

Table 9.1- Important nutrients for the liver

THE LIVER AND THE BILIARY TRACT

Common symptoms/signs: fatigue, depression, irritability, jaundice, increased liver size (hepatomegaly), nausea, headache, pain (usually referred/radiating in the right shoulder), skin rashes or aggravation of previous skin lesions; other signs and symptoms will be presented within the clinical description of a particular disease

ASSESSMENT

MEDICAL	NUTRITIONAL
1. Clinical picture, based on symptoms and signs; 2. Physical examination: of liver size, of pain location, etc.; 3. Laboratory tests: bilirubin, liver enzymes, etc.; 4. X-ray: detection of calcifications in the liver and/or biliary tract; 5. Ultrasound: detects biliary tract problem and liver masses; 6. MRI: used for tumours identification; 7. Cholecystogram: introduces a contrast agent to identify gall bladder and biliary tract abnormalities; 8. Liver biopsy: to assess changes at cellular level.	1. Liver function assessment: based on presence of symptoms and signs and by liver clearance tests; (see below under Tests) 2. Digestive system status; assessment, as a malfunctioning digestive system will lead into malnutrition and immune system overload; 3. Colon function assessment, as a slow transit will lead into constipation and increased toxicity; 4. Immune system status assessment, as an impaired immune system will not eliminate toxins properly; 5. Toxicity level assessment, by hair analysis or urine analysis; 6. Assessment of toxic exposure (smoking, coffee, environmental and/or occupational toxins; 7. Assessment of toxic dietary exposure: increased saturated fat, trans fatty acids presence, sugar overload, additives, etc.;

Table 9.2- Assessment of liver functions

LIVER FUNCTIONS

1. BILE SECRETION (production)

Bile is a carrier in which many substances are eliminated from the body. Bile is produced in the liver, but stored in the gall bladder. Bile is necessary for fat digestion, for fat soluble vitamins absorption, and for conversion of beta carotene into vitamin A.

All by-products of liver detoxification will be eventually released into the bile, which carries them to the intestines, where the bile and its toxic load are absorbed by fiber and excreted. Most of the bile acids are reabsorbed and recycled.

Bile composition:

- Bile acids: the liver synthesizes them from cholesterol; glycine and taurine are needed for their secretion; help with fats solubility, making them more accessible to absorption;
- Bilirubin (from catabolism/breaking down of hemoglobin);
- Cholesterol and phospholipids (lecithin).

2. MAJOR METABOLIC ORGAN: processes every class of nutrients:

- Regulation of carbohydrate metabolism and glycogen production;
- Cholesterol synthesis and metabolism control;
- Fat synthesis and production of lipoproteins;
- Formation of urea (end product of protein metabolism), albumin (the protein that holds the water in the blood stream), clotting factors, enzymes.

3. CARBOHYDRATE METABOLISM REGULATOR:

- *Glycogenesis:* conversion of glucose to glycogen (storage form of glucose);
- *Glycogenolysis:* breaking down of glycogen into glucose when energy is needed;
- *Gluconeogenesis:* synthesis of glucose from non-carbohydrates, like fatty acids or amino acids.

4. HORMONES DEGRADATION: as widely used hormones are not able to perform their function properly (hormones go through" wear and tear" too), they are transported to the liver for degradation and disposal; also, converts T_4 (thyroxin) into T_3 (triiodothyronine).

5. BLOOD FILTER: of various toxins

- toxins that come from the gut, either because of constipation or because of gut flora's action on undigested food;
- microbial toxins, either the ones released by the gut microbial flora or the ones that are released into the circulation after the immune system acted upon microorganisms and destroyed them.

6. MAJOR DETOXIFICATION ORGAN

- Liver cells detoxify drugs, toxins and alcohol of various origins (see *Detoxification* below).

7. GTF SYNTHESIS: glucose tolerance factor is created in the liver from chromium and glutathione; GTF acts with insulin in blood sugar regulation.

ASSESMENT OF LIVER FUNCTION/TOXICITY

1. **Medical history and symptoms/signs present**

    - History of liver disease;
    - Environmental and /or occupational exposure to various toxins;
    - Use of drugs and/or chronic medication;
    - High intake of alcohol and/or smoking;
    - High intake of food additives, preservatives and highly processed foods;
    - High intake of saturated fat and/or refined carbohydrates;
    - History of digestive system problems/abnormalities (dysbiosis, parasites);
    - History of allergies.

2. **Medical laboratory investigations:** bilirubin and liver enzymes (when positive, they establish the presence of the disease process; when negative, but some factors listed under **1.***(Medical history and symptoms/signs present)* above are present, that means that there is no disease yet, but that does not exclude an imbalance).

3. **Assessments of phase I and II detoxification**, by ingestion of various substances (caffeine or acetaminophen) followed by timely measurements (for caffeine, for example, saliva levels are measured).

> **NOTE**: as we can see, whereas some forms of assessments of liver function are not necessary in our realm of complementary alternative modalities, the ones listed under **1.** definitely are. Our aim is to assess and identify imbalances before the disease process is established. Truly, the liver detoxification and support, which serve vital body functions, are more than accessible and not difficult to approach. All it takes is patience, compliance (at least some) and knowledge of nutrition.

DETOXIFICATION

**reduction of toxicity*

Whereas the liver is the major detoxification organ, other organs and systems play also important roles.

OVERVIEW OF THE DETOXIFICATION SYSTEMS*

ORGAN/ ORGAN SYSTEM	DETOXIFICATION APPROACH	TYPES OF TOXINS REMOVED
LIVER	Filtering of the blood	Microorganisms, by-products of the microorganisms metabolism, immune complexes
	Bile secretion	Cholesterol metabolism by-products, hemoglobin breakdown products
	Phases of detoxification	Drugs, degraded hormones, pesticides, irritants, nicotine
INTESTINES	Excretion through feces	Toxins from gut bacterial flora
		Fat soluble toxins

ORGAN/ ORGAN SYSTEM	DETOXIFICATION APPROACH	TYPES OF TOXINS REMOVED
KIDNEYS	Excretion through urine	Many toxins after they were acted upon and turned water-soluble by the liver
SKIN	Skin is a miniexcretory system through sweat	Fat soluble toxins: heavy metals

Table 9.3-Overview of detoxification systems

*the major detoxification organs are the liver, intestines and kidneys; skin and lungs are detoxifying , too, but to a lesser degree.

Simply put, the body will neutralize toxins (via the liver) then eliminate them via urine or feces. In the following, we will approach the **liver detoxification** systems.

Phases of Liver Detoxification

PHASE I: neutralizes some chemicals, on one hand, and on the other, alters some toxins to a chemically active form to be dealt with in phase II.
To accomplish all of that, the liver uses a group of enzymes called **cytochrome P450.** This group acts upon toxins by either making them weaker or making them water soluble, which allows for elimination through the kidneys.

Unfortunately, as the liver's detoxification enzymes are working overtime, some free radicals may be released. Glutathione, an antioxidant produced by the liver, will step in and neutralize them. Ideally, we should improve as much as possible the phase I of liver detoxification, so the chemicals/toxins can advance towards phase II to be destroyed.
(*cross reference table below)*

PHASE II: alters the weakened toxins sent by Phase I by attaching some various chemicals to them, and in doing so, renders them either neutralized or easily eliminated via the gut. This process is called *conjugation.* Phase II has six major chemical pathways. I will list them here, for information purposes, as to what type of nutrients are needed for each process.

- **Glutathione conjugation:** (cysteine, glutamic acid and glycine are needed for glutathione synthesis); turns fat soluble toxins from heavy metals, solvents and pesticides into water soluble forms, easily excreted by kidneys;
- **Amino acid conjugation:** Glycine, taurine, glutamine, and arginine combine with various toxins and neutralize them;
- **Methylation:** needs methionine which inactivates estrogen and estrogen metabolites;
- **Sulfation:** Methionine and cysteine are needed to detoxify drugs, food additives, gut bacterial toxins, thyroid hormone metabolites, neurotransmitters metabolites (metabolites are substances resulting from metabolic processes);
- **Acetylation:** vitamins B1, B5 and C are needed to allow combination of sulfa drugs (antibiotics) with acetyl CoA for neutralization;
- **Glucuronidation:** limonene (in citrus peel) supports this process, that allows most commonly prescribed drugs, aspirin, and food additives to be eliminated

NUTRIENTS NEEDED FOR THE PHASES OF LIVER DETOXIFICATION

PHASE	NUTRIENTS
PHASE I	• Brassica family foods (cabbage, broccoli, Brussels sprouts); • Citrus fruits*; • Vitamins C and B's;
PHASE II	
Glutathione conjugation	• Glutathione rich foods (asparagus, walnuts, avocado); • Brassica family; • Vitamin C and vitamin B_6;
Amino acid conjugation	• Adequate protein intake;
Methylation	• Methionine; • Vitamins B_6 and B_{12}; • Folic acid;
Sulfation	• Sulfur containing foods (garlic, onions, broccoli);
Acetylation	• Vitamins B's and C.
Glucuronidation	• Sulfur rich foods; • Citrus fruit.

Table 9.4-Phases of liver detoxification: nutrients needed

*Do not use too many grapefruits if you have reason to believe that your liver is excessively overloaded, as it may slow down phase I.

MAINTAINING GOOD LIVER HEALTH

1. Ensure proper digestion and elimination;
2. Avoid environmental stressors;
3. Increase water and fiber intake;
4. Avoid excessive alcohol, saturated fat and refined sugar;
5. Diet and nutrients:

FOODS	SUPPLEMENTS
• Sulphur containing foods: Garlic, onion, legumes, eggs • Fiber: pears, bran, apple • Cabbage family: broccoli, Brussels sprouts, cabbage • Artichoke, beets, carrots, dandelion, turmeric	• Good multivitamin/mineral formula • Antioxidants • Vitamin B complex, Calcium. • Lipotropic agents (promote bile flow): Choline, methionine, vitamins B_6, folic acid, and B_{12}

Table 9.5- Maintaining good liver health: foods and supplements

LIVER DETOXIFICATION: PRINCIPLES AND PROTOCOLS

1. The first step in liver detoxification approach is to **remove dietary, environmental and lifestyle stressors** (as much as possible; by stressors we mean alcohol, coffee, smoking, environmental toxins, etc.); we can recommend the best foods and supplemental measures, but if the body continues to be bombarded with toxins, then there is not much that we can achieve.

2. The second step is to **improve the diet**; avoid all liver dietary stressors, and increase intake of fruits, vegetables, legumes, fish and nuts; do not forget increased water intake; do use the foods that have been listed above under Liver Support.

3. While you are working along with your client on steps number 1 and 2, employ a very simple and effective method: **lemon water cleanse.** Use a glass of pure, room temperature water in which you squeeze a few drops of fresh lemon juice (lime juice is as good). Drink it first thing in the morning. Wait for 30 minutes before you eat or drink anything else. Do not take any vitamins or other pills with your lemon water, and do not squeeze the lemon in fruit juice (as the liver will start working on that instead of detoxifying). The reason behind this cleanse is that the liver accumulates toxins in bile overnight, and the lemon juice stimulates gall bladder contractions, allowing the bile to flow into the duodenum. Do start your cleanse with only a few drops of lemon. If the liver is even slightly overloaded, you may end up having "side effects of detoxification". If everything goes well for 3-4 days, you can add more lemon drops to your daily lemon water. The final quantity varies with the person's tolerance.

4. **Dandelion root tea** greatly supports liver detoxification. Have a cup a tea everyday. Dandelion leaf tea will support the kidneys detoxification. **Milk thistle tea** is very helpful in regeneration of the liver tissue.

5. **Supplements:**

   - Good multivitamin and mineral formula, as prescribed;
   - Vitamin B complex, 50 mg/day;
   - Vitamin C with bioflavonoids, 1-2 g/day;
   - Vitamin E, 400 IU/day.

6. **Other measures:**

   - **Fasts** are frequently used by people who wish to detoxify; there are many types of fasts, from water fasts, to juice fasts, to combinations of juices and vegetables fasts, and so on; they are very helpful, but keep in mind that every client is different and apply your approach to the case (a hypoglycemia case should not fast, for example). Even short termed fasts are helpful (some people do it for a half a day only);
   - **Lymphatic drainage**, by rubbing vigorously the outside of the thighs (helps drainage from the large intestine); rubbing the inside of the thigh will stimulate the drainage of small intestine;
   - **Epsom salts** or sea salt and baking soda baths are helpful for detoxification.

CLINICAL FEATURES OF LIVER DISEASE

A. JAUNDICE

**yellowing of the skin and some mucosal membranes, due to excess bilirubin*

Etiology:

- Hepatocellular dysfunction (for example, hepatitis, drug toxicity, cirrhosis);
- Hemolysis (destruction of red blood cells);
- Biliary tract obstruction (by stones or tumours).

Clinical aspect:

- Mild jaundice without dark urine suggests hemolysis (because bilirubin did not go through a specific chemical reaction in the liver, named *conjugation*);
- Jaundice with dark urine (the dark coloration of urine precedes jaundice);
- Nausea and vomiting preceding jaundice indicate acute hepatitis or obstruction;
- Pruritus (itching; pathogenesis is unclear).

B. HEPATOMEGALY

**enlargement of the liver*

Etiology:

- Acute hepatitis;
- Fatty liver;
- Cyrrhosis;
- Tumours.

♦ LIVER DISEASES

A. FATTY LIVER (HEPATIC STEATOSIS)

**increased fat accumulation in the hepatocytes (liver cells)*

Etiology:

- Alcoholism, obesity or diabetes;
- Inborn metabolic disorders (of glycogen, homocysteine, etc.);
- Drugs (corticosteroids, tetracycline).

Clinical aspect: non-remarkable; the fatty liver is found on physical examination or on ultrasound (hepatomegaly); the liver does not hurt, unless the capsule that surrounds it is overly stretched. Lately, fatty liver in non-alcoholic obese females has become quite frequent.

Nutrition and holistic approach:

- Avoid all saturated fat and refined sugar intake;
- Avoid alcohol, coffee, drugs, toxin exposure;

- Employ all liver detoxification measures listed above;
- Increase fruits and vegetables intake;
- High fiber, low refined carbohydrates diet;
- Obesity approach, if appropriate;
- Get regular exercise;

Food therapy:
- Eat onions and garlic, as they reduce cholesterol levels;
- Oats contain inositol, which contributes to lowering plasma lipid levels;
- Grapefruits and grapefruit juice help fat breakdown;
- Apples, red peppers and turmeric seem to decrease cholesterol levels as well;
- Some say that walnuts intake helps decrease fats levels.

Supplements:
- Vitamin B complex, 50-100 mg/day, as some of the B vitamins (like B_5) are lipotropic factors, improving fat transport and utilization;
- Vitamin C and bioflavonoids, 2-4 g/day, or up to bowel tolerance, as it promotes the fat break down;
- Vitamin E, 400-800 IU/day, as it prevents cholesterol oxidation;
- A good multivitamin and multimineral formula containing a strong lipotropic complex (choline, lecithin, inositol);
- Flax seed oil, one tablespoon/day.

Others:
- Garlic is very beneficial, in diet and in supplement form (minimum of 4000 mcg. allicin /day; (*allicin is the sufur containing active compound*);
- Ginger and cayenne reduce blood cholesterol.

B. CIRRHOSIS

**irreversible diffuse fibrosis (scarring) of liver tissue*

Normal liver function is greatly impeded, as only parts of the liver function properly

Etiology:
- Alcohol (80% of cases);
- Hepatitis;
- Autoimmune;
- Drugs and toxins.

Clinical features:
- Anorexia, fatigue, fever/chills;
- Jaundice, bruising, muscle wasting, weight loss;
- Abdominal distension;
- Hepatomegaly, ascitis (water accumulating in the abdominal cavity).

Nutrition and holistic approach:

- Employ all general measures listed under Liver support;
- Eliminate ALL liver stressors;
- The diet should focus on fruits and vegetables intake, fish and nuts; avoid legumes, as, in some cases, seem to be stressing a compromised liver;
- Avoid meat and meat products;

Food therapy:

- Carrots, red beets and artichokes are liver-friendly foods;
- Kefir and yogurt are easily digested;
- Quark helps rebuild the liver tissue;

Supplements:

- Good multivitamin and mineral formula, as prescribed;
- Choline, 1 g/day, which slows down fatty accumulation in the liver;
- Vitamin B complex, 100 mg/day, as it is involved in all energy pathways;
- Vitamin C with bioflavonoids, 1-3 g/day, as an antioxidant and detoxifier.

Other measures:

- Milk thistle is well known for its liver regeneration properties;
- Dandelion root, yellow dock and licorice are good liver and blood tonics and detoxifiers;
- Black radish promotes bile flow;
- Stinging nettle is a liver purifier;
- Essential oils of chamomile, juniper, lemon or orange, in carrier oil could be either massaged into the abdomen or added to a bath.

C. HEPATITIS

**inflammation of the liver*

ACUTE VIRAL HEPATITIS:

	Hepatitis A	Hepatitis B	Hepatitis C
Etiology	Hepatitis A virus	HEP B virus (hepadna virus)	Flavivirus ("post-transfusion hepatitis")
Transmission route	Fecal-oral (by ingestion)	Blood or blood products Sexual transmission	Blood transfusion
Signs/ symptoms	Fever, jaundice, dark colour urine; NO CHRONIC SEQUELLAE (complications); NO CARRIER STATE	2 month incubation; fever, nausea, pain on the higher right side of the abdomen, jaundice, dark urine; relapses rarely; can progress to carrier state or chronic hepatitis; predisposes to liver cancer and cirrhosis	May be asymptomatic for years; 6 weeks incubation; fever, nausea, pain on the higher right side of the abdomen, jaundice, dark urine; relapses commonly; may progress to chronic carries state; predisposes to liver cancer

	Hepatitis A	Hepatitis B	Hepatitis C
Diagnosis	• Clinical picture • Laboratory tests: liver enzymes, antibodies		

Table 9.6-Acute hepatitis

ACUTE HEPATITIS IS A MEDICAL CONDITION: our approach is supportive; chronic hepatitis cases benefit more from our care

Nutrition and holistic approach for chronic hepatitis:

- Encourage bed rest for the acute phase; drink plenty of nourishing fluids (soups, juices);
- Eliminate all dietary and environmental liver stressors;
- Avoid excessive meat consumption and dairy products;
- Employ liver detoxification protocol as listed above;

Food therapy:

- Black radish juice, artichoke juice and watercress juice are great liver tonics;

Supplements and others:

- Vitamin C with bioflavonoids, 1-3 g/day;
- Good formula multivitamin and mineral levels, with vitamin B_{12} and folic acid;
- Licorice supplementation, as prescribed, as it protects the liver and it has antimicrobial and immune supporting properties;
- Milk thistle supplementation, as prescribed, as it helps regenerate the liver tissue.

◆ BILIARY TRACT DISORDERS

A. CHOLELITHIASIS (GALL BLADDER STONES):

hard stone-like masses in the gallbladder or in the biliary tract;* arise when there is an imbalance among bile components, and one or more components precipitate (clump together); the stone grows after that by ***accretion* (deposits of layers of more precipitated bile components).

STONES COMPOSITION:

- Pure cholesterol
- Pure pigment (bilirubin)
- Mixed
- Entirely mineral

Etiology:

- Abnormal bile composition (too much cholesterol or too much pigment, etc.);
- Blockage of the bile duct, which leads into precipitation of the components;
- Infections and/or inflammations of the biliary tract, which lead to stagnation and accumulation of one element or the other;
- Hereditary component.

Risk factors:

- Females over 30 years;
- Obesity, due to increased cholesterol synthesis;
- Food sensitivities, as they overburden the liver and may create inflammation and swelling of the bile ducts, increasing the risk of bile components precipitation; eggs, pork, onion, milk and coffee seem to be the frequently encountered culprits;
- High fat diet;
- Drugs (*cholesterol lowering drugs*, by decreasing the blood cholesterol while increasing the bile cholesterol*, *estrogen, BCP* (birth control pills); the last two greatly burden the liver detoxification pathways);
- Gastrointestinal tract disease, as it interferes with bile components reabsorption and creates an imbalance among bile constituents.

*the blood cholesterol levels are not the same as the bile cholesterol.

Clinical aspect:

- Acute upper abdominal pain, sometimes in the center of the upper abdomen, radiating in the right shoulder and sometimes between the shoulder blades;
- Nausea and/or vomiting;
- If there is blockage, jaundice may appear;
- Associated inflammation of the gall bladder (cholecystitis).

Diagnosis:

- Clinical aspect;
- Ultrasound.

THE BILIARY COLIC IS A MEDICAL EMERGENCY!!

Nutrition and holistic approach

Our approach will apply to the chronic presence of gallbladder stones:

- Identify and approach the etiologic factors;
- Decrease intake of refined sugar, as it increases the risk for increased lipid levels;

- Increase fiber intake, as it promotes the elimination of a compound (*deoxycholic acid,* produced by the gut bacteria action on bile acids) which increases the cholesterol insolubility in the bile, therefore creating conditions for its precipitation;
- Decrease legumes intake, as they contain *saponins*, which increase the accumulation of cholesterol in bile;
- Avoid coffee, as it stimulates gallbladder contractions;

Food therapy:
- Vegetarian diets seem to be protective against gallstones;
- Artichoke and rhubarb stimulate bile flow;
- Increase fish intake, as it seems to have a stabilizing effect on the cholesterol.

Notes on gallbladder flushes*:*

Some authors suggest that liver and gallbladder classical flushes with olive oil and lemon juice are not recommended, as they stimulate the contraction of gallbladder with potential lodging of the stones in the biliary tract, which will require emergency surgery. I completely agree with this concern, as I have seen this happening; this does not mean that the principle of the flush is wrong; just be cautious when you apply it and do not recommend it when stones are present. Nothing wrong with using olive oil in salads, though.

Supplements:
- Vitamin C, 1-2 g/day, as it reduces cholesterol stones formation;
- Vitamin E, 400 IU/day, as an antioxidant;
- Lecithin, as prescribed, as lecithin increases the cholesterol solubility within the bile, not allowing it to precipitate;

*bile acids supplementation may be employed; results will vary

Other measures:
- Milk thistle may dissolve gallstones;
- Dandelion and turmeric promote the bile flow;
- Boldo decreases bile thickness;

Notes on removed gallbladder:

- As there is no bile accumulation to support the fat digestion (bile is still produced by the liver, but it just continuously drains into the intestines), avoid fatty meals, as they will definitely overburden the digestion process;
- There are quite a few preparations on the market promoting bile constituents (in most of the cases, it is ox bile) and also bile acids supplementation; these could be taken along with meals;
- Pancreatic enzymes with a good lipase component may be beneficial;
- Ensure proper liver function, as elimination of toxins via bile, while taking place, may be slowed down;
- Milk thistle, dandelion root and turmeric are helpful, by promoting bile flow and, consequently, proper detoxification.

B.CHOLECYSTITIS

**inflammation of the gallbladder resulting from sustained obstruction by gallstones*

Clinical presentation:

- Severe constant epigastric (upper middle region of the abdomen) or pain in the upper right region of the abdomen;
- Systemic (general) signs: low grade fever, tachycardia;
- Palpable gall bladder.

Diagnosis:

- Leukocytosis (high number of white blood cells: infection markers);
- Elevated bilirubin, liver enzymes;
- Ultrasound.

Complications:

- Mucus accumulation in gall bladder with possible obstruction of the bile ducts;
- Gangrene and perforation.

THIS IS A MEDICAL EMERGENCY!!

CHAPTER 10

MUSCULO-SKELETAL DISORDERS

The way we move and the strength with which we move depend very much on the health of the musculoskeletal system. Actually, this system is composed by two separate systems: the skeletal system, composed by bones and joints and the muscular system, which comprises all muscles attached to the skeleton (skeletal muscles).

Unfortunately, a multitude of factors can affect the health of our musculoskeletal system: physical effort, position, nutritional imbalances and trauma. In the following chapter we will describe the most common conditions of the musculoskeletal system and the measures that we can take in order to have healthy bones, joints and muscles.

THE SKELETAL SYSTEM: bone composition and necessary nutrients

The composition of the bones:

1. Calcium

Deficiency caused by:

- Coffee, alcohol, and smoking: create a negative calcium balance;
- Soft drinks intake increase calcium excretion (due to their phosphorus content);
- Sugar overload: increases urinary excretion of calcium;
- Vitamin D deficiency;
- Liver, kidney or small intestine disorders (important in vitamin D metabolism);
- Dysbiosis, Candidiasis, Inflammatory Bowel Disease, Celiac disease, Leaky Gut (impede nutrient absorption);
- Low estrogen levels (incorporation of calcium in bones depends on the estrogen levels);
- Hyperparathyroidism (increased levels of parathyroid hormone will result in continuous breaking of the bone tissue);
- Hypochlorhydria (low stomach acid levels): absorption of calcium depends on it being ionized by the stomach acid.

2. The protein matrix - *osteocalcin,* which is a calcium-binding protein

Deficiency caused by:

- Vitamin K deficiency decreases osteocalcin production;
- Hypoproteinemia (due to kidney diseases);
- Dysbiosis and other digestive system problems (impaired absorption);
- Lack of intake;
- Liver conditions (results in impaired proteins metabolism).

3. Proteoglycans and Glucosaminoglycans: proteins and polysaccharides that strengthen the bone by forming a network (cross linking) between collagen fibers.

- Magnesium and Silicon are required because they are responsible for the cross linking of the collagen fibers;
- Vitamin C is vital for collagen fibers production.

IMPORTANT NUTRIENTS FOR THE MUSCULO-SKELETAL SYSTEM

Nutrient	Role
Vitamin C	Collagen fibers formation
Magnesium	Cross linking of collagen fibers; relaxes muscular tonus
Vitamin K	Important for the osteocalcin production
Vitamin B complex	Necessary for the energy production
Calcium	Vital in muscle contraction
Vitamin D	Vital for calcium absorption
Bioflavonoids	Enhance vitamin C absorption
Copper	Helps in collagen formation
Iron	Deficiency results in fragile bones
Phosphorus	Needed for bone formation
Arginine	Important in muscle metabolism, by maintaining a proper nitrogen balance
Cysteine	Helps in the production of collagen
Lysine	Helps build muscle protein

Table 10.1- Important nutrients for the musculo-skeletal system

Common signs and symptoms: bone pain, gait (abnormality in walking), muscle pain and weakness: joint pain, joint swelling, restricted ROM (range of motions), bone deformities, muscle spasms.

ASSESMENT OF THE MUSCULO-SKELETAL FUNCTION

MEDICAL ASSESSMENT	NUTRITIONAL ASSESSMENT
1. Clinical aspect: based on symptoms and signs; **2.** Evaluation of bone function: gait analysis(how a person walks), serum calcium and phosphorus, x-ray films, angiography, bone scanning and MRI(magnetic resonance imaging); **3.** Evaluation of joint function: arthrography, arthroscopy, MRI, synovial fluid analysis;	**1.** Macro and micronutrient deficiencies and excesses as listed in the table above; **2.** Hypochlorhydria: may be responsible for impeded calcium absorption (calcium needs to be ionized by stomach acid for absorption); **3.** Impeded liver function: improper metabolism of macro and/or micronutrients resulting in deficiencies; **4.** Improper lower digestive tract function (Dysbiosis, Candidiasis, etc) may impede digestion and/or absorption of nutrients;

MEDICAL ASSESSMENT	NUTRITIONAL ASSESSMENT
4. Evaluation of muscle function: physical examination, serum creatine kinase*, electromyogram, muscle biopsy.	**5.** Immune system status: firstly, if status is low, the immune system may require more proteins and shunt them away from the muscles; secondly, it allows for development of circulating immune complexes that can deposit in joints, creating the premises for autoimmune diseases (i.e.:rheumatoid arthritis).

Table 10.2-Assessment of the musculo-skeletal function

*if increased, shows damage of the muscle fiber

MUSCULOSKELETAL DISORDERS

♦AUTOIMMUNE AND DIFFUSE CONNECTIVE TISSUE DISORDERS

A. RHEUMATHOID ARTHRITIS (RA)

*****_chronic, symmetric, erosive synovitis of peripheral joints._ Age of onset: 20-40; joints typically involved are hands, feet, wrists, ankles and knees.

Etiology:

- Autoimmune: antibodies developed against joint tissue components (unknown what triggers the immune reaction)

Other theories:

- **Genetic factors:** 70% of RA cases have a specific genetic marker; also it seems that RA is encountered often in children of parents with RA; the environment (lifestyle, diet) plays a great role in the development of disease, though;
- **Leaky gut:** because of increased intestinal permeability, it allows circulating toxins to leak out of the intestines into the blood stream where they act as antigens; the immune system may create antibodies against them and the coupling of the antigens with the antibodies will create immune complexes which have a tendency to deposit in the join tissue;
- **Viral theory**: which, at this point, is just a hypothesis.

Pathogenesis:

- Hallmark (means characteristic): hypertrophy of the synovial membrane with destruction of the articular cartilage and subchondral bone (the bone tissue underneath the cartilage);

Clinical manifestations:

- Fatigue, low grade fever, weakness, weight loss;
- Inflammatory process begins in the small joints and then progresses to the other joints;
- Morning stiffness longer than one hour;

- Pain on motion or tenderness of at least one joint;
- Swelling of small joints of hands or wrists;
- Restricted movement;
- Deformities;
- Arthritis of three or more joints;
- Symmetric arthritis (involvement of the same joint on both sides of the body);
- Rheumatoid nodules (under the skin, on bony prominences);
- Extra-articular involvement: episcleritis, nodules, pulmonary fibrosis, Hashimoto thyroiditis;

*the joint signs must be continuous for at least six weeks for diagnosis purposes

Complications:

- Joint deformities;
- Subluxations;
- Tendon sheath involvement;
- Ruptured cysts.

Diagnosis:

- Laboratory: increased inflammatory markers, **Serum rheumatoid factor** present;
- X-ray changes: soft tissue swelling, erosions, joint space narrowing.

Medical treatment

- Corticosteroids;
- NSAID: non steroidal anti-inflammatory drug;
- Gold injections;
- Surgery.

Nutritional and holistic approach:

- Identification and appropriate approach of food sensitivities: as their presence results in overloading of the immune system and may create the conditions for autoimmunity;
- Management of dysbiosis and/or Leaky gut;
- Liver cleanse and detoxification: it is vitally important to have proper liver function; nutrients metabolism depends on it. Also, a healthy liver will be able to eliminate toxins properly, taking the load off the immune system, therefore allowing it to properly dispose of immune complexes;
- Immune system support and slow building; do not use boosting, as RA is considered an autoimmune disease;
- Elimination of the most common allergens, like wheat and dairy, very limited consumption of beef and pork, elimination of foods of the *Nightshade family* (potatoes, tomatoes, eggplant and peppers) and a diet rich in fruits, vegetables and fiber and low in refined sugar and saturated fat would be extremely beneficial for cases with RA;
- Check the Hydrochloric acid status as it may be responsible for insufficient protein digestion with consequent Leaky gut;

Food therapy:

- It seems that foods like celery (reduces body's acidity), dandelion (liver protection), berries (antioxidants) and fish (anti-inflammatory effect) are very beneficial for arthritis.

Supplements:

- Omega 3 fatty acids, necessary to reduce inflammation: two tablespoons/day;
- Vitamin C with bioflavonoids for immune system support, neutralization of inflammation and collagen fibers support: 1-3 grams/day;
- Selenium (200mcg/day) and Vitamin E (400IU/day) have a beneficial effect in diminishing inflammation, as they act favorably on the prostaglandin pathway;
- Manganese, 15mg/day, as it seems to be low in cases with RA and it seems to improve symptoms when given;
- Zinc, 30-45 mg/day, as it seems to improve the symptoms;
- Niacinamide, 500 mg three times/day proved to be quite beneficial in alleviating the symptoms of RA sufferers; do have the liver enzymes checked every 6 months, as its consumption may result in liver toxicity; do not give such doses to cases with impaired liver function;
- Glucosamine sulfate, as it supports the health of the joint;
- Bromelain (for its anti-inflammatory properties).

Other measures:

- Clients reported that pain gets better when they wear a copper bracelet;
- Suggest DGL (deglycyrrhizinated licorice) to cases on NSAID: it protects the stomach lining;
- Botanicals: Curcumin and Ginger (have anti-inflammatory effects), feverfew and White willow are antirheumathic herbs; Siberian ginseng seems to be useful in relieving arthritis symptoms;
- Bergamot and myrrh oil reduce inflammation;
- Massage with oil of black pepper may reduce stiffness; lavender oil and chamomile oil have similar results and also relieves pain;
- Physical therapy: heat applications, cold packs for acute flare-ups, massage, are very beneficial;
- Adapt an exercise program to the client's condition (presence of flare-ups would require gentle massage and mild passive exercises);
- Stress management and support groups.

B. SYSTEMIC LUPUS ERYTHEMATOSUS (SLE)

**inflammation in several organ systems affecting the connective tissue and the production of autoantibodies; more frequent in women; age of onset: 13-40.*

Etiology:

- Altered immunity: presence of autoantibodies acting by cytotoxic reaction or immune complexes deposits;
- Heredity: some cases have a common antigen;
- Viral theory;
- Drugs related: intake of BCP (Birth control pills), anticonvulsivants, antiarrhytmics.

Clinical aspect:
- Malar rash: "butterfly rash" on face;
- Sometimes discoid rash (round patches);
- Oral/nasal ulcers;
- Arthritis: symmetric, involving two or more small or large peripheral joints;
- Serositis (serous membranes are affected-peritonitis, pericarditis);
- Headaches, seizures, neuropathy.

Diagnosis:
- Clinical criteria (not all signs and symptoms have to be present for diagnosis);
- Laboratory criteria: proteinuria (elimination of proteins via urine), anemia, leucopenia (low WBC), thrombocytopenia (low thrombocytes), ANA (*antinuclear antibody*; this is a specific antibody for this disease);
- Other features: conjunctivitis, vasculitis, depression.

Medical treatment:
- Avoidance of UV light which affects the condition;
- NSAID;
- Antimalarials;
- Topical steroids for rash;
- Systemic corticosteroids;
- Cytotoxic agents;
- Immunosuppressant drugs.

Nutritional and holistic approach (this is one of those conditions that requires increased attention, being an autoimmune condition; our approach will be mostly supportive):
- Mild liver support and detoxification;
- Immune system support (use the approach described under *The immune system,* use lower nutrient dosages, never boost the immunity!);
- Digestive system support (to improve nutrient absorption);
- Adrenal support, as this person is more than likely to be an adrenal fatigue case because of the chronicity of the situation;
- Identify and eliminate food sensitivities, as they may overload the immune system even further;
- An alkaline diet will help improve the well being of a lupus case (it seems that chronic conditions are acidic in nature);
- Follow the dietary advice mentioned under *Rheumatoid arthritis.*

Supplements:
- DHEA, 10-25 mg/day has been cited to be able to improve the symptoms of the condition;
- Flax seed oil or fish oil on a daily basis: one tablespoon;
- Vitamin E, 400-800Iu/day;
- Zinc, 30mg/day;
- Vitamin B_6 in increased dosages (even 500mg/day have been cited by various sources!);
- Digestive enzymes with bromelain.

*all the above-mentioned nutrients have been redeemed useful in clinical trials.

Other measures:

- Basil can provide relief from the arthritic pain;
- Yucca, Feverfew, White willow, have anti-inflammatory properties;
- Chamomile, Lemon balm and Passion flower have relaxing effects, helping the person deal with the condition;
- Chamomile, Lavender and Juniper oil have anti-inflammatory and soothing effects;
- Chamomile compresses, Aloe Vera gel and Calendula may help sooth the rash.

C. ANKYLOSING SPONDYLITIS (AS)

**chronic autoimmune rheumatic disease, that tends to affect young males, characterized by progressive bony sclerosis starting in the sacroiliac joints; onset before age 40.*

Etiology theories:

- Autoimmune; presence of HLA-B27 (Human Leukocyte Antigen), which is characteristic for the disease;
- Hereditary: family history is common;
- Intestinal infection, which allows the microorganism's capsule to form antibodies against HLA-B27;
- Increased intestinal permeability, which allow circulating toxins to overload the immune system.

Clinical features:

- Low back pain and stiffness;
- Asymmetrical large joint involvement;
- Ligament inflammation, where it attaches to the bone;
- Flexion contraction of hip;
- Limb joints usually spared;
- Extra-articular manifestations: acute anterior uveitis (eye disease), aortitis (aorta inflammation), nephropathy;
- Better with hot showers and mild physical activities;
- Worse when twisting the body, early in the morning and lying down.

Diagnosis:

- Clinical aspect and physical examination;
- X-ray: joint sclerosis, bony fusion, "bamboo spine" (almost bony fusion).

Medical treatment:

- Heat applications;
- Exercises;
- Surgery;
- NSAID.

Nutritional and holistic approach: *follow the principles of treatment under Rheumatoid arthritis, as it is very similar*

♦DEGENERATIVE ARTHRITIS

A. OSTEOARTHRITIS (DEGENERATIVE JOINT DISEASE) (OA)

**deterioration of articular cartilage;"wear and tear" arthritis*; incidence has increased lately; affects mostly the hands and the weight bearing joints (knees, hips and spine).

Etiology:

- Genetic predisposition;
- Abnormal physical forces leading to altered joint function and damage (trauma);
- Altered bone and joint biochemistry;
- With age, there is a deterioration of the articular cartilage, even in the absence of trauma;
- Hypochlorhydria: by creating the premises for leaky gut, and dysbiosis and/or candidiasis; both may be responsible for maldigestion and malabsorption, therefore, needed repair nutrients are not provided;
- Joint inflammation, which alters the homeostatic mechanisms at joint level creating the premises for alteration and degeneration of joints elements.

Pathophysiology:

- Catabolism of cartilage (breaking down) is higher than cartilage synthesis;
- Loss of water exposes underlying bone;
- Abnormal local bone metabolism;
- Synovitis secondary to articular damage.

Classification
- → **Primary**: occurs with aging, due to decreased reparatory processes at joint level
- → **Secondary**: post-traumatic, mechanical, post-inflammatory, endocrine metabolic disorders (hypothyroidism)

Diagram 10.1- Osteoarthritis classification

Clinical manifestations:

- Over age 40;
- Signs and symptoms localized to affected joints;
- Pain is insidious and progresses over years;
- Flare-ups and remissions may occur;

- Joint pain with motion, relieved by rest;
- Asymmetric;
- Short duration of stiffness after immobility;
- Deformity, angulations;
- Limited ROM (range of motions);
- Any joint can be affected, mostly shoulder, elbow, wrist and ankle.

Evaluation:

- Laboratory inflammatory markers: normal in OA;
- X-ray: narrowing of joint space, bony erosions, osteophytes (bony growths).

Medical treatment: weight loss, exercise, diet, symptomatic, surgical.

Nutritional and holistic approach:

- Identify food allergies;
- Liver support and detoxification;
- Digestive system support: hypochlorhydria, leaky gut, dysbiosis approach, if necessary;
- Weight loss, if necessary, as the excess weight bears down on the affected joint;
- Eliminate nightshades (tobacco is one of them, among others; this plant family contains some substances called alkaloids that inhibit cartilage repair mechanisms and are pro-inflammatory);
- Choose an alkaline diet, rich in fibers, low in sugar and saturated fats.

<u>Supplements:</u>

- Antioxidant complex and vitamin C: reduces the risk of cartilage loss and prevents further deterioration;
- Glucosamine sulphate, 500 mg three times per day: provides glucosaminoglycans that are a normal part of the bone and joint structures; decreased glucosamine will allow the cartilage to lose its flexibility; while here, let us make a note on the chondroitin sulphate supplementation: its absorption, on its own, is much less than the one of glucosamine sulphate; also, in the human body, it turns into glucosamine, so our advice is to either take it along with glucosamine sulphate or not take it all; do not replace glucosamine sulphate with chondroitin sulfate;
- Niacinamide, 500 mg three times a day: has been proven to increase joint mobility;
- SAM (S-acetyl methionine): if deficient, the cartilage loses its shock absorbing properties;
- Vitamin E, 400 IU/day: inhibits the cartilage break down;
- Vitamin B_5 is involved in cartilage growth;
- Vitamin A, (5000 IU/day), B_6, (50 mg/day), Zinc,(30 mg/day): are involved in cartilage formation;
- EFA: flax seed oil one tablespoon/day.

<u>Other measures:</u>

- Physical therapies: exercise, diathermy, hydrotherapy, are all beneficial and improve joint function;
- Botanicals: Yucca, Feverfew, Devil's claw, Ginger, Curcumin;

- Topically: menthol based preparations (Tiger balm) and/or capsaicin preparations (cayenne) help relieve pain;
- Oils of white camphor, allspice, chamomile, juniper, lemon and myrrh may prove helpful.

♦INFECTIONS OF BONES AND JOINTS

A. INFECTIOUS ARTHRITIS

**infection of the joint cavity*

Routes of spread:
- Hematogenous (by blood);
- Direct spread from adjacent (nearby) infections;
- Inoculation (either trauma or rarely, medical procedures).

Etiology: various micro organisms: S.aureus, N.Gonorrhea, M.Tuberculosis, etc

History:
- Severe pain;
- Acute sepsis: fever, chills, dehydration, lethargy;

THIS IS A MEDICAL EMERGENCY!!

Clinical manifestations:
- Fever, malaise (feeling of discomfort, not feeling well);
- Local joint tenderness, swelling, heat;
- Neonates (newborns) get pseudo paralysis;
- Unable or willing to move joint.

Evaluation
- Blood cultures;
- Joint aspirate for cultures, ESR, WBC, C reactive protein, (the last three are inflammatory markers), glucose.

Medical treatment:
- Analgesics (pain relievers);
- Antibiotics;
- Surgery.

Nutritional and holistic approach:
*keep in mind that this is an acute condition that will require appropriate aggressive treatment, or the infection can spread; we are just supporting the body while recovering:
- All necessary cleanses are to be employed;
- Recommend an alkaline diet; low sugar and fat intake, increased fruits and vegetables;
- Immune system boosting, as described under *The immune system;*
- Probiotic supplementation, if they are on antibiotic protocol.

B. OSTEOMYELITIS
**bone or bone marrow infection(looks like an abscess inside the bone tissue).*

Etiology: bacterial, viral or fungal

Transmission: hematogenous or by inoculation

Forms:
- Acute: fever, chills, pain,

THIS IS A MEDICAL EMERGENCY!!

- Chronic: infection that persists more than 6-8 weeks.

Clinical aspect:
- Local tenderness, swelling, decreased joint motion

Diagnosis: elevated ESR, increased WBC, X-Ray, bone scan.

Medical and holistic treatments: as described above, cross reference *Infectious arthritis*

♦CRYSTAL-INDUCED CONDITIONS

GOUT
**hyperuricemia (increased uric acid), monosodium urate crystals deposits in tissues and joints, leading to an inflammatory reaction; recurrent episodes of acute arthritis; common in males.*
*uric acid is the final breakdown product of purine's (nucleic acids) metabolism.

Etiology:
- Dietary excess (organ meats, sardines, alcohol, especially beer, meat);
- Primary or genetic (either increased synthesis of uric acid or reduced ability to excrete it);
- Secondary to another disease process: kidney disease or excessive cells breakdown.

Pathophysiology: derangement in purine metabolism.

Clinical manifestations:

- Pain involving lower extremities;
- Inflammation of big toe;
- Recurrent attacks;
- Urate crystals deposits in the tissue surrounding the joint and in other tissues;
- Uric acid kidney stones.

Evaluation

- Increased uric acid levels in blood;
- Joint aspirate (identifies urate crystals in the joint fluid);
- Radiology.

Medical treatment:

- Analgesics, symptomatic, dietary considerations, antihyperuricemic drugs.

Nutritional and holistic approach:

- Liver and kidney cleanse and detoxification;
- Treatment of obesity and diabetes mellitus, as they seem to predispose to an attack;
- Decrease sugar intake, as it increases uric acid production;
- Decrease fat intake, as it decreases uric acid excretion;
- Increased fluid intake, as it contributes to urine dilution and further elimination of unwanted substances;
- Greatly restrict foods rich in purines: organ meats, meats, sardines, anchovies, dried legumes, spinach, asparagus;
- Excessive alcohol may elicit an attack by releasing lactic acid;
- Beer has a high content of purines;
- Milk seem to be a source of an enzyme (xantine oxidase) which can increase uric acid levels;

Food therapy:

- Cherries or cherry juice (even canned cherries) decrease uric acid levels;
- Raw potato juice: may increase uric acid excretion;
- Charcoal tablets may reduce uric acid levels.

Supplements:

- Quercetin, 200-400 mg three times a day, as it may inhibit uric acid production;
- Flax seed oil: one tablespoon/day;
- Folic acid, 25mg three times a day: inhibits the enzyme responsible for uric acid production.

Other measures:

- Bromelain, Devil's claw, curcumin;
- Raw apple and cucumber juice may help relieve the severity and incidence of attacks;
- Celery seed tea is cleansing and helps eliminate excessive uric acid;

- Crushed cabbage leafs in a local compress may alleviate the pain;
- Massage the sore joint with lavender, frankincense and grapeseed oils;
- Other oils that can be used: pine, rosemary or juniper.

♦DEFICIENCY DISEASES

A. OSTEOMALACIA AND RICKETS

Rickets: appears in children; due to vitamin D deficiency; calcium absorption is low and bones are unmineralized.
Osteomalacia is vitamin D deficiency in adults, associated with bone calcium deficiency.

Etiology:

1. Vitamin disorder:
   - Not enough sun exposure;
   - Decreased vitamin D availability, due to intake deficit;
   - Malabsorption;
   - Liver or kidney diseases.
2. Aluminum exposure, which impairs bone mineralization;
3. Anticonvulsive drug therapy.
4. Hypothyroidism.

Clinical aspect

Rickets	Osteomalacia
• Skeletal deformities, bowlegs • Prone to fractures • Disturbed growth • Rachitic rosary (prominent rib joints) • Hypocalcemia	• Less serious than rickets • Diffuse skeletal pain • Prone to fractures • Muscle weakness • Gait disturbance

Table 10.3- Clinical aspect of Rickets and Osteomalacia

Diagnosis:

- Clinical aspect;
- Laboratory findings: low serum calcium and phosphorus, decreased calcium in urine;
- Radiology.

Medical treatment: according to the cause.

Nutritional and holistic approach:

- Hypochlorhydria approach, if necessary;
- Encourage sun exposure (even 20-30 minutes a day is sufficient in the winter time);

- Identify and approach possible malabsorption causes: dysbiosis, leaky gut, intestinal parasites, candida, etc.;
- Identify and approach food sensitivities, as they may elicit inflammation at gut level with subconsequent malabsorption problems;
- Identify and approach liver and/or kidney conditions, which may impede on vitamin D metabolism;
- Avoid excess carbohydrates, pop (contains phosphorus), excess meat; all these wash out calcium from the body;
- Increase mushrooms intake (unless health conditions require a different approach), as they are a very good source of non-animal calcium.

Supplements:

- Fish oil supplements, as prescribed;
- Calcium supplementation, according to age (1-1.2 g/day in adults and 400-800 mg/day in children);
- Magnesium supplementation (1:2 with calcium);
- Multivitamin/multimineral formula.

B. OSTEOPOROSIS:

**age-related condition characterized by decreased bone mass and destruction of the protein matrix of the bone;* deterioration of bone tissue with consequent increase in bone fragility and susceptibility to bone fractures

Risk factors and etiology:

- Small caucasian or asian female, family history of osteoporosis;
- Estrogen-related bone mass: early menopause, amenorrhea;
- Advanced age;
- Nutritional imbalances: decreased magnesium, boron, silicon, vitamins C and K;
- Secondary to medical disease: stomach, bowel, liver, kidney;
- Diet, smoking, alcohol, caffeine: increase urinary excretion of calcium;
- Minimal weight bearing physical activity: which affects bone mass.

Classification:

→ **Primary**: within 20 years after menopause

→ **Secondary**: endocrinopathies (hyperparathyroidism) malignancy (multiple mieloma), gastro-intestinal diseases, drugs (steroids) RA, renal diseases, poor nutrition

Diagram 10.2- Osteoporosis classification

Pathophysiology: bone resorption is greater than bone formation/remodelling

Clinical manifestations:

- Commonly asymptomatic;
- Usually affects the spine, hips and ribs;

- Pain, mostly backache;
- Collapsed vertebrae resulting in height loss;
- Fractures: hip, vertebrae, upper arm, wrist, Dowager's hump (collapse fracture of vertebral bodies in mid-dorsal region);
- The resultant immobility after falls may be responsible for the development of additional problems: pulmonary or urinary infections, depression.

Diagnosis:
- Laboratory: calcium, phosphate;
- Densitometry (shows bone mass).

Medical treatment:
- Prevention and lifestyle modifications: weight bearing exercises, increased calcium intake, vitamin D supplementation, avoid risk factors;
- Measures to decrease further bone loss: HRT (Hormone replacement therapy), calcium, calcitonin.

Nutrition and holistic approach:
- Think prevention, even in early adulthood: exercise, decrease factors that promote calcium excretion and increase calcium intake, in synergy with other nutrients as mentioned below, under *Supplementation*;
- Take appropriate measures to identify and treat: hypochlorhydria, gut absorption problems, liver and/or kidney conditions;
- Employ a diet rich in fruits, vegetables, grains, fish, and low in excess refined carbohydrates, meat, pop;
- Avoid alcohol and smoking;
- Increase intake of magnesium rich foods, as it seems that this plays a great role in prevention of osteoporosis;
- Increase intake of green vegetables, as they are a source of vitamin K1, which converts osteocalcin to its active form;
- Increase intake of phytoestrogens (plant estrogens), as they appear to enhance the deposition of calcium in bones via calcitonin enhancement.

Supplements:
- Calcium, 800-1200 mg/day;
- Vitamin D, 400 IU/day;
- Magnesium, 400-600 mg/day;
- Multivitamin/multimineral formula that contains vitamin K, boron and silicon.

Other measures:
- Drink three cups of comfrey leaves a day (promote rapid healing of broken bones);
- Bone pain can be helped by taking white willow or meadowsweet, which are analgesic herbs;
- Herbs that contain calcium: nettle, parsley, dandelion leaves, kelp and horsetail;
- Estrogenic herbs: calendula, ginseng, false unicorn root, sage, hops;

- If bruising present, use witch hazel compresses; calendula applications help speed up healing;
- Oils of bergamot, chamomile, lavender and rosemary will help ease pain; do not apply on broken skin.

♦NONARTICULAR RHEUMATISM

A. NECK PROBLEMS

A1. WHIPLASH
**sudden force causes a violent twisting or/and bending of neck in one direction, followed by the muscle contraction*

A2. TORTICOLLIS
**involuntary contraction/spasm of the neck muscles (sternocleidomastoid) causing rotational tilting of the head*

Etiology
- Idiopathic (not known);
- Exposure to cold/draft;
- Trauma;
- Medical conditions: tumors, CNS infections.

Clinical aspect:
- Pain, spasm, tension, unilaterally;
- Abnormal head position;
- Affected ROM.

Medical treatment:
- Physical therapy, massage;
- Antispasmodic medication, benzodiazepines.

Nutritional and holistic approach: this is not a condition easy to approach nutritionally; the results very much depend on the cause and on severity of the condition; the measures listed below are just supportive
- Drink celery juice to ease nerve pain;
- Local heat may help with muscle relaxation;
- Light and careful massage, on its own or using oils of camphor, chamomile, blue gum eucalyptus or lavender;
- Magnesium supplementation 400-600 mg/day, as it may promote muscle relaxation;
- Increase intake of magnesium rich foods;
- Coenzyme Q10 and germanium rich foods may help by increasing tissue oxygenation.

B. LOW BACK PAIN

pain in the low lumbar and/or lumbosacral region, that can be accompanied or not by pain radiating down on the back of the legs(uni or bilateral); prevalence increases with age;

Lumbago: pain in the lumbar area
Sciatica: neuralgia (nerve pain) along the sciatic nerve

Etiology:
- Muscular strain: physical effort, position, weight;
- Trauma;
- Musculoskeletal diseases: OA, AS;
- Poor sleep, psychological problems, stress;
- Disk herniation.

Clinical aspect:

- Pain in the above mentioned areas;
- Acute form: comes with various degrees of restricted movements;
- Chronic form: pain and affected ROM;
- Pain radiating on the sciatic nerve territory;
- Muscle spasm, stiffness;
- Possible "pins and needles" sensation.

Medical treatment:
- Physical therapy: heat application, massage, rest;
- Analgesics.

Nutritional and holistic approach (supportive measures, adapted to the cause of the condition)
- Relaxation techniques, stress management;
- Approach the cause, if appropriate;
- Rub fresh lemon over the affected area (not the juice).

<u>Supplements:</u>
- Magnesium supplementation, if muscle contracture present;
- Vitamin B complex with additional B_6, if sciatica present.

<u>Other measures:</u>
- Mustard poultice or mustard essential oil help relieve pain;
- Cramp bark cream massaged into the area helps relieve the spasms;
- Massage with ginger and black pepper oils is beneficial when acute pain present;
- Beneficial herbs: St John's wort, white willow, devil's claw;
- Elderberry is a known folk remedy for sciatica;
- Lavender, chamomile or thyme essential oils may be used in a bath, to help relieve the symptoms;

- Chamomile, lemon balm, valerian, passion flower: help with stress related and sleep problems.

C. INTERVERTEBRAL DISK HERNIATION (SLIPPED DISK)
**protrusion of part of nucleus pulposus (a semifluid mass of fine fibers in the middle of an intervertebral disk).* Most commonly affected are the lumbo-sacral disks.

Etiology: trauma and/or degenerative disk disease

Pathophysiology: ligament and posterior capsule of the disk are torn, nucleus pulposus protrudes, and the nerve is compressed.

Clinical aspect

- Pain distribution depends on lesion location; pain is worse on straining (coughing, sneezing);
- Impaired ROM;
- Impaired temperature and touch sensation in the respective dermatomes;
- Possible muscular weakness and atrophy, according to the severity of herniation.

Evaluation and treatment:

- X-ray: CT scan, MRI;
- Traction, compression, local heat, symptomatic relief.

Nutrition and holistic approach:

- Local heat applications;
- Rest;
- Diet emphasizing magnesium rich foods;
- Decrease intake of saturated fats;
- Celery juice helps relieve the pain;
- Stress management, support groups.

<u>Supplements:</u>

- Magnesium supplementation;
- Glucosamine sulfate supplements;
- Coenzyme Q 10 and germanium rich foods increase cellular oxygenation;
- Vitamin B complex with additional B_6.

<u>Others:</u>

- Gentle massages and applications of mustard, lavender, black pepper or chamomile oils;
- Helpful herbs: willow, cramp bark, chamomile, devil's claw.

♦SPRAINS AND STRAINS OF TENDONS AND LIGAMENTS

STRAIN: tendon tear
SPRAIN: ligament tear
Avulsion: complete separation of the tendon/ligament from its bony insertion

Etiology: trauma, RA, SLE

Pathophysiology: local inflammatory reaction for 4-5 days followed by collagen formation and vascular fibrous tissue formation.

Clinical aspect:
- Intense localized sharp pain;
- Affected ROM;
- Tissue swelling.

Evaluation and Treatment: stress x-ray, arthroscopy

Medical treatment: rest, immobilization, surgical approach when needed, pain relief

Nutrition and holistic approach: see below, under *Tendinitis and Bursitis*

♦TENDINITIS AND BURSITIS

Tendinitis: painful inflammation of tendons
Bursitis: painful inflammation of bursae

Etiology: trauma, cristal deposits, postural misalignment
Pathophysiology: inflammatory local changes, bleeding, and edema, calcium deposits
Clinical manifestations:
- Localized to one joint;
- Local pain worse with active motion.

Evaluation: Physical examination, arthroscopy, MRI

Medical treatment: rest, immobilization, symptomatic relief, physical medicine techniques

Nutrition and holistic approach: applies to ligament and tendon sprains and strains and to tendonitis and bursitis with a few exceptions, mentioned at the appropriate time:
- RICE: rest, immobilization, compression, elevation;

- Massage (except for the sprains and strains in acute phase);
- Alkaline diet, to reduce inflammation.

Supplements:
- As mentioned previously: magnesium, vitamin C, bioflavonoids, coenzyme Q10, germanium, glucosamine sulphate;
- Immune system boosters, for tendonitis and /or bursitis, which are inflammatory conditions (do not forget garlic and EFA's).

Other measures:
- Devil's claw and willow will reduce inflammation;
- Black pepper, chamomile, mustard, juniper oils will help relieve pain when massaged in the area.

♦FIBROMYALGIA
**chronic, diffuse musculoskeletal pain with characteristic tender points and disturbed sleep*; shares features with CFS (chronic fatigue syndrome)

Etiology	Unknown; possible viral etiology; Cause of pain is low levels of serotonin; functional changes occur according to sleep depravation;
Clinical presentation	**Major criteria:** generalized aches or stiffness of at least three anatomical sites, for three months; six or more reproducible tender points; exclusion of other disorders that may cause similar symptoms; **Minor Criteria:** fatigue, headache, sleep disturbances, neurological complaints, joint swelling, IBS, numbing, tingling.

Table 10.4-Fibromyalgia : clinical presentation

Diagnosis: on clinical aspect alone; all three major criteria required and four or more minor criteria

Medical treatment:
- Physical therapy, massage, relaxation;
- Antidepressants, analgesics, anti-inflammatory medication;
- Corticosteroids in some cases.

Nutrition and holistic approach:
- Identify and approach any imbalance that may apply an additional strain on the body: food sensitivities, immune system conditions;
- Ensure the health of the digestive system, as proper nutrient absorption is essential;
- Support the health of liver and kidneys;
- Ensure proper sleep (as in length, timing, depth);
- Employ stress management and relaxation techniques;
- Increased intake of foods rich in tryptophane, as it is the serotonin precursor;
- Avoid the nightshade family, as it contains pro-inflammatory alkaloids;

- Increase intake of methionine containing foods, as methionine is involved in melatonin metabolism (meat, fish, poultry, eggs, wheat germ sunflower deeds, avocado);
- Use an alkaline diet, to minimize the eventual inflammatory status.

Supplements:
- Comprehensive, quality multivitamin and multimineral formula;
- Magnesium, 200-250 mg three times per day;
- Glucosamine sulphate;
- Coenzyme Q10, 100 mg/day, to increase tissue oxygenation;
- Vitamin B complex, 100 mg/day, very important in supporting the energy production pathway;
- Flax seed oil or fish oil supplements;
- Vitamin C, 2-3 g/day.

Other measures:
- Appropriate exercise;
- Massage with chamomile, white camphor, ginger, lavender essential oils;
- Feverfew, white willow, devil's claw, meadowsweet help with pain and inflammation;
- St john's wort is an antidepressant and an antiviral herb;
- Massage temples or take a bath with oils of: lavender, lemon balm, grapefruit, jasmine or orange blossom essential oils to relieve stress and depression.

♦HAND CONDITIONS

CARPAL TUNNEL SYNDROME

**median nerve entrapment at wrist;* female: male prevalence ratio 4:1

Etiology:
- Secondary to repetitive trauma;
- Wrist injury.

Clinical manifestations:
- Patient awakes at night with pain/numbness relieved by shaking, rubbing;
- Decreased sensitivity testing;
- Advanced cases: wasting/weakness of muscles innervated by median nerve.

Evaluation: clinical, history, physical examination.

Medical treatment: conservative and/or surgical, analgesics, antiinflammatories.

Nutrition and holistic approach:
- Take appropriate measures to ensure the functioning of all detoxification pathways;

- Avoid oxalic containing foods, which accentuate joint problems (asparagus, beets, beet greens, rhubarb, spinach, cabbage, parsley);
- Avoid excessive salt intake which may increase water retention with consequent increased pressure on the involved nerve;
- Avoid use of yellow dye#5, which interferes with vitamin B_6 metabolism ;
- Employ rest and wear comfortable clothes (tight sleeves or elastic around the wrist may induce edema with pain caused by increased pressure on the nerve);
- Increase intake of fresh fruits and vegetables; pineapple is anti-inflammatory.

Supplements:

- Multivitamin/multimineral complex;
- Vitamin B_6, 25 mg three times a day (to improve nerve's function) with additional vitamin B_2 (converts vitamin B_6 in its active form);
- Coenzyme Q10, as prescribed.

Others:

- Alternating hot (three minutes) and cold (thirty seconds) hand bath to increase local circulation;
- St. John's wort: to improve nervous transmission;
- Devil's claw, willow, feverfew: natural antiinflammatories;
- Local muscle massage with relaxing oils: chamomile, lavender, juniper, camphor.

CHAPTER 11

NERVOUS SYSTEM DISORDERS

The Nervous System is a wonderful structure designed to allow rapid internal communication. Remember what you do when you see a car speeding towards you? Or when you touch a hot stove? You react immediately. Special structures called receptors will transmit information (a car is coming, or the stove is hot) via nerves to your CNS, (Central Nervous System) which will interpret the information received and it will issue a command, via other nerves, to the effector organ (you contract your muscles to either jump out from in front of the car or to take your hand away off the hot stove). To accomplish these, your nervous system uses various chemicals (neurotransmitters) and ions (sodium, potassium, etc).

Let us begin with a brief description of neurotransmitters.

NEUROTRANSMITTERS

BRAIN	PERIPHERY*
• **Norepinephrine: maintenance of arousal, mood regulation; • ***Dopamine: emotional response, complex movements; • Serotonin: sleep, temperature regulation, sensory**** perception; • GABA: inhibitory effect, movement control; • Acetylcholine: memory and cognitive function.	• Norepinephrine: sympathetic nervous system function; • Acetylcholine: acts at neuromuscular junction; • Serotonin (produced by many cells, like thrombocytes): induces vasoconstriction.

Table 11.1-Neurotransmitters

*In the blood stream

For ** and *** tyrosine is a common precursor

****applied to senses

Biochemistry of neurotransmitters:

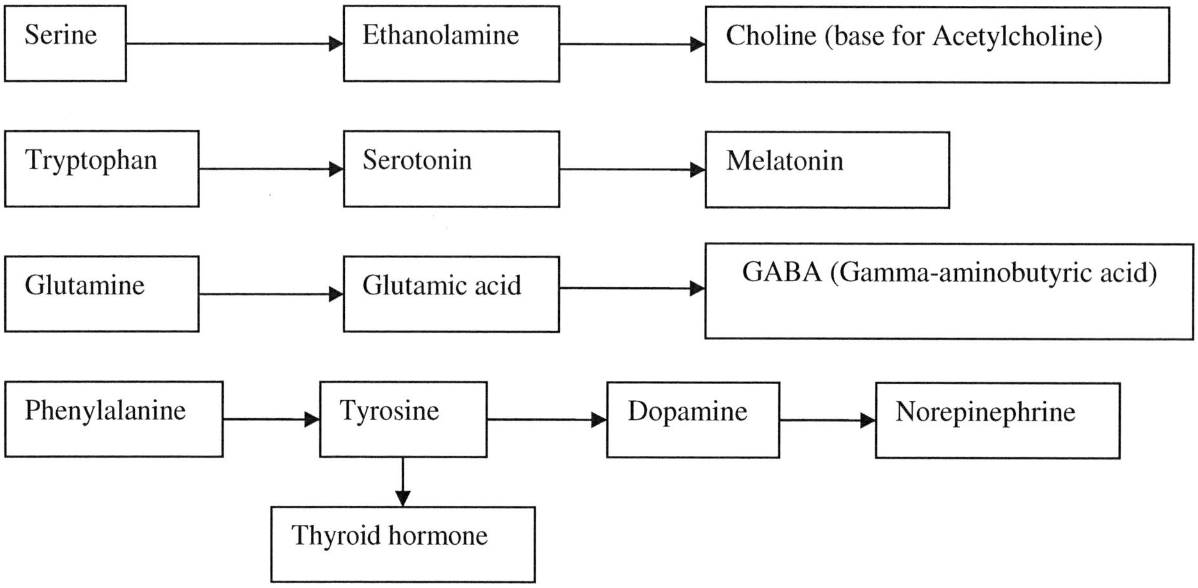

Diagram 11.1-Biochemistry of neurotransmitters

IMPORTANT NUTRIENTS FOR THE NERVOUS SYSTEM

Nutrient	Function
Vitamin B Complex	Supports nerve function; energy pathway nutrient
Vitamin B1	Important in cognition
Vitamins B_3, B_6	Brain function Vitamin B_6: indicated in Parkinson
Vitamin B_{12}	Prevents nerve damage, by keeping myelin sheath intact
EFA	Vital for brain cell function; myelin sheath formation
Vitamins B_5, B_{12}	Choline production
Lecithin	Formation of choline and inositol
Calcium, magnesium	Nerve conduction
Coenzyme Q10	Increases cellular oxygenation
Boron	Enhances brain function and promotes alertness
Manganese	Maintains healthy nerves
Potassium/Sodium	Nervous impulse transmission
Glutamine	Brain fuel

Table 11.2-Important nutrients for the nervous system

SYMPTOMS OF IMBALANCE:

◪**CNS:** irritability, apathy, insomnia, hypersomnia, headache, loss of balance, hyperactivity, lack of concentration, depression, illusions, hallucinations, delusions, obsessions.

◪**PNS**: paresthesia ("pins and needles"), anesthesia (lack of feeling), pain, tingling, numbing.

NEUROLOGIC DEFICIT

→ *Motor:* movement impairment (lack of movement, diminished movement)

→ *Sensory:* applied to sensations (tingling, lack of sensations, etc)

Diagram 11.2- Types of neurological deficit

ASSESSMENT OF THE NERVOUS SYSTEM FUNCTION

MEDICAL	NUTRITIONAL
1. Clinical aspect: headaches, dizziness, loss of balance, irritability, etc.; 2. Physical examination: testing of motor function (strength), testing of sensory function (touch, temperature, pain, etc), assessing balance; 3. Laboratory investigations: CSF analysis; 4. Imaging investigations: x-ray films, computer tomography, MRI, angiography, brain scan, electroencephalogram.	1. Assessment of nutritional abnormalities as listed in the table above; 2. Carbohydrate metabolism: the brain will react to low carbohydrate status by exhibiting symptoms and signs of hypoglycemia; 3. Liver toxicity status assessment: clinic and by complimentary medicine tests;a toxic liver will allow toxins with potential neurotoxicity to be released in the blood stream; 4. Food allergies status, as their presence will overload the immune system (which will not be able to do its"clean-up" function appropriately; 5. Various tests: fatty acids profiling (a low fatty acids status has been linked with impeded nervous system function), Heavy Metal toxicity testing (heavy metals can induce the apparition of neurologic symptoms and signs), and hair analysis.

Table 11.3- Assessment of nervous system function

NERVOUS SYSTEM CONDITIONS

♦ HEADACHE (H/A)

**pain of the structures of head and neck*; the brain itself is insensitive to pain; it can also be a symptom of other organs diseases: ear, nose, sinuses, teeth, jaw, neck muscles or systemic disease (these systemic disease types of headaches are called *Toxic state headaches* and are due to toxemia, septicemia, alcoholism, infections).

Headache
- → **Primary** (benign): migraine, tension headache, and cluster headache
- → **Secondary** (serious): H/A is a symptom of an underlying disease (meningitis, temporal arteritis, tumor)

Diagram 11.3- Headache classification

A. MIGRAINE

**recurrent attacks of vascular (characterized by a throbbing, pounding pain) headache, often severe, may be accompanied by nausea, vomiting, and visual disturbances, etc*; more prevalent in women

- □ Common migraine (85% of cases): without aura;
- □ Classical migraine (15% of cases): accompanied by aura.

Etiology:

- Stress, lack of sleep, atmospheric pressure changes, fatigue;
- Various medications (this is *rebound headache*, caused by excessive use of painkillers);
- Hormonal factors: PMS, menopause;
- Dietary factors: cheese, red wine, chocolate, coffee, are the most frequent triggers;
- Food sensitivities;
- Increased liver toxicity;
- Caffeine withdrawal.

Pathogenesis:

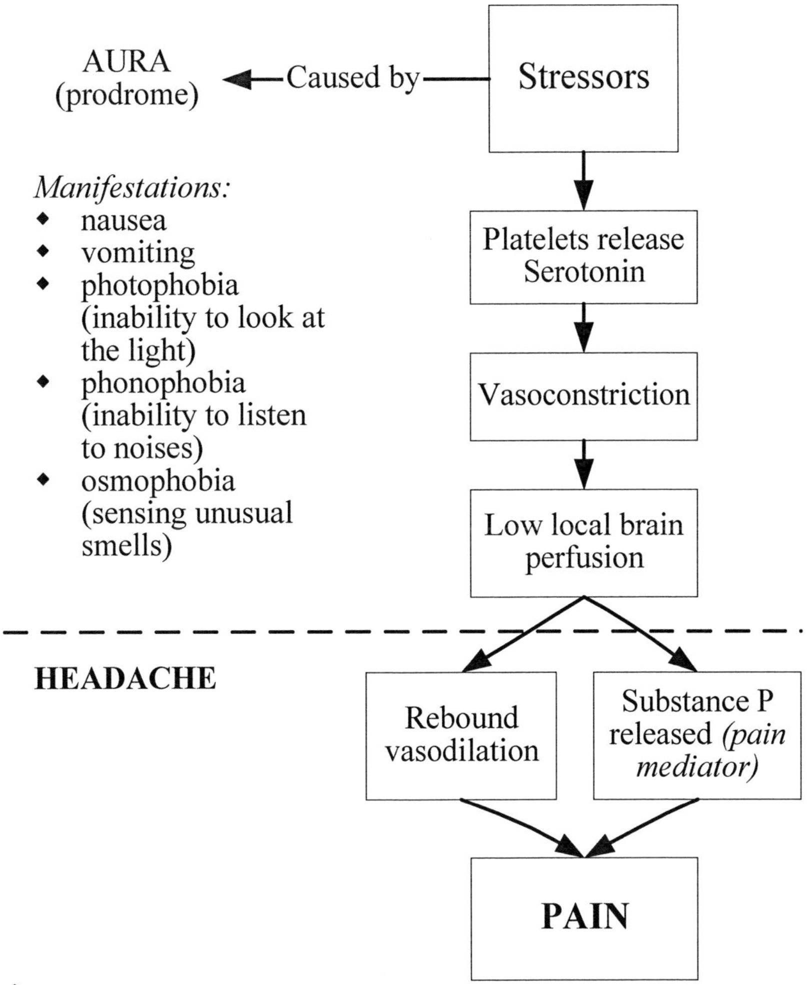

Diagram 11.4-Pathogenesis of headache

Clinical aspect:

- Usually unilateral, throbbing;
- Gradual onset (it can last from a few hours to a few days);
- Worse with movement, noises, light, coughing;
- Better with rest, darkness, cold compresses applications;
- Interferes with ADL (activities of daily living).

Medical treatment: avoid triggers, analgesics, physiotherapy.

Nutrition and holistic approach:

- Identify food sensitivities;
- Avoid known stressors (red wine, cheese, chocolate, beer contain *tyramine,* which stimulates histamine release in certain individuals, causing vasodilation and pain);

- Sustained liver detoxification and support;
- Avoid saturated fats which will feed into the inflammatory pathway;
- Increase intake of alkaline foods;
- Garlic inhibits platelet aggregation (serotonin is released by clumping together of the platelets,);
- Increase intake of foods rich in magnesium;
- Stress management techniques;
- Employ proper sleep and a positive attitude.

Supplements:

- Magnesium, 200 mg three times a day, to relax the smooth muscle of the blood vessels;
- Vitamin B_6, 25 mg three times a day, seems to be useful in histamine related headaches;
- Quercetin, 100 mg three times/day and vitamin C, 2g/ day, in divided doses, stabilize mast cell membrane, reducing the release of histamine;
- Flax seed oil, one tablespoon/day.

Other measures are very useful:

- Hydrotherapy (treatment with water): cold applied to head and heat applied to feet, to allow blood to rush from head downwards, relieving the pain;
- Peppermint or lavender oils applied on temples and forehead are extremely helpful;
- Useful herbs: feverfew (you will achieve great results if you take this herb on a long term basis; please, consult a herbalist), chamomile, peppermint, linden;
- To relieve stress, use chamomile, lemon balm, passion flower or valerian.

B. CLUSTER HEADACHE

**uncommon, male prevalence higher than the female one, more frequent in middle age men*

Etiology:

- Presumably, histamine related headache, triggered by high intake of amine rich dietary agents: wine, beer, cheese, coffee, chocolate;
- Triggered also by stress and lack of rest.

Clinical aspect:

- Clusters of short headache periods (lasting from minutes to a few hours), severe, non-throbbing;
- Some cases present with unilateral pain, eye redness and increased nasal secretion;
- Lasts for one or two hours every day, for weeks to months;
- The attack may return after a few months;
- It is not accompanied by an aura, so the onset is difficult to assess.

Medical treatment: various types of pain relievers, corticosteroids, O_2 inhalation.

Nutritional and holistic approach: please, see above under Migraines.

C. TENSION TYPE HEADACHE

**very common, females more affected than males*

Etiology:

- Postural;
- Cervical spine abnormalities leading to muscle contraction;
- Stress, anxiety, depression.

Clinical aspect:

- Non throbbing, dull, strong, bilateral, usually occipital headache;
- Aura not present;
- Can occur on a daily basis;
- It can last from hours to several days.

Medical treatment: counseling, removal of triggers, physiotherapy, massage, relaxation, NSAID's

Nutrition and holistic approach:

- Identify and take appropriate measures to deal with food sensitivities, as they will overburden the liver detoxification pathway (with consequent headache);
- Consult with a chiropractor or osteopath, if appropriate;
- Improve position of head, neck and upper back to avoid muscle contracture;
- Stress management, relaxation, meditation;
- Local massage.

Supplements:

- Multivitamin/multimineral formula, to support the general health;
- Magnesium, 200 mg three times/day, as it helps with muscle contraction;
- Vitamin B complex as an antistress formula, 50-100mg/day.

Other measures:

- Oils of lavender, chamomile, grapefruit, peppermint and orange blossom help relieve stress and tension;
- Oils of white camphor, blue eucalyptus, peppermint and ginger have muscle relaxant properties;
- Lemon balm, chamomile, passion flower and linden are relaxing herbs.

◆SEIZURE DISORDERS

***seizure**: *acute alteration of behaviour and/or EEG changes as a result of abnormal activity of cerebral neurons*

Etiology:

- Idiopathic (occurring without known cause);
- Brain damage: at birth or post encephalitis;
- Infections and febrile disorders;
- Cerebral trauma;
- Cerebral tumors;
- Vascular: intracranial hemorrhage, brain infarcts;
- Drugs (ethanol withdrawal, neuroleptics, and amphetamines).

A. EPILEPSY

*_an indication of an abnormality in brain function_

▲**Generalized** (Grand mal and petit mal): common, due to an electrical discharge across the brain surface, bilaterally; the difference stays in intensity of the discharge:

- *Grand mal:* begins with aura of olfactive hallucinations, gastric discomfort, limb jerking, right before the attack; then the seizure follows with a shout, loss of consciousness, foaming at the mouth, muscle contraction;
- *Petit mal:* uncommon, in children; short lasting loss of consciousness; child interrupts activity and stares.

▲**Partial seizure**: is localized; aura of a very short duration (fear, anger, hallucinations of smell, music, taste), followed by a period in which the person stares, then automatism starts (swallowing, chewing, lip smacking); upon recovery, accompanied by headache.

Symptoms vary with the affected area of the brain.

Diagnosis:

- Extensive laboratory analysis to exclude organic causes of seizures;
- Brain scan, MRI;
- EEG.

Medical treatment: anticonvulsivants; family education.

Nutrition and holistic approach:

- If the cause of seizures is known and approachable from a nutritional point of view, apply the appropriate protocol;
- Employ appropriate liver detoxification protocols, as circulating neurotoxins may accumulate in the brain tissue and accentuate the problem;
- Limit folic acid intake if clients take anticonvulsivants like Phenytoin;
- Manganese deficiency in pregnancy may result in seizure disorder of the new born;
- Ketogenic diet: high in fats and low in carbohydrates and proteins seems to improve the status of an epileptic client; the mechanism of action is unknown;
- Assess heavy metal toxicity, as it may mimic a seizure disorder;

- Increase the health of the gut, as to avoid the circulation of toxins;
- Avoid sage consumption; it seems to increase the number of episodes.

Supplements:

- Vitamin B complex, 1oo mg twice a day;
- Vitamin B_5, 300 mg daily;
- Magnesium, (400-600 mg/day), calcium, (800-1200 mg/day) and zinc, (30 mg/day) seem to prevent attacks;
- Taurine seems to control seizures-take as prescribed;
- Coenzyme Q10, 30 mg/day ;
- Vitamin C and bioflavonoids, 2 g/day.

Other measures:

- Stress management, appropriate exercise regimen;
- Vervain and valerian may help diminish the severity and frequency of attacks;
- Oils to avoid: sage, fennel, hyssop, wormwood.

♦ SLEEP DISORDERS

**disturbances that result in affected sleep (either too much or not enough) or abnormal sleep behavior*

*sleep occurs on a nightly basis every 90-120 minutes(sleep stages); the periods of deep sleep (the ones that allow us to feel rested) become longer and longer as we go from one sleep stage into the next one.

A. INSOMNIA

**difficulty in falling asleep (sleep-onset insomnia) or in staying asleep(sleep-maintenance insomnia)*

Etiology:

- Irregular sleep schedule;
- Use of stimulants late at night; also, increased fluid intake;
- Medical conditions: sleep apnea, chronic fatigue syndrome, presence of pain and/or discomfort due to various medical reasons;
- Psychologic/psychiatric conditions: stress, worry, anxiety, depression, etc.;
- Decreased levels of taurine (due to a defect in its metabolism);
- Tryptophan deficiency;
- Nocturnal hypoglycemia (low blood glucose will allow for release of glucagons and cortisol, which are brain stimulants).

Medical treatment: avoiding stimulants, establishing regular sleeping patterns, exercise, relaxation, sleep inducing medication.

Nutrition and holistic approach

- Identify the etiology and apply the approach accordingly;
- Hot foot bath with mustard power taken before bedtime helps;

- Lettuce is considered a mild sleeping aide;
- Sleep on a pillow that contains dried lavender;
- Increase intake of tryptophan rich foods.

Supplements:

- Calcium , 500 mg at bedtime;
- Vitamin B_1, 100mg/day (vitamin B_1 deficiency may decrease serotonin availability);
- Vitamin B_6,50mg/day and magnesium, 250-300mg/day, taken along with niacin before bedtime (cofactors in the process of conversion of tryptophan to serotonin);

Other measures:

- Warm bath with chamomile and lavender infusion before bedtime;
- Teas of chamomile, lavender, lemon balm, catnip or valerian help;
- Essential oils of chamomile, lavender or rose: either a few drops in the bath tub, or applied on the pillow.

B. SLEEP APNEA

**group of sleep disorders in which sleep is interrupted for more than 10 seconds at a time, more than 20 times in an hour*; causes decreased levels of oxygen in the blood.

Etiology

- Usually due to obstruction (upper respiratory passages);
- Central (decreased activity of the respiratory center);
- Increased frequency in obese cases.

Clinical aspect:

- Frequently interrupted sleep;
- Morning headache, drowsiness;
- Possible cardiac complications: arrhythmia, tachycardia, etc.

Medical diagnosis: overnight polysomnography (records the sleep pattern with all interruptions).

Medical treatment: CPAP (nasal continuous positive airway pressure); will take care of the obstructive aspect; good results in most of the cases.

Nutrition and holistic approach: general dietary and supplemental support.

C. RESTLESS LEG SYNDROME (RLS)

(*one of the PARASOMNIAS—abnormal sleep):
**common; irresistible urge to move the legs; family history*

Etiology:

- Presence of nocturnal myoclonus (repeated leg muscle contractions during sleep);
- Folic acid deficiency;

- Iron deficiency (with or without anemia; assessment based on ferritin levels, which are low in RLS).

Nutrition and holistic approach:
- If low ferritin (storage form of iron) present, supplement with iron ;
- Folic acid, 10-30mg/day;
- Calcium and magnesium supplementation with at least 500-600 mg calcium and adequate magnesium levels;
- Gingko biloba, 80 mg three times a day.

♦ CEREBROVASCULAR DISEASES

A. ISCHEMIC SYNDROMES

**lack of blood to a certain brain territory*

□**Transient Ischemic attack (TIA):** stroke syndrome characterized by neurological symptoms lasting for minutes to hours, followed by recovery.

□**Ischemic stroke:** lack of blood to a given brain territory leading to cerebral infarction (the tissue dies because of lack of oxygen); it can be caused by **embolism** (a sudden blocking of an artery due to a blood clot or any foreign material, like fat or atherosclerotic plaque) or **cerebral thrombosis** (blockage by a blood clot); clinical appearance varies with the area of the brain that is affected by the stroke.

Risk factors:
- High blood pressure;
- Diabetes mellitus;
- Hypercholesterolemia;
- Obesity;
- BCP use;
- Increased homocysteine levels.

B. HEMORRHAGIC SYNDROMES

HEMORRHAGIC STROKE: sudden onset of neurological symptoms due to hemorrhage (bleeding) in the brain tissue; no TIA precedes it; the onset is upon activity, it is rapidly progressive, starts with a high intensity sudden headache

Medical investigations and treatment are complex and employ extensive measures: CT scan, MRI, comprehensive laboratory testing, medication, resuscitation, surgery, etc.

Nutrition and holistic approach:

First of all keep in mind that this is one of those health conditions where prevention is the key, as the treatment is very difficult and the outcome varies greatly.

Consequently, focus on management of the above mentioned risk factors. In a case like that, when it comes to approach, we can mostly support the general health:

- Focus on an alkaline diet, increased fiber, increased fish intake;
- When high levels of homocysteine present, folic acid and vitamins B_{12} and B_6 offer protection;
- Rosemary and yarrow are circulatory tonics; use for prevention;
- Gingko biloba helps with recovery after a ischemic stroke;
- Use a good multivitamin/multimineral formula, with care; adjust dosages as necessary (as vitamins C and E and fish oil are all blood thinners and may interfere with your client's medication).

◆ CNS INFECTIONS

*these are MEDICAL EMERGENCIES

A. MENINGITIS

**inflammation of meninges of the brain*

Etiology:

- *Primary:* bacterial, viral, fungal infections (affect the meninges directly)
- *Secondary* infection (from a foci located elsewhere in the body: pneumonia, abscesses, etc)

A1. Bacterial infections have unfavourable prognosis.

Clinical aspect: intense headache, neck stiffness, malaise, high temperature, high-pitched cry and bulging fontanelles in babies and infants. CSF is purulent.

A2. Viral meningitis has a much better prognosis

Clinical aspect: headache, malaise, fever, neck stiffness

B. POLYOMYELITIS

**infection by poliovirus leading to various clinical syndromes; damage of the anterior horn cells*

- **Acute**: hyperesthesia (increased sensitivity) and paresthesia, headache, neck pain, positive meningeal signs (that show that the meninges is affected), fever, asymmetric flaccid limb paralysis;
- **Chronic**: progressive or static.

Polyomyelitis cases may results in deformities, as the virus can affect medulla and cerebellum, creating coordination problems.

C. ENCEPHALITIS
**inflammation of brain;* could be severe, resulting in necrotizing encephalitis or could present as focal areas of suppuration, abscesses and necrosis.

Medical treatment: intense antibiotic therapy, antiinflammatories, supportive measures.

Nutrition and holistic approach (supportive of the conventional treatment):

- Light, nutritious diet (heavy eating will result in the body's energies being shunted away from the healing process into digestion);
- Probiotic supplementation, as they will be on an antibiotic protocol;
- Garlic, as prescribed, as a natural antibiotic;
- Multivitamin and multimineral formula, for general support;
- Immune system boosting.

♦ CRANIAL NERVES DISORDERS

***Nutrition and holistic approach** for the following conditions will be presented under *Neuropathies*

A. TRIGEMINAL NEURALGIA: bursts of severe pain due to idiopathic disturbance of trigeminal nerve(the nerve that innervates the mastication/chewing muscles and the mandible); acute, brief attacks of severe, shooting pain along the nerve; no sensory or motor abnormalities.

B.BELL'S PALSY: unilateral paralysis of facial nerve (innervates the muscles of facial expression, lacrimal and salivary glands; unilateral facial muscles weakness and decreased taste; jaw or ear ache; sudden onset and recovery in 1-7 weeks.

♦ DISORDERS OF THE PERIPHERAL NERVOUS SYSTEM

A. NEURALGIA: *any nerve pain;* shooting pain along the nerve's trajectory; any nerve problem will refer in the area that the nerve enervates and it will manifest as either pain or/and sensory symptoms, and muscle weakness/wasting, in advanced cases (due to lack of nervous activation).

Etiology:

- Inflammation of the nerve sheath;
- Injury;
- Entrapment by a contracted muscle;
- Intervertebral disk herniation;
- Repetitive trauma.

B. NERVE INJURY: usually posttraumatic (accidents, surgery, dental procedures).
In some nerve injuries, there is no actual damage to the nerve, but it still fails to function; recovery in up to a few days.
Other injuries result in various effects:

- When the axon is disrupted, but the nerve sheath is intact, there is recovery, but it is slow (1mm/day); nutritional support is very important for these cases;
- When the nerve is completely severed, the treatment is surgical.

C. NEUROPATHIES: *disturbances of the peripheral nervous system*; sensory loss associated or not with muscle weakness

- Axon affected: diabetes, uremia, toxicity;
- Myelin sheath affected: Guillain-Barré syndrome.

□**Guillain-Barré syndrome:** acute, progressive inflammatory polyneuropathy characterized by muscle weakness and sensory loss;

THIS IS A MEDICAL EMERGENCY!!

*an infection, vaccination or surgery may precede it; demyelinating neuropathy

Clinical aspect:

- Symmetric weakness and paresthesia starting in legs and progressing in arms;
- Various degrees of dysfunction;
- Improvement generally after a few months.

The **medical treatment** for the cranial nerves neuralgia and for the peripheral nervous system conditions varies according to the cause and with the gravity of the condition.
(antibiotics, corticosteroids-*except Guillain Barré-*, antiinflammatories, analgesics, etc.)

Nutritional and holistic recommendations for the conditions listed above:

- If appropriate, address the cause of the condition;
- Celery juice relieves neuralgic pain;
- Multivitamin and multimineral formula;
- Vitamin B complex, 50-100mg/day;
- Warm chamomile compresses applied to the area will help relieve the pain;
- Essential oils of peppermint, chamomile, lavender, rosemary, either applied as a light massage or in a bath are helpful;
- St. John's wort helps with the pain.

Additional nutritional and holistic recommendations for **Guillain-Barre**: immune system support, valerian and/or oats, as calming agents; essential oils of chamomile, Melissa, lavender and rosemary support the nervous system.

♦ DISORDERS OF MOVEMENT

A. HUNTINGTON'S CHOREA

*Chorea: involuntary, irregular jerky movements;
* Genetic etiology; no cure; death after 10-20 years of evolution;
*Associated with low levels of neurotransmitters: GABA and acetylcholine.

Clinical aspect:

- Chorea starts initially at hands level, affecting the fine movements;
- Progressive intellectual deterioration;
- Ultimately, the client loses his/her physical and mental abilities.

Medical treatment: none known, so far.
General **supportive nutritional** therapy recommended

B. PARKINSON'S DISEASE (SHAKING PALSY)

**idiopathic, slowly progressive, irreversible degenerative disease;* onset between 40-70 years; affects men more than women; it has been suggested that toxic damage to the brain and free radical damage may be causative factors

Pathogenesis: loss of dopamine in a part of the brain that causes loss of control over voluntary movement.

Clinical aspect: TRAP

- **T**remor (at rest, "pill-rolling"; voluntary movement can stop or diminish it);
- **R**igidity (stiffness, immobile facial expression);
- **A**kinesia/bradykinesia (loss of movement, respectively, less movement);
- **P**ostural instability (gait (manner of walking), falls).

Medical treatment: Levodopa, which supplies dopamine to the brain; this drug and vitamin B_6 interfere with each other.

Nutrition and holistic approach:

- Avoid any source of free radicals;
- Mild but steady liver and colon cleanse; body detoxification;
- Approach of dysbiosis, candidiasis, parasitosis, or any other source of circulating toxins;
- Very low protein diet in the morning and in the evening, which seems to allow Levodopa to be better absorbed;
- Antioxidant rich diet is recommended.

Supplements:

- Methionine seems to relieve some of the symptoms (found in animal products, sunflower seeds, egg yolks);
- Good quality multivitamin and multimineral formula;
- Additional antioxidants: vitamin C, 2-4g/day and vitamin E, 400IU/day;
- Flax seed oil, 1-2 tablespoons/day;
- Phenylalanine supplementation, as prescribed, as phenylalanine is a precursor for dopamine
- Vitamin B complex, 50-100mg/day; take away from medication time, if they have been prescribed Levodopa;
- Gingko biloba: increases blood flow to the brain;
- Ginseng and oats boost the nervous system's function.

♦ DEMYELINATING DISEASES

MULTIPLE SCLEROSIS

**gradual, progressive loss of the myelin sheath (demyelination in patches),* resulting in various neurological signs and symptoms; remission/relapse pattern.

Etiology: multifactorial

- Viral theory (it seems that clients with MS have antibodies present in their CSF);
- Autoimmune disease: presumably, there are antibodies against the myelin sheath protein component; not yet proven;
- Diets high in gluten, milk and/or dietary fat seem to have a higher incidence of multiple sclerosis;
- Decreased capacity to neutralize free radicals, due to reduced activity of an antioxidant enzyme (glutathione peroxidase); the result is increased lipid peroxidation (fats altered by free radicals);
- Heavy metal toxicity, especially mercury; it seems that mercury has a certain degree of brain affinity and it can deposit in the brain tissue, mirroring MS symptoms.

Clinical aspect:

- Usually, insidious (slow) onset: some sensory and/or motor symptoms/signs;
- The disease progresses on a remission relapse pattern;
- Motor impairment: clumsiness, leg dragging, weakness, unsteadiness;
- Sensory impairment: tingling, numbing;
- Visual impairment: blurring, fogginess, pain (because of a serious condition called *optic neuritis*), sometimes double vision;
- Vestibular impairment: lightheadedness, dizziness;
- Genito-urinary involvement: incontinence, loss of bladder function.

Not all symptoms/signs are present at the same time, in the same case. It seems that cases that have visual impairment have a better prognosis (unproven theory).

Diagnosis:
- Clinical aspect;
- MRI: shows pathognomonic (characteristic) lesions;
- CSF analysis.

Medical treatment: limited to corticosteroids, immunomodulatory and symptomatic drugs.

Nutrition and holistic approach:
- Liver cleanse and detoxification;
- Identify any possible source of toxins (food allergens, dysbiosis, parasitosis, etc), and approach it therapeutically, as circulating toxins may greatly add to the burden of a MS client;
- Adrenal gland sustained support;
- If heavy metal toxicity present, employ the approach suggested in appendix B;
- Stress management, relaxation, support groups, massages;
- SWANK diet is a successful diet that allows only 10grams saturated fat/day; increase fish intake, vegetables, fruits; low saturated fat foods.

Supplements:
- Take EFA supplementation, both in a omega 3 and omega 6 form (which will displace the saturated fat molecules from the brain cell membranes); they also have an anti-inflammatory effect;
- Antioxidant supplementation (choose a good formula that contains vitamin E ,400-800 IU/day and selenium , 200 mcg/day);
- Vitamin B_{12}, 2 mg/day; injectable forms are very helpful;
- Digestive enzymes, as MS has been linked with increased levels of circulating immune complexes;
- Good multivitamin and multimineral formula.

Other measures:
- Gingko biloba, 40 mg three times/day;
- Nervine herbs and /or essential oils of: chamomile, lavender, melissa;
- Oat bath; add lavender flowers;
- Encourage exercise to the best of your client's possibilities.

CHAPTER 12

OPHTHALMOLOGIC, EAR, NOSE AND THROAT DISORDERS

Vision, hearing, smell and taste are called *Special senses*, because their receptors are different from any other receptor structures in the body. The eye receptors are called *photoreceptors*, because they are stimulated by light. The hearing receptors are called *mechanoreceptors*, because they are stimulated by movement. The smell and taste receptors are called *chemoreceptors*, because chemical substances stimulate them.

Nevertheless, the special senses are fascinating structures and nutrition plays a great role in supporting their health. Let us begin with *The eye* and the sense of vision.

THE EYE

NUTRITIONAL IMBALANCES

Nutrient	Role
Vitamin A	Vitally important for vision.Protects the mucus membranes of the eye
Vitamin B complex	Important for all energy pathways
Vitamin B6	Deficiency can lead to conjunctivitis
Vitamin C	Antioxidant; collagen fibers formation
Bioflavonoids	Enhance vitamin C absorption

Table 12.1- The eye: nutritional abnormalities

Common signs and symptoms of eye conditions:

- Redness of conjunctiva, increased lacrimation, various discharges (watery, purulent, etc.);
- Redness of sclera, visible blood vessels;
- Decreased visual acuity, either in the daytime or/and night time;
- Visual abnormalities: seeing spots;
- Photophobia (abnormal visual intolerance to light), pain, visual defects.

ASSESSMENT

MEDICAL ASSESSMENT	NUTRITIONAL ASSESSMENT
1. Clinical assessment: of the signs and symptoms listed above 2. Ocular examination: of conjunctiva, eyelids, cornea, pupil; assessment of visual fields (how much you can see up, down, left and right; 3. Ophthalmoscopic examination: examines the internal structures of the eye (retina, fundus, optic disc-the place where the optic nerve leaves the eye); 4. Tonometry: the measurement of the intraocular pressure; diagnosis of glaucoma; 5. B-mode ultrasonography: used to assess retinal tumors, retinal detachments, foreign bodies; 6. Slit-lamp examination: to detect opacities.	1. Assessment of nutritional signs and symptoms of imbalances as listed above 2. Malabsorption assessment (presence of leaky gut, dysbiosis, etc), which will impede on nutrient absorption; 3. Liver function assessment: as liver problems will impede nutrients metabolism and transport.

Table 12.2- Assessment of the eye function

EYE CONDITIONS

♦ INFLAMMATORY AND INFECTIOUS CONDITIONS

A. CONJUNCTIVITIS

**conjunctiva inflammation*

Forms

- ***Acute*:** caused by viruses, bacteria or allergy;
  Clinical aspect: redness, watery discharge, ocular irritation, eyelids are stuck together upon awakening;

  *one aspect is gonococcal conjunctivitis, which could occur during a gonorrhoeal genital infection.
- ***Chronic:*** similar causes to those of the acute form, but the evolution is much milder and usually the discharge is either absent or in decreased amount.

Medical treatment: applies to the cause: antibiotics, anti-inflammatory drugs, antihistaminic drugs

Nutrition and holistic approach

- Firstly, assess the cause and apply your protocol accordingly; bacterial and viral conjunctivitis will require immune system boosting, whereas allergic conjunctivitis (characterized by redness, itching, watery discharge, upon presence of allergen) will require immune system building, not boosting;
- Liver and digestive system cleanse and detoxification;
- Apply cold whole wheat bread to the inflamed eye, as it is soothing and it is a rich source of vitamins B;
- Mix filtered, clean water with a small quantity of honey; use as eyewash.

> **Important !:** various local preparations exist on the market; caution your client on the aseptic (cleanliness) aspect; do not touch the dropper to the eye structures; always wash hands before administering the preparations; use only pre-prepared eye drops, as they have to respect the manufacturer's aseptic conditions

<u>Supplements</u> (oral and topical)

- Immune system support, as described in the *Immune system* chapter;
- Eye drops with vitamin C with or without vitamin A seem to help in cases of viral and allergic conjunctivitis: use only as prescribed and never use a higher dosage without consulting with the practitioner, as vitamin C may cause transient stinging;
- Eyewashes of the following herbs are very useful: chamomile, fennel seeds, elderflower or eyebright; make a chamomile tea; refrigerate the tea bag for a few hours; apply the cold bag, as a compress on the inflamed eye.

B. STYE

**abscess around the root of an eyelash; usually caused by bacteria;* may spread to nearby follicles;

Clinical aspect: redness, pain, swelling, and pain.

Medical treatment: antibiotic therapy.

Nutrition and holistic approach:

- Immune system boosting;
- Warm bread poultice applied to the stye will help bring out the infection;
- Dab the stye (carefully, so no preparations go in the eye) with a drop of tea tree oil or a drop of calendula tincture;
- Chamomile or eyebright, either as washes or compresses are anti-inflammatory.

♦ CATARACT

*opacity of the lens

Etiology:

- Aging (protein coagulation at lens level);
- Radiation exposure;
- Systemic disease (diabetes);
- Systemic medication (corticosteroids).

Clinical aspect:

- Painless, progressive vision loss (depends on the size and location of opacity)
- Change in colour and detail perception

Diagnosis: ophtalmoscopy and slit-light examination;

Medical treatment: surgery, if frequent eyeglasses changes do not help.

Nutrition and holistic approach:

- Decrease intake of milk products, as galactose may promote cataract formation;
- Increase antioxidant intake, in food form and as supplements.

Supplements:

- Riboflavin, 30-50 mg/day (as it seems that vitamin B_2 is found in the retina of the eye and its low levels have been linked to increased incidence in cataract formation-on animal studies);
- Quercetin ,500 mg/day, which reduces sorbitol accumulation (it seems that sorbitol—*a sugar alcohol found in apples, pears and peaches*—may play a role in cataract formation);
- Zinc, 15-30mg/day, mostly used in senile cataracts, as it seems to be a cell membrane stabilizer of the ocular tissue;
- Vitamin C, 2-3 grams/day, as it prevents oxidative damage and it prevents sorbitol accumulation;
- Vitamin E, 400 IU/day and Selenium, 200-300 mcg/day have been proven quite protective against cataract formation.

♦ MACULAR DEGENERATION

**degeneration of macula* (a physiologic depression of retina, next to the optic disk; involved in central vision)

Etiology: age related, oxidative damage.

Clinical aspect: visual distortion, progressive loss of vision; these cases usually maintain good peripheral vision and colour sense.

Medical treatment: laser photocoagulation.

Nutrition and holistic approach:

- Low fat diet abundant in antioxidants seems to be protective;
- Increased intake of lutein rich foods (found in spinach and collard greens) ,as lutein is a major component of the macular pigment;
- Increased taurine rich diet, as taurine seems to be the most abundant aminoacid in the retina;
- Zinc, 30 mg/day, as it seems that slows the rate of visual loss in senile macular degeneration;
- Vitamin E, 400 IU/day, Selenium, 200 mcg/day, Vitamin C, 2 g/day and Vitamin A, 5000-10000 IU/day, as all of them play an important role in retinal health;
- Bilberry extract and Gingko biloba: showed improved visual status in cases with macular degeneration.

♦ GLAUCOMA

* *increased intraocular pressure*

Acute form: pain, redness, the eye is hard to touch, marked visual impairment;

THIS IS A MEDICAL EMERGENCY!!

as it can lead to blindness.

Chronic form: slowly progressive, starts with peripheral vision loss and progresses to central vision loss.

Nutrition and holistic approach for chronic glaucoma:

- Chronic glaucoma can improve upon identification and elimination of allergies;
- Vitamin C, to bowel tolerance seems to improve the condition and reduce intraocular pressure;
- Chromium, which increases the focusing power;
- Bioflavonoid complex, as prescribed, as they support vitamin's C function, aid in collagen formation and prevent free radical damage;
- Theoretically, magnesium may help as it relaxes the vasculature's smooth muscle and thus it may improve the blood flow;
- EFA's, as fish oils seem to have beneficial effects in reducing the intraocular pressure;
- Coenzyme Q10, as prescribed, as it improves oxygenation;
- Gingko biloba and Bilberry extract.

THE EAR

NUTRITIONAL IMBALANCES

CONDITIONS/SIGNS/SYMPTOMS	NUTRITIONAL ABNORMALITIES
Vertigo	Magnesium deficiency
Dark earwax	EFA deficiency
Cracks behind ears	Decreased zinc levels
Diagonal ear lobe crease	In males, associated with cardiovascular diseases

Table 12.3- The ear: nutritional abnormalities

Common signs and symptoms;

- Pain (otalgia);
- Discomfort, discharge;
- Increased ear wax amount;
- Tinnitus (noise in the ear);
- Dizziness;
- Vertigo (abnormal sensation of spinning/rotation with balance difficulty);
- Decreased hearing acuity, hearing loss.

ASSESSMENT

MEDICAL ASSESSMENT	NUTRITIONAL ASSESSMENT
1. Clinical aspect, based on symptoms and signs; 2. Otoscopic examination: assesses the aspect of external auditory canal (for wax presence, foreign bodies or otitis externa) and the tympanic membrane (for color, bulging, perforation, discharge); 3. Hearing tests, to assess the type of hearing loss (as to the cause: ear related conditions or the acoustic nerve/auditory cortex involvement); 4. Audiometry: the method that assesses how much hearing loss is present; 5. Vestibular apparatus testing: to assess the cause of vertigo/dizziness.	1. Assessment of nutritional abnormalities, as listed above; 2. Malabsorption assessment (presence of leaky gut, dysbiosis, etc), which will impede on nutrient absorption; 3. Liver function assessment: as liver problems will impede nutrients metabolism and transport; 4. EFA status

Table 12.4-Assessment of ear function

EAR CONDITIONS

♦ TINNITUS

**presence of sounds (hissing, ringing, popping) experienced in one or both ears in the absence of acoustic stimuli*

Etiology:

- not well known; it can appear on its own or it may be a symptom of any underlying ear disease; allergies and carbohydrate intolerance seem to increase the likelihood of the condition; decreased vitamin B_{12} levels have been considered as causing tinnitus in some cases; Chinese medicine says that tinnitus means that the essence, the strength of life is diminished.

Nutrition and holistic approach (should apply to the case, according to the etiology, if known):

- Identify and approach allergies;
- Eliminate sugar and refined carbohydrates;
- Assess vitamin B_{12} status and take appropriate approach, if necessary;
- Increase antioxidant rich foods and also increase bioflavonoids intake;
- Increase magnesium intake;
- Zinc supplementation seems to help;
- Feverfew seem to prevent the attacks;
- Essential oils of rosemary, cypress, lemon and rose, massaged on the skin of scalp, neck and chest.

♦ MENIERE'S DISEASE

**disorder characterized by vertigo, eventual hearing loss, tinnitus and feeling of fullness in the ear*

Etiology:

- Unknown; disturbed carbohydrate metabolism, allergies, impaired blood flow to the brain , exposure to loud noises, free radical damage and TMJ (temporo-mandibular joint) syndrome, manganese deficiency, hypercholesterolemia –all these factors have been considered as possible etiologic aspects.

Nutrition and holistic approach: will depend on the cause of the condition, if known

- Identify and approach allergies;
- Identify and approach carbohydrate metabolism problems;
- Focus on a bioflavonoid and antioxidant rich diet;
- Flax seed oil, at least one tablespoon/day;
- Gingko biloba and coenzyme Q10, to improve circulation and respectively cellular oxygenation.

♦ OTITIS

A. OTITIS EXTERNA

**outer ear canal infection/inflammation*

Etiology: bacterial, viral, fungal; swimmer's ear is caused by an infection with a microorganism called Pseudomonas aeruginosa.

Clinical aspect: pain, discomfort, discharge; lymphadenopathy may be present as well;

Nutrition and holistic approach:

- Immune system boosting;
- Roasted onion compress or warm bread poultice can be topically applied, as it will draw out the infection and relieve the pain;
- Warm garlic oil and mullein oil, a few drops applied in the ear canal will help alleviate the infection;
- Ear canal washes with infusions of chamomile, elderflower and goldenseal; also, tea tree oil wash is very helpful.

B. OTITIS MEDIA

**middle ear infection*

Etiology:

- Infection (bacterial, viral, fungal) of the middle ear, or from the nearby organ systems (quite frequently, otitis media is a consequence of respiratory tract infections);
- Allergies: this aspect has been involved in the etiology of otitis media quite frequently lately; as allergic reactions proceed (mostly to food; milk allergy is a common cause of otitis), the inflammatory reaction that accompanies them will create the conditions for swelling of the middle ear mucosa and/or fluid accumulation; unfortunately, when there is fluid in the middle ear, one of the therapeutic measures is *myringotomy*, which involves the placement of a tube through the tympanic membrane to release the fluid; scarring and further infections are known consequences of this procedure.

Clinical aspect: pain, pressure, fluid build-up, and later, possible hearing loss.

Nutrition and holistic approach:

- Identify and approach allergies (recurrent ear infection has been associated with using a milk formula, for example);
- Immune system boosting, as in diet and supplements;
- Vitamin A, 10000-20000 IU/day, for a few days, then decrease the dosage to 5000-10000 IU/day;
- Vitamin C, 2-4 grams/day, or up to bowel tolerance;
- Bioflavonoid complex, as prescribed;
- Zinc, 30-50 mg/day.

Topically:

- Garlic oil and mullein oil in warm applications;
- Infusions of chamomile, Echinacea and/or goldenseal are excellent ear washes; they can be also used as local warm compresses;
- Essential oils of chamomile, tea tree or clove are helpful when massaged around the ear and down the neck on the affected side.

NOSE AND SINUSES

NUTRITIONAL IMBALANCES

CONDITION/SIGNS/SYMPTOMS	NUTRITIONAL IMBALANCES
Anosmia (lack of smell)	Zinc deficiency
Epistaxis (bleeding from the nose)	Decreased vitamin C and bioflavonoids status, also sign of vitamin A toxicity
Polyps(any growth or mass protruding from a mucous membrane);	Food sensitivities
Salute sign (appears in children; rubbing of the tip of the nose in an upward fashion with the palm of the hand; due to the presence of nasal itching);	Food sensitivities

Table 12.5- The nose and sinuses: nutritional abnormalities

Common symptoms and signs: anosmia, redness of the nasal mucosa, excessive elimination of various forms of discharges (watery, purulent, etc), frontal headache;

ASSESSMENT

MEDICAL ASSESSMENT	NUTRITIONAL ASSESSMENT
1. Clinical aspect as described above 2. Illumination of nasal mucosa: to assess inflammatory signs, septum deviation, etc.; 3. Illumination of sinus cavities 4. Radiologic examination	1. Assessment of nutritional imbalances as listed above 2. Allergic terrain testing 3. Immune system status assessment 4. Liver and digestive system status assessment

Table 12.6- Assessment of the nose and sinuses

NOSE AND SINUSES CONDITIONS

A. EPISTAXIS *(nosebleed)*

Etiology:
- Trauma, injuries, nose picking, drying of the mucous membranes;
- Secondary to local infections: rhinitis, sinusitis;
- Local tumors;
- Arteriosclerosis, hypertension, liver diseases, blood disease.

Treatment: will vary with the etiology.

Nutrition and holistic approach: (before employing any nutritional protocol, make sure that there is no medical or surgical condition that is responsible for the epistaxis)
- Lemon is known to stop bleeding; put a drop or two on the end of a cotton ball and apply intranasally;
- When you experience a nosebleed, pinch your nose and lean forward; this will often diminish the bleeding;
- Vitamin C, 2-3 grams/day associated with a good bioflavonoid complex, as they improve vascular fragility (when blood vessels rupture easily);
- Multivitamin and multimineral formula with vitamin A, as vitamin A is supportive of mucous membranes;
- Essential oil of lavender applied locally will encourage healing.

B. RHINITIS

**inflammation of the nasal mucosa*

Etiology: infectious (viruses or bacteria) or allergic (usually environmental allergens).

Clinical aspect:
- Swelling of the nasal mucosa;
- Nasal discharge (watery in allergic rhinitis, thick, yellow and/or purulent in bacterial rhinitis; viral rhinitis is frequently accompanied by watery, then thick discharge);
- Nasal obstruction.

Treatment: will vary with the cause

Nutrition and holistic approach: will depend on the cause of the condition
- Use a humidifier, as a dry mucosa will be easily affected by disease;
- Avoid milk products and refined carbohydrates;
- Identify and approach an allergic terrain.

<u>Supplements:</u>
- Vitamin C, 2-3 grams/day, or up to bowel tolerance;

- Quercetin, if allergy is present, 400-500 mg/day, as it stabilizes mast cells membranes and prevents degranulation; vitamin C has a similar effect;
- Vitamin A, 5000-10000 IU/day, as it supports the nasal mucosa health;
- Zinc, 30-50 mg/day;
- Bioflavonoid complex, as prescribed, as it supports vitamin C absorption.

Others:

- Mustard seed foot bath; chamomile tea inhalations; ginger tea and coriander seeds may help relieve the congestion;ginger, onion or sage tea with a pinch of cayenne will have the same effect;
- Either eat or take garlic supplements;
- Essential oils of lemon, chamomile, eucalyptus, thyme and mint are decongestants (relieve nasal congestion).

C. SINUSITIS

**inflammation of the sinuses*

Etiology: infectious (viral or bacterial) or allergic (exposure to environmental allergens)
*in most of the cases, the infectious etiology is secondary to a nearby infection (usually respiratory or dental).

Clinical picture: frontal or maxillary headache, abundant nasal discharge, possible nosebleeds and/or sense of smell.

Nutrition and holistic approach:
For the general approach and supplementation, see *Rhinitis*

Other measures:

- Horseradish, lemon and honey may help relieve the congestion;
- Steam inhalation works very well: either plant infusions of chamomile, thyme, peppermint or elderflower, or essential oils of lavender, eucalyptus or tea tree could be used.

THROAT DISORDERS

A. PHARYNGITIS

**inflammation of the pharynx mucosa*

Etiology: infectious (bacterial or viral) or irritative (caused by environmental pollutants like smoke or dust inhalation).

Clinical aspect: sore throat, difficulty swallowing, burning sensation, hoarseness, possible lymphadenopathy, if infection is the cause; possible earache.

Nutrition and holistic approach will depend on the etiology; an allergic etiology will require appropriate protocol, as described in *Allergies*.

For common pharyngitis:

- Immune system boosting; does not apply in allergic conditions;
- Salt water or honey water; red sage, goldenseal or calendula gargles;
- Ginger root, honey and lemon juice;
- Steam inhalation of lavender or thyme;
- Essential oils of lavender or tea tree oils in a carrier oil, massaged into the neck.

B. TONSILLITIS

*_inflammation of pharyngeal tonsils_

Etiology: infectious (viral or bacterial); rarely, complications as quinsy (an abscess behind the tonsils) may develop

Clinical picture:

- Headache, malaise, general weakness, fever;
- Sore throat with pain on swallowing and difficulty swallowing;
- Lymphadenopaty.

Nutrition and holistic approach:

- Immune system boosters, as in diet, supplements and herbs;
- Eat garlic liberally or take garlic supplements;
- Ginger root, lemon and honey have a soothing effect;
- Blackcurrant tea or hot juice will relieve the pain;
- Mullein and marshmallow have soothing effects;
- Drink teas of chamomile, elderflower, yarrow and limeflowers, to reduce the inflammation;
- Essential oils of thyme, lavender or tea tree in carrier oil either massaged into the neck or in a vaporizer are helpful.

C. LARYNGITIS

*_inflammation of the mucosa of the larynx, usually involving the vocal cords as well_

Etiology:

- **Acute**: infectious;
- **Chronic**: irritation from smoking, airborne pollutants or overuse of vocal cords (singers and teachers).

Clinical aspect:

- Dry, irritating cough;
- Hoarseness **attention to this sign;** in the absence of the etiological factors for laryngitis, it may be a sign of a laryngeal or mediastinal tumour;

- Possible discomfort on swallowing.

Nutrition and holistic approach:

- If the etiology is infectious, use immune system boosters;
- For the chronic/irritative aspect, use soothing agents, as described below;
- Increased antioxidant food intake, especially vitamin C rich foods;
- Flax seed oil, 1-2 tablespoons/day;
- Warm honey water with lemon is soothing;
- Red sage and echinacea gargles help diminish the inflammation;
- Marshmallow or slippery elm are demulcents (soothing agents);
- Essential oils of geranium, rosemary or tea tree in a glass of water, as a gargle;
- Lavender or tea tree oils in carrier oil can be massaged into the neck area.

CHAPTER 13

THE ENDOCRINE SYSTEM

The Endocrine system is the second controlling system of the body, after the Nervous system. The nervous system acts very fast and uses chemical substances that are called **neurotransmitters**, whereas the endocrine system acts much slower, using chemical messengers called **hormones**, which continuously regulate all functions of the body.

Remember what happens when we are scared? Your Sympathetic Nervous System will stimulate the adrenal medulla to release norepinephrine, which in turn is responsible for the clinical manifestations of " the fight or flight" response. A given hormone always acts on a target cell or organ.

The Major Endocrine Glands and their Hormones

Gland	Hormone	Action
Pineal	Melatonin	Daily rhythm/sleep
Thymus	Thymosin	Involved in Immune response (Lymphocytes T mature in thymus)
Posterior Pituitary	Oxytocin	Contraction of uterus
	ADH (antidiuretic)	Regulates the water balance by retention of water by kidneys
Anterior Pituitary	GH (growth hormone)	Stimulates growth Protein and glucose sparing hormone
	PRL (prolactin)	Stimulates milk production
	TSH (Thyroid stimulating hormone)	Stimulates the thyroid gland to secrete its hormones
	ACTH (adrenocorticotropic hormone)	Stimulates adrenal cortex to produce its hormones
	FSH (Follicle Stimulating Hormone)	Stimulates production of ova and sperm
	LH (Luteinizing Hormone)	Stimulates ovaries and testes to produce their own hormones
Thyroid	T3 (triiodothyronine) and T4 (thyroxine)	Stimulate the body's metabolism
	Calcitonin	Involved in blood calcium regulation: decreases blood calcium levels by depositing it into the bone
Parathyroid	Parathyroid hormone	Increases blood calcium levels, by breaking down the bone tissue when blood calcium levels are too low
Pancreas	Glucagon	Increases blood sugar levels, by breaking down glycogen
	Insulin	Decreases blood sugar levels, by introducing the glucose molecules into the cells

Gland	Hormone	Action
Adrenal Medulla	Adrenaline and Noradrenaline*	Involved in stress response
Adrenal Cortex	Aldosterone	Involved in water balance, by sodium reabsorption at kidney level
	Cortisone	Increases blood glucose levels Anti-inflammatory effect
	Androgens	Precursors for sex hormones
Ovaries	Estrogens and Progesterone	Responsible for ova production and development of secondary sex characteristics
Testes	Testosterone	Responsible for sperm production and development of secondary sex characteristics

Table 13.1- The major endocrine glands and their hormones

*also known as Epinephrine and Norepinephrine

BASIC NUTRIENTS FOR THE ENDOCRINE SYSTEM

Nutrient	Role
Vitamin B_5	Adrenal hormones synthesis
Vitamin C	Stress hormones synthesis
Vitamin B_3	Deficiency leads to low blood sugar; Sex hormones synthesis.
Vitamin B_6	Acts as a mild diuretic, therefore useful in PMS approach; Very useful for the approach of diabetic neuropathy.
Biotin	Deficiency may cause high blood sugar; therefore it may reduce blood glucose levels in diabetes.
Vitamin B_{12}	Indicated in diabetic neuropathy and retinopathy; also in infertility.
EFA, vitamins E and B complex	Support the health of the pituitary gland.
Iodine and selenium	Support the thyroid gland.
Potassium	Deficiency results in glucose intolerance.
Taurine	Useful for cases with hypoglycemia.
Tyrosine	Part of the thyroid hormone.

Table 13.2-Important nutrients for the endocrine system

Common symptoms/signs: various, according to the condition

ASSESSMENT

MEDICAL ASSESSMENT	NUTRITIONAL ASSESSMENT
1. Clinical picture: based on the presence of signs/symptoms; **2.** Physical examination: objectively assesses the modifications at organ level; **3.** Laboratory testing: to assess hormonal values and also precursors; **4.** Imaging techniques: CT scan, x-ray, MRI.	**1.** Clinical picture: based on the presence of signs/symptoms; **2.** Carbohydrate metabolism assessment: presence of hypoglycemia; carbohydrate addiction; **3.** Liver function assessment; **4.** Digestive system function assessment; **5.** BBT (Basal Body Temperature): to assess subclinical hypothyroidism.

Table 13.3-Assesment of the endocrine system

ENDOCRINE SYSTEM DISORDERS

♦ PITUITARY GLAND DISORDERS

A. ANTERIOR LOBE DISORDERS

HORMONE	PATHOLOGY
Growth Hormone	**CHILDHOOD** → *Low:* Dwarfism; → *High:* Gigantism **ADULT**: **Acromegaly:** growth of soft tissues, thick skin, large bones, coarse features, osteoarthritis, hypertension *Etiology*: pituitary adenoma, rarely carcinoid tumors
Prolactin	• Raises in response to stress; • Hypoprolactinemia: inability to lactate; • Hyperprolactinemia*:* galactorrhea*.
FSH LH	Low hormonal secretion: hypogonadism**, amenorrhea (lack of menses), impotence, loss of body hair, testicular atrophy, failure of pubertal development.

Table 13.4-Pituitary gland: anterior lobe disorders

*lactation, in men or in women who do not breastfeed
**decreased functional activity of either ovaries or testis

B. POSTERIOR LOBE DISORDERS

Diabetes Insipidus

**temporary or chronic condition due to deficiency of ADH (vasopresin)*
**this disease has nothing to do with blood sugar levels; it has been named Diabetes because of the characteristic symptoms (see below).*

Etiology: genetic predisposition or secondary to disease (tumors, vascular lesions, trauma or infections).

Clinical aspect:
- Polyuria (increased urination);
- Polydipsia (increased thirst);;
- Dehydration.

Medical treatment is usually hormone therapy.

Nutrition and holistic treatment is just generally supportive of the conventional medicine treatment:
- Multivitamin and multimineral formula;
- Vitamin C, 2 g/day;
- Flax seed oil ,1-2 tablespoons/day;
- Vitamin B complex, 50 mg/day;
- Stress management.

◆ THYROID GLAND DISORDERS

Synthesis and release of the thyroid hormone:

Iodine (from food and water) + **Tyrosine** = **T_3** (triiodothyronine) and **T_4** (Thyroxine)

The T_3 and T_4 released from the thyroid gland reach the bloodstream, where they are bound to a specific transport protein, TBG (*Thyroxin binding globulin*); at tissue level, TBG releases the thyroid hormones and only T_3 and T_4 are available in the periphery (remember, "*periphery*" means the blood stream) to exercise their action and also for measurement purposes;

T_3 and T_4 synthesis is under control of TSH. When thyroid hormone levels are low in the bloodstream, TSH will stimulate the thyroid gland to produce more hormones. Consequently, when T_3 and T_4 are high in the bloodstream, TSH secretion will be suppressed and the thyroid gland, not prompted by TSH anymore, will slow down the hormone production.

TESTS OF THYROID FUNCTION:

- Circulating thyroid hormones: T_3 and T_4;
- TSH (low in hyperthyroidism and high in hypothyroidism);
- Radioactive iodine uptake;
- Thyroid anatomy-by palpation;
- Fine needle aspiration for cytology (cell aspect);
- Thyroid scan;
- Thyroid antibodies.

A. HYPERTHYROIDISM (Thyrotoxicosis)
condition characterized by hypermetabolism and elevated blood levels of thyroid hormones

A1. Grave's disease (Diffuse toxic goiter)

**Hyperthyroidism of autoimmune etiology (antibody against the thyroid TSH receptor, which results in continuous stimulation of the thyroid gland)*; chronic evolution with remissions and relapses; runs in families, with female prevalence;

Clinical aspect:

- Tachycardia (fast heart rhythm), warm, moist skin;
- Nervousness, increased activity, weight loss;
- Palpitations, fatigue, insomnia;
- Eye signs: stare, exophthalmia (eyes are bulging), lid lag (takes a while to close the eyes), lacrimation, irritation.

Diagnosis: intensive laboratory testing, immunologic testing.

A2. Toxic Nodular Goiter

**glandular enlargement with multiple foci of intense hormone formation.*
*increased T_3 and T_4 levels, decreased TSH level

Nutrition and holistic approach for Hyperthyroidism

- Foods belonging to the Brassica family (cauliflower, broccoli, Brussels sprouts, cabbage, mustard greens, spinach and turnips) suppress the thyroid function and are to be consumed; they are called *goitrogenes;*
- Sustained liver detoxification, as the body's metabolic rate increases and the liver is exposed to overloading;
- The digestive process accelerates as well, so proper nutrition is very important; employ an alkaline diet with low saturated fat intake, low refined carbohydrates intake;
- Avoidance of stressors.

Supplements:

- Do not boost the immune system;
- Vitamin C, 2 g/day;
- Multivitamin and multimineral complex, as prescribed;
- Vitamin B complex, 50 mg/day;

- Vitamin E, 200-400 IU/day; do not exceed these dosages, as vitamin E may stimulate the thyroid gland;
- Flax seed oil, 1-2 tablespoons/day.

Others:
- Stress management, as this case will be exposed to high stress levels;
- Bugleweed is a antithyroid herb;
- Mild relaxing teas as chamomile and melissa may be helpful;
- Essential oil of geranium is balancing for the thyroid gland; use in the bath or for a gentle massage.

B. HYPOTHYROIDISM (MYXEDEMA)
**the clinical response to thyroid hormone deficiency*

PRIMARY: probably autoimmune; defect at thyroid gland level; usually associated with a firm goiter; T_3 and T_4 will be low (as the thyroid gland does not function properly) and TSH will be high (because of low levels of thyroid hormones, TSH will be released to stimulate the thyroid gland to produce more hormones); 95% of cases are primary.

SECONDARY: the problem belongs to the hypothalamus-pituitary axis, and not to the thyroid gland; T_3 and T_4 will be low, because there is not enough TSH to stimulate the thyroid gland; TSH will be low as well.

Etiology:
- **Iodine deficiency** (will impede the thyroid hormones synthesis; also, because there is not enough iodine, the thyroid cells, stimulated by TSH to produce more and more hormone, will eventually swell up, causing the apparition of goiter);
- **Use of goitrogens,** which depress the thyroid function by blocking iodine utilization;
- **Autoimmune (Hashimoto):** antibodies bind to the thyroid gland, impeding the thyroid hormone synthesis;
- **Nutrient deficiency**: Vitamins C, B_2, B_3, B_6, A, E and zinc are necessary for thyroid hormone synthesis; also, selenium is part of an enzyme that helps T_4 turn into T_3;
- **Mercury toxicity,** as it seems that mercury may attach to the thyroid hormone receptors on the cells of the body and block the thyroid hormone utilization;
- **Adrenal fatigue:** as the stress hormones have the same amino acid as a base as the thyroid hormone (*tyrosine*), adrenal fatigue may shunt away tyrosine from the thyroid hormone production into stress hormone synthesis;
- **Free radical damage**, as it may interfere with nutrients absorption, metabolism and utilization.

Clinical aspect:
- Fatigue, weakness, difficulty losing weight;
- Depression;
- Constipation, coldness of extremities, thin, dry hair;
- Possible goiter (as in Hashimoto).

Diagnosis: measurement of hormones levels.

Subclinical hypothyroidism: may manifest the signs and symptoms of hypothyroidism without abnormalities of the thyroid hormones; it is an imbalance that stands a good chance for correction. The assessment of subclinical hypothyroidism uses a method called BBT (Basal Body Temperature);

BBT method: set your thermometer on your night table at night time; as soon as you wake up in the morning, reach gently (fast movements would jump start the thyroid), take the thermometer and set it under your armpit; measure the temperature for three weeks, as shorter intervals may present with false positives or negatives; record the results daily; the normal basal temperature should be between 97.6 and 98.2 degrees Fahrenheit. Constant lower temperatures than the ones listed previously would indicate subclinical hypothyroidism.

Medical treatment: involves hormone replacement therapy, with thyroid hormone.

Nutrition and holistic approach: will be approached according to the identifiable cause; keep in mind that these clients will be on thyroid replacement therapy in one form or another and use caution in applying your recommendations; usually, the thyroid hormone therapy will be one of the following: either synthetic thyroid hormone or desiccated natural thyroid (which contains all thyroid hormones, and not just thyroxin):

- Avoid all dietary stressors (food additives, excessive fat, etc), also stress, generally, as the liver will be overloaded (the liver is already slow because of slow metabolism);
- Identify and approach allergies (which set a burden on the body, by stressing the immune system) and digestive system problems (as they will eventually lead into malabsorption);
- Avoid goitrogenic foods or cook them (they seem to lose their goitrogenic properties upon cooking);
- Use of plenty of fruits and vegetables, which are rich in fiber;
- Seafood contains high amounts of iodine; use with caution because of possible heavy metal toxicity;
- Garlic contains iodine, so eat liberally;
- Do not boost the immune system when an autoimmune condition is present.

Supplements:

- Kelp, 2 g/day, as it contains high amounts of iodine;
- L-Tyrosine, 500 mg once or twice daily;
- Vitamin C, 1.5-2 g/day; supports tyrosine's absorption; do not exceed these dosages, as it may interfere with thyroid hormones synthesis;
- Vitamin B complex, 100 mg/day, necessary for the cellular respiration process;
- Multivitamin and multimineral complex containing all nutrients necessary for the thyroid function, as listed in *Etiology.*

Other measures:

- Essential oil of Geranium balances the thyroid gland;
- Using chamomile, lemon balm and passion flower may help with relaxation.

◆ ADRENAL GLAND DISORDERS

Let us take a look at the pathophysiology of the adrenal gland. Whereas the adrenal medulla and the adrenal cortex secrete different hormones, certain conditions will over stimulate the entire gland.

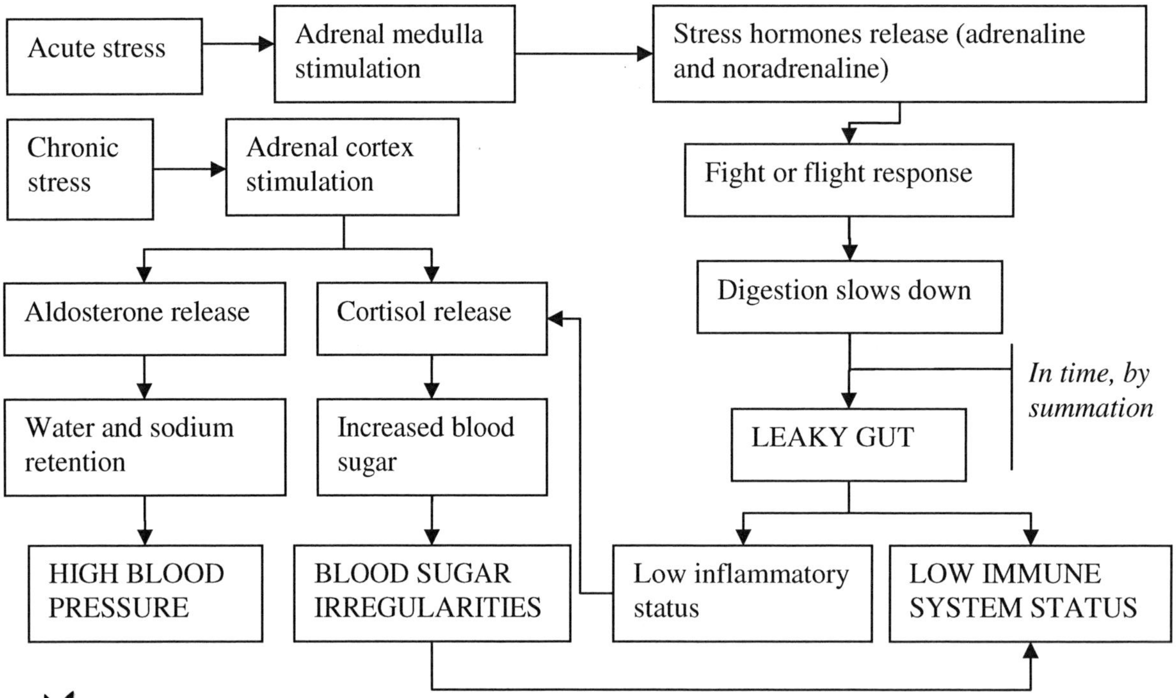

Diagram 13.1- Pathophysiology of the adrenal gland

A. ADRENAL CORTICAL HYPOFUNCTION: ADDISON DISEASE

**adrenal cortex hypo function; chronic failure to secrete aldosterone and cortisol; slow onset and chronic course*

PRIMARY: diseases of the adrenal gland.
SECONDARY: low ACTH stimulation, which implies a pituitary pathology.

Etiology:
- Autoimmune;
- Tuberculosis, tumor, inflammation;
- Rarely, post drug administration.

Clinical aspect: tiredness, weight loss, decreased blood pressure, mineral imbalances, dehydration.

B. ADRENAL CORTICAL HYPERFUNCTION

B1. Cushing's syndrome

**hormonal hyper secretion of cortisol*

Etiology: adrenal or pituitary tumor; administration of excess ACTH.

Clinical aspect: Obesity of trunk, moon face, muscular weakness, menstrual irregularities .

B2. Conn's syndrome

**increased aldosterone secretion, usually caused by an adrenal tumor*

Clinical aspect: High blood pressure (due to water and sodium retention), arrhythmia, cramps.

C. ADRENAL MEDULLA HYPOFUNCTION: ADRENAL FATIGUE

**disturbed adrenal hormonal balance; adrenal fatigue is an imbalance*

Etiology:

- Constant stress levels;
- Excessive use of stimulants and immune system suppressors; lack of sleep;
- Presence of chronic diseases;
- Malnutrition;
- Perturbed liver function (which affects the nutrient metabolism);
- Low inflammatory status (arthritis, leaky gut, etc), which continuously stimulates cortisol release and ultimately suppresses the immune system;
- Chronic medication, especially the ones that suppress the immune system, like corticosteroids.

Clinical aspect:

- Fatigue, weakness, inability to concentrate;
- Low resistance to disease, sleep disturbances (often insomnia);
- Cold extremities, depression, nervousness;
- Salt craving (because of continuous stimulation of the adrenal cortex as well, aldosterone levels will eventually decrease, followed by decreased blood volume with consequent low blood pressure; salt craving will require water intake, which will increase blood volume and ultimately, the blood pressure);
- Orthostatic hypotension: blood pressure is measured firstly when the client lies down, then upon sudden change to an upright position; normally, blood pressure levels should increase slightly, because the sudden move results in adrenaline release; a client with adrenal fatigue will not be able to respond quickly with adrenalin release and his/her blood pressure will stay the same, or, in severe cases, it may even drop slightly.

> **Note** that some of the symptoms are very similar to those encountered in hypothyroidism cases; this happens because tyrosine (necessary for adrenal hormones synthesis) is being shunted away from the thyroid gland, and the result is a tendency to low thyroid function

Nutrition and holistic approach:

- Apply your treatment according to the cause of the condition;

- Identify and approach: allergies, low immune system status, low liver and/or digestive system status;
- Avoid stimulants;
- Increase fruits, vegetables and fish intake;

<u>Supplements:</u>

- Vitamin C, 2-3 g/day;
- Vitamin B complex , 50-100 mg/day;
- Additional vitamin B_5, 100-300 mg/day;
- Zinc, 30-50 mg/day;
- Magnesium, 200-400 mg/day.

**all of the above-mentioned nutrients are very important in adrenal hormones synthesis*

- Use Ginseng to restore vitality; Ginseng is usually considered a male tonic (according to TCM);
- Use Licorice, which supports the health of the adrenal gland; licorice is usually considered a female tonic (TCM);both of the above mentioned herbs belong to a category called *Adaptogenes,* which means that they help the body adapt to stress;
- Use chamomile, lemon balm and passion flower as a mixed tea; it is very helpful in relieving stress and anxiety.
- Essential oils of lavender, chamomile, orange and lemon balm are quite calming.
- Try to encourage a positive attitude.
- Meditation, massages, relaxation techniques, breathing exercises: they are all very helpful.

♦ DISORDERS OF THE CARBOHYDRATES METABOLISM

What happens when you have two nice sugar doughnuts early in the morning?
Let's just assume, for the sake of the argument that you are young and basically healthy. Well, your blood sugar levels (**glucose**) will raise very quickly, as the refined carbohydrate that the doughnut is made of gets digested and absorbed very fast. All of a sudden, your blood sugar is high and you need to do something about it (remember, this is a physiological change).

Insulin, from the pancreas will be called in to help and it will remove the sugar molecules from the blood stream and introduce them into the cells, where they are used for energy purposes (via the Krebs cycle). Insulin can do its work thanks to the receptors for insulin, located on the surface of the body cells. If the receptors are sensitive, the intake of glucose by the cells occurs without any surprises.

Mechanism of blood sugar metabolism

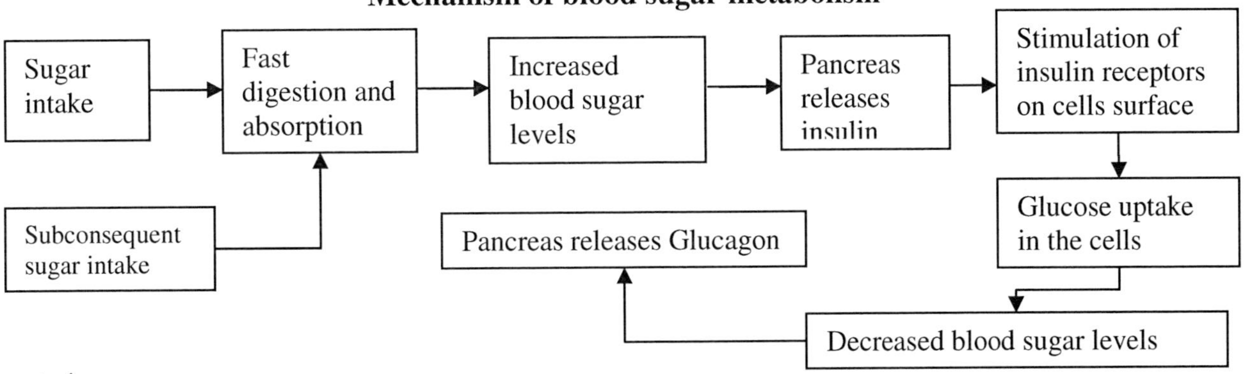

Diagram 13.2-Mechanism of blood sugar metabolism

There is glucose in the cells now, but not too much left in the blood stream. The brain is the organ that seems to suffer most from lack of glucose and it will react by the means of headache, dizziness, a feeling of "space out". This is called "**reactive hypoglycemia**". Well, obviously, you will need some more sugar intake. If the choice is again *-let's say-*a source of refined carbohydrates (a chocolate bar or, why not, two more doughnuts), then the events described above will happen again, in the same sequence.

More to this story, when a person does not eat for hours, another hormone called **Glucagon** will be released from the pancreas, and it will break down some glycogen reserves in order to provide some glucose for the cells, for energy.

Over time, your pancreas will become tired from excessive stimulation and insulin respectively glucagons may be delayed in their release. Another unwanted consequence of this continuous stimulation is decreased sensitivity of the insulin receptor.

Mechanism of blood sugar irregularities

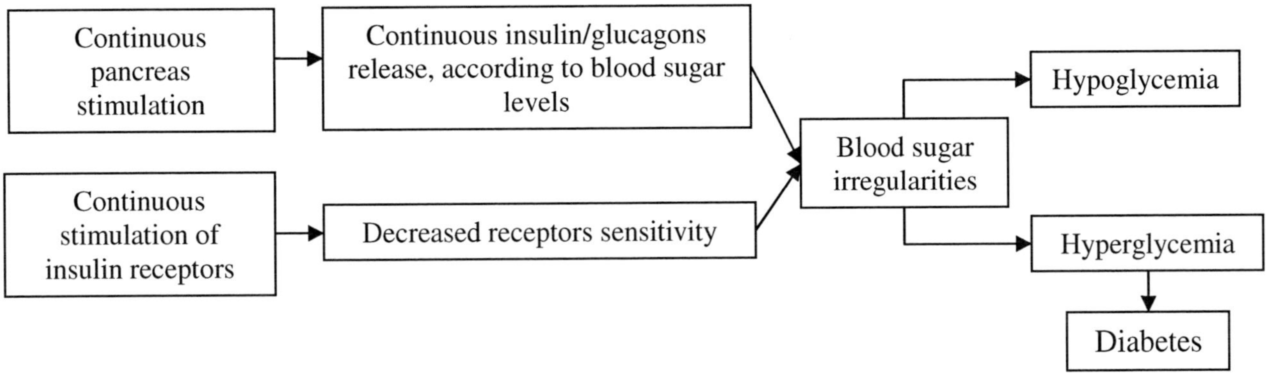

Diagram 13.3-Mechanism of blood sugar irregularities

Ultimately, the sugar will pool out in the blood stream, not being able to be utilized by the cells, and you will become tired, as the base for energy production is missing from the cells. These are the premises for creating blood sugar irregularities and the pathological base for hypoglycemia and later on, diabetes.

A. DIABETES

**increased blood sugar levels resulting from insulin impairment, either in secretion or in action*

There are two types of diabetes:

1. **Type 1**: IDDM (Insulin dependent diabetes mellitus);
2. **Type 2**: NIDDM (Non-insulin dependent diabetes mellitus).

Comparison of type 1 and type 2 diabetes

	Type 1:IDDM	**Type 2: NIDDM**
Etiology	• Idiopathic • Autoimmune (antibodies against the pancreatic cells) • Possible viral etiology	Genetically linked Diet related • Obesity • Increased dietary fat • Chromium deficiency • High intake of refined carbohydrates
Onset	Before age 30	After age 30, but it could be present in children and adolescents, as well
Pathogenesis	Complete destruction of insulin-producing cells in the pancreas	• Abnormal insulin secretion • Increased insulin resistance in target tissues • Hyperglycemia
Risk factors	• Personal history of autoimmune diseases	• Obesity • Family history of diabetes • Prior abnormal glucose tolerance • Hypertension • Hyperlipidemia
Body appearance	Typically normal to wasted	Typically overweight
Clinical aspect	Mostly common; classic triad: • Polyuria (excessive urination) • Polydipsia (excessive thirst • Polyphagia (excessive hunger)	Also, generally: fatigue, nausea
Pharmacological therapy	Insulin required	Combination of ± insulin and /or oral hypoglycemic agents

Table 13.5 –Comparison of type 1 and type 2 diabetes

DIABETES NEEDS CONSTANT MONITORING!!

Diabetes complications

Acute complications	Chronic complications*
1. Hypoglycemia • Too much insulin intake • Missing a meal • Over exercise	1. Atherosclerosis: seems that it is a result of lipoprotein glycosylation; affected LDL can not fit into the cholesterol receptors
2. Diabetic ketoacidosis • Lack of insulin leads into ketoacids accumulation • Can lead to coma	2. Diabetic neuropathy: loss of peripheral nerves function, resulting in tingling, numbness, pain, muscle weakness
3. Non ketogenic hyperosmolar syndrome • Due to dehydration, pneumonia, burns, stroke, recent surgeries	3. Diabetic retinopathy: visual impairment, due to modifications of the retinal blood vessels
	4. Diabetic nephropathy, which affects the blood vessels at kidney levels
	5. Diabetic foot ulcers, due to small peripheral vessels being affected and not being able to supply oxygen to the cells

Table 13.6-Diabetes complications

*Two theories play an important role:

1. **Glycosylation of proteins** (binding of glucose to proteins), which can affect the normal protein structure; also glucose can bind to the protein part of the lipoproteins, interfering with lipid transport and creating enough modifications at vascular level, that the occurrence of atherosclerosis is very possible.
2. **Sorbitol accumulation**: in the normal body, sorbitol (byproduct of glucose metabolism) breaks down into fructose; in a diabetic case, the blood sugar control is impeded and sorbitol accumulates inside the cells (of the lens, peripheral nerves, pancreas and retinal blood vessels), disturbing the normal metabolic processes.

Diagnosis:

1. Clinical aspect;
2. Measurement of fasting blood sugar levels, which will show increased values;

3. GTT (Glucose Tolerance Test); the case is suggested to have increased carbohydrate intake, followed by measurements of the blood sugar levels; if the body can cope by normal means (insulin release), then the test is negative;
4. The Glucose-Insulin tolerance test, which measures the insulin sensitivity; some cases with normal GTT show abnormalities of the insulin sensitivity;
5. Hb A_{1c} (glycosylated hemoglobin); based on the fact that glucose attaches to the hemoglobin chain and a red blood cell lives for about 120 days; therefore, this test measures the blood sugar control for the previous 1-3 months.

Medical treatment applies to the diabetes type, as listed previously in the comparison table.

Nutrition and holistic treatment is supportive in type 1 diabetes and is very helpful in type 2 diabetes; this author has seen marvellous results in the management of diabetes type 2, based on dietary approach and supplementation. **Careful monitoring of blood sugar levels is a must!!**

- Very important to keep the body functioning as well as possible; do identify stressors and approach them; food allergies approach; sustained liver detoxification and support; optimal digestive system's health; obesity approach;
- HCF diet (High complex carbohydrate, high fiber diet); the glucose molecules contained in the complex carbohydrates structures are enclosed within cells and are associated with fiber. Thus their digestion will take a longer time and their absorption will be gradual, allowing for much steadier levels of blood sugar, and, ultimately, for much better blood sugar control;
- Increased fiber intake, as it slows down the carbohydrates absorption and improves glucose uptake by cells and tissues;
- Do have a glycemic index table (standard value of 100 is based on the increased levels of blood sugar after 100 g glucose ingestion) and use mostly foods on the low glycemic index side;
- Fructose (sugar in fruits) has been on the interdiction tables for a long time; whereas we do not suggest a diet abundant in fruits, please keep in mind that small amounts of fruits, spaced out in time, may be actually beneficial, as the fructose is slow to be absorbed (fructose and galactose-*milk sugar*- turn into glucose at liver level) and it seems to enhance insulin sensitivity;
- Low fat diet, as cardiovascular complications are frequent consequences of diabetes;
- Do not use juicing, as the glucose molecules will be absorbed very fast;
- Always eat a carbohydrate with a protein, as it allows for much steadier blood sugar levels; food combining does not work in diabetes cases;
- Onions and garlic seem to regulate blood sugar levels and are protective of the cardiovascular system;
- Alfalfa seems to improve blood sugar control;
- 1/8 teaspoon of ground cinnamon, taken at mealtime may greatly increase insulin sensitivity;
- Watercress and horseradish have beneficial effects on the pancreas;
- Potassium rich foods seem to increase insulin sensitivity;
- Bitter melon and Jerusalem artichoke are helpful in lowering the blood sugar levels;
- Brewer's yeast (nutritional yeast; it is grown on hops) contains chromium and vitamins B.

Supplements:

- Chromium , 200 mcg/ day, as it balances blood sugar levels;

- Vitamin C , 2 g/day, as it reduces sorbitol accumulation and it has an inhibitory effect on protein glycosylation; we need insulin in order to facilitate vitamin C's uptake in the cells;
- Vitamin B complex with at least 50 mg vitamin B_3, which seems to improve blood sugar control and it has been used to lower cholesterol, as well; lately, niacinamide has been recommended for this purpose;
- Vitamin B_6, 50 mg/day, as it may prevent diabetic neuropathy;
- Vitamin E , 400-800 IU/day, as it improves the activity of insulin and protects against long term complications of diabetes;
- Magnesium, 500 mg/day, as it seems to be deficient in diabetic cases and it has shown to prevent diabetic retinopathy;
- Bioflavonoid complex, 1-2 g/day, as they promote insulin secretion and have a protective role against sorbitol accumulation;
- Zinc, 30-50 mg/day, as it is involved closely in the metabolism of insulin;
- EFA's, as omega 3 offers protection against cardiovascular complications and enhances insulin secretion and omega 6 protects against diabetic neuropathy.

Other measures:

- Fenugreek seeds regulate blood sugar levels;
- Bilberry extract and blueberries are useful in the diabetic retinopathy approach;
- Gingko biloba is useful in the approach of diabetic neuropathy;
- Gymnema sylvestra is a herb that seems to enhance blood sugar control;
- Stinging nettle, dandelion and licorice root are helpful in balancing blood sugar levels.

B. HYPOGLYCEMIA

**Low blood sugar levels*

*refer to the blood sugar metabolism described previously

Synopsis of hypoglycemia mechanisms

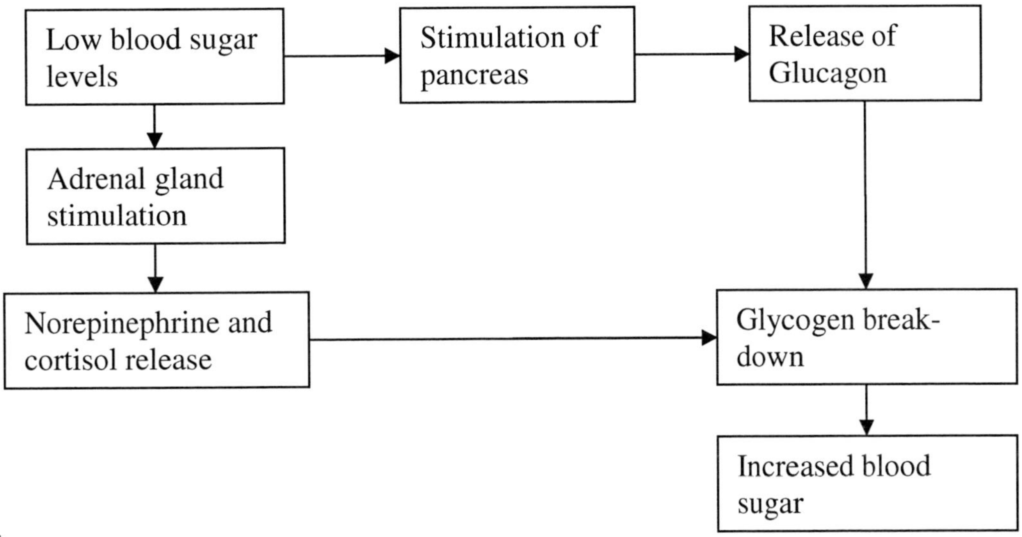

Diagram 13.4 –Synopsis of hypoglycemia mechanisms

As you will observe, blood sugar irregularities will end up over-stimulating not only the pancreas, but the adrenal gland as well. One of the consequences of this mechanism could be adrenal fatigue.

Etiology:

- Abnormal carbohydrate metabolism due to a diet too rich in refined carbohydrates;
- Carbohydrate addiction;
- Medical conditions leading into fasting hypoglycemia, as described below;

Types of hypoglycemia:

1. **Reactive**: hypoglycemia symptoms develop 3-5 hours after a meal;
2. **Fasting:** is a consequence of excessive insulin injections, pancreatic tumors, extensive liver damage, etc.

Clinical aspect:

- Headache, dizziness, irritability;
- Depression, blurred vision, sweating (usually, the sweat feels on the cold side).

Side effects of hypoglycemia:

- Tendency to PMS-C (premenstrual syndrome associated with cravings, increased appetite, headache, fatigue);
- Precipitation of migraines;
- Abnormal blood sugar control may lead to cardiovascular consequences;
- Low blood sugar levels have been linked in some individuals with aggressive behavior.

Diagnosis:

- Clinical aspect;
- Blood sugar levels measurement;
- GGT;
- Hypoglycemic index, which takes into consideration how low blood sugar levels can go and involves mathematic calculations.

Nutrition and holistic approach for Hypoglycemia

- Please, employ all general and dietary measures outlined under *Diabetes;*
- Approach the health of the adrenal gland;
- Eat smaller meals, spaced out every 3-4 hours;
- Use foods on the low side of the glycemic index;
- Avoid alcohol intake, as it interferes with glucose utilization by the body; alcohol abuse may result in hypoglycemia;
- Onion, garlic and brewer's yeast regulate blood sugar levels.

<u>Supplements:</u>

- Chromium, 200 mcg/day, as it regulates blood sugar levels;
- Vitamin B complex, as it supports the nervous system, so easily affected by hypoglycemia;
- Vitamin C and bioflavonoids, as they seem to reduce the incidence of hypoglycemia;
- Spirulina, as prescribed, between meals, as it seems to stabilize blood sugar levels.

Other measures:

- Ginseng helps regulate blood sugar levels and it supports the adrenal gland;
- Chinese lotus seed seem to be able to regulate blood sugar levels.

DISORDERS OF THE LIPID METABOLISM

The risk for cardiovascular disorders increases substantially upon presence of abnormal lipid metabolism and/or transport. We will approach most of the cardiovascular disorders in the *Cardiovascular disorders* chapter. Here we will explain the pathophysiology of the lipid metabolism, as hyperlipidemia is one of the major causes of cardiovascular disorders.

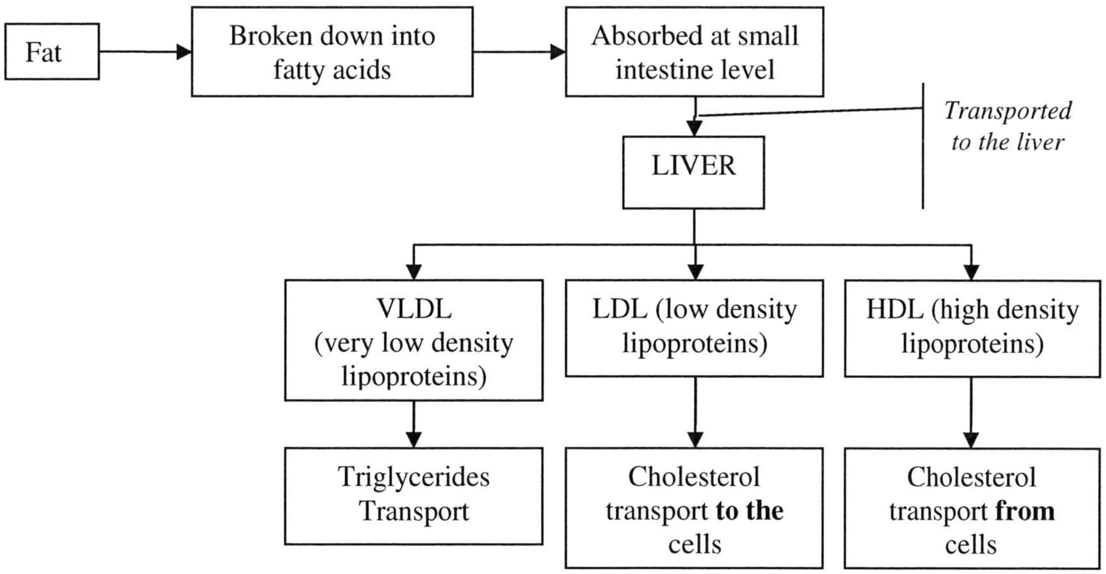

Diagram 13.5 –The physiology of the lipid metabolism

Because VLDL and LDL transport fats to the cells of the body, their elevated levels have been associated with increased risk for cardio-vascular disease (which means that the body takes up lots of fat, either for deposit or for repair; some say that elevated cholesterol levels are an image of how much "patching up" the body needs, as cholesterol is a patching material).

Elevated levels of HDL have been associated with lower risk for cardiovascular disease, because cholesterol molecules and cholesterol metabolites are being returned to the liver, for further degradation and disposal. Of more importance is the cardiac risk factor, as depicted by the LDL to HDL ratio. Certain levels will be suggestive of various degrees of cardiovascular risk.

*Lp (a): lipoprotein (a); is a plasma lipoprotein with a structure similar to the one of LDL, but with an additional damaging factor, an adhesive protein, called **apolipoprotein;** this substance is much more damaging than LDL itself, because it "glues" itself easily to the walls of the arteries and can create damage.

♦ HYPERCHOLESTEROLEMIA

**elevated cholesterol levels in the plasma;* risk factor for cardiovascular diseases like arteriosclerosis, high blood pressure, coronary artery disease

Etiology:

1. Dietary and lifestyle factors;
2. Genetic predisposition (*Familial hypercholesterolemia*: defect in the LDL receptor in the liver, which fails to inform the liver to stop making cholesterol as the LDL is saturated and ready for transport);
3. Liver diseases or liver overload;
4. Low thyroid function, which will decrease the metabolic rate of all processes.

Medical treatment employs various cholesterol lowering drugs; unfortunately, they may be hepatotoxic and carcinogenic

Nutrition and holistic approach for **Hypercholesterolemia** is very helpful:

- Liver detoxification, cleanse and support;
- Identification of body stressors and appropriate management, as they pose a threat of overloading the liver;
- Eat a diet low in saturated fat;
- Increase intake of fish;
- High fiber, low refined carbohydrates diet;
- Obesity approach, if appropriate;
- Get regular exercise;

Food therapy:

- Eat onions and garlic, as they reduce cholesterol levels;
- Oats contain inositol, which contributes to lowering plasma lipid levels;
- Grapefruits and grapefruit juice help fat breakdown;
- Apples, red peppers and turmeric seem to decrease cholesterol levels ;
- Some say that walnuts intake helps decrease fats levels.

Supplements:

- Niacin, as inositol hexaniacinate, 500 mg three times a day (liver function monitoring is very important);
- Vitamin B complex , 50-100 mg/day, as some of the B vitamins (like B_5) are lipotropic factors, improving fat transport and utilization;
- Vitamin C and bioflavonoids, 2-4 g/day, or up to bowel tolerance, as it promotes the fat break down and supports the health of the arterial wall (collagen formation);
- Vitamin E, 400-800 IU/day, as it prevents cholesterol oxidation;
- A good multivitamin and multimineral formula containing a strong lipotropic complex (choline, lecithin, inositol);
- Flax seed oil, one tablespoon/day.

Others:

- Garlic is very beneficial, in diet and in supplement form (minimum of 4000 mcg allicin- *sufur containing active compound-*/day);
- Ginger and cayenne reduce blood cholesterol and inhibit platelet aggregation(which is a risk factor for atherosclerosis);
- Gugulipid-*an extract of the mukul myrrh tree of Indian descent-* seems to improve the liver metabolism of LDL cholesterol;
- Hawthorne prevents arterial build-up.

CHAPTER 14

INTEGUMENTARY SYSTEM

This system is composed of the *skin* and *skin annexes* (glands, hair, nails). It has multiple functions in the body:

- Isolation;
- Protection;
- Vitamin D synthesis;
- Miniexcretory system (fat soluble toxins like DDT and heavy metals are excreted through sweat).

TYPES OF SKIN LESIONS

PRIMARY **Skin changes that did not go through natural evolution or manipulation (no bleeding or scratching, for example)**		**SECONDARY** **Result by modifications of natural evolution (bursting of a vesicle) or by manipulation (scratching)**	
LESION	**ASPECT**	**LESION**	**ASPECT**
MACULE	Flat, small, discolored (freckles)	SCALES	Dry, flaky skin lesion, irregular (seborrheic dermatitis)
PAPULE	Small, elevated lesion larger than 10mm(wart)	CRUSTS (SCABS	Dried serum, pus or blood
PATCH	Large macule, larger than10mm (vitiligo)	EROSION	Loss of epidermis only
PLAQUE	Elevated (raised), firm, rough, larger than 1cm (psoriasis)	ULCERS	Loss of epidermis and part of dermis; concave
NODULE	Palpable, solid lesion, firm (cysts)	EXCORIATION	Linear hollow area caused by scratching
VESICLE	Raised, superficial, fluid filled, less than 1cm(shingles)	SCARS	Areas of fibrous tissue replacing normal skin
BULLA (BLISTER)	Vesicle larger than1cm	LICHENIFICATION	Rough, thickened epidermis (chronic dermatitis)
PUSTULE	Superficial, raised, pus filled (acne)	FISSURE	Linear crack or break from epidermis into dermis
WHEALS (HIVES)	Transient, raised lesions (Urticaria)		

Table 14.1- Types of skin lesions

PRURITUS (ITCHING): a sensation that requires relief by scratching or rubbing

Etiology:

1. Skin diseases: scabies, urticaria, insect bites, atopic dermatitis, malaria;
2. Systemic conditions (pruritus in the absence of skin lesions): billiary obstruction, uremia, lymphoma, leukemia, drug reactions, and allergies.

IMPORTANT NUTRIENTS FOR THE INTEGUMENTARY SYSTEM

Nutrient	Role
Vitamin A	Supports health of skin
Vitamin B complex	Involved in energy production
Vitamin B_2	Helps oxygen usage by the cells of skin and its appendices
Vitamin B_3	Important in skin's circulation
Biotin	Used in the treatment of " cradle cap"/ seborrheic dermatitis
Inositol	Very important for the growth of the hair
Vitamin C	Collagen formation; antioxidant
Vitamin E	May reduce scarring
EFA	Skin's lubrication and moisture
Calcium	Deficiency found in eczema
Copper	Important in collagen formation
Iron	Deficiency results in brittle hair
Potassium	Deficiency results in dry skin
Silicon	Important for formation of skin, nails and hair

Table 14.2- Important nutrients for the integumentary system

Common symptoms/signs: see above described skin lesions; itching; rashes

ASSESMENT OF SKIN DISEASES

MEDICAL ASSESSMENT	NUTRITIONAL ASSESSMENT
1. Clinical aspect: view of the skin integrity, description of lesions, location; all these factors can point the diagnosis in the right direction; every skin disorder has a particular clinical representation; 2. Skin biopsy: diagnosis of cellular structure (benign versus malignant); 3. Gram stain: a method of identifying what type of microorganism is involved in the etiology of a skin lesion, by using	1. Liver toxicity or liver disease: whereas skin diseases are not a result of liver problems, keep in mind that any skin condition, particularly allergic and/or inflammatory conditions, will be exacerbated (flare-ups) when the liver does not function properly and toxic products that accumulate in the blood stream are not eliminated; 2. Dysbiosis (imbalanced bacterial flora in the gut), candidiasis, parasitosis and leaky gut: they are not responsible for the skin diseases themselves, but for the accutizations (flare-ups). Also, rashes that do not have a clear and obvious cause may be due to increased internal toxicity. A malfunctional digestive system will not allow for proper absorption (which results in *malnutrition, low nutrient status, low immune system function,* followed by improper elimination of

MEDICAL ASSESSMENT	NUTRITIONAL ASSESSMENT
a special dye; 4. Culture: skin secretions and scrapes can be cultured on special mediums in order to identify the type of microorganism involved; 5. Wood's lamp examination: will show fungus a bright yellow-green color; 6. Patch and scratch test: used to identify allergies; 7. Skin scraping: application of potassium hydroxide on skin scraping may identify the presence of fungi;	stressors) nor for proper elimination (which will increase the quantity of circulating toxins that will reflect in skin aspect); 3. Hypochlorhydria (low stomach acid) will allow for large protein molecules to create the premises for Leaky Gut; an excessively permeable intestinal wall will allow for substances that should be eliminated to travel to the blood stream and overload the immune system and the liver's detoxification pathways.

Table 14.3- Assessment of the integumentary system

Treatment note:
As a general rule, skin conditions will greatly benefit from internal and external (topical) treatment. Any topical application should be tested on skin previously to application on the lesion: *apply a small amount of the substance that is to be tested on a stamp size area on the front of the arms. Wait for 24 hours. The substance can be used if no discomfort, redness, pain, swelling or itching is present on the tested area.*

SKIN DISORDERS

♦BACTERIAL INFECTIONS OF THE SKIN

A. CELLULITIS

**non suppurative (absence of pus) infection of skin and subcutaneous tissue*

Etiology: infectious, by exacerbated skin bacteria (Staphylococcus, Streptococcus).

Clinical aspect:
- Pain, tenderness, swelling, redness with poorly defined borders;
- Fever, chills.

Medical Treatment:
- General antibiotics;
- Topical (local) antibacterial agents.

Nutrition and holistic approach: (keep in mind that this condition may be a medical emergency; do send your client to be seen by a medical doctor; the nutritional approach will not replace the allopathic treatment, but it will support it)*:*

- Liver and digestive system cleanse and support;
- Immune system support.

Supplements:

- Vitamin C, 3g/day, according to bowel tolerance;
- Antioxidant complex, as prescribed;
- Vitamin A, 5000 IU/day; vitamin E, 400 IU/day;
- Zinc, 30-45 mg/day;
- Flax seed oil, one tablespoon/day;
- Bromelain-based digestive enzymes;
- Probiotics, if on antibiotic protocol.

Others measures:

- Goldenseal compresses (either tincture diluted in water: one part tincture to five parts water, or tea applications).

B. CUTANEOUS ABSCESS

**localized collection of pus causing swelling and redness*

Etiology: bacterial (usually Staphylococcus aureus); usually following local trauma

Clinical aspect:

- Localized swelling in various locations of the body;
- Redness, pain;
- Pus collection;
- Restricted or loss of function, depending on the involved area.

Medical treatment:

- Antibiotics;
- Surgical approach; it is being said that where there is pus, it should be expressed and eliminated; consequently, for localized pus collections, the elective treatment is excision.

Nutrition and holistic approach (supportive, but not replacing the medical treatment)*:*

- Liver, digestive system, blood and immune system cleanse and support, as presented in the previous chapters.

Supplements:

- Vitamin C with bioflavonoids , 2-4 g/day, or up to bowel tolerance;
- Vitamin A , 5000 IU/day;
- Zinc, 50mg/day;

- EFA, Bromelain;
- Coenzyme Q10, to increase tissue oxygenation;
- Germanium (trace element); also increases tissue oxygenation; found in garlic, onions and Shiitake mushrooms;
- Garlic, as a very potent natural antibiotic.

Other measures:

- Local applications of anti-inflammatory herbs: goldenseal, tea tree;
- Applications of honey or hot cabbage leaves may draw out the infection;
- Warm compress with essential oils of chamomile, lemon, lavender or thyme will help draw out the infection, as well

♦ FUNGAL SKIN INFECTIONS

A. DERMATOPHYTES

ATHLETE'S FOOT

Etiology: Fungal, caused by *Tinea pedis.*

Clinical aspect:

- Chronic: non pruritic, scaling, pink keratosis (thickening) of skin on soles and sites of foot;
- Acute: vesicles, redness, scales, maceration; sometimes a flare up of a chronic lesion.

Diagnosis:

- Clinical aspect;
- Direct microscopic examination;
- Wood's lamp examination.

Medical treatment: topical antifungals (**Attention:** protein deficiency will increase the potential for long-term toxicity and immune system depletion).

Nutrition and holistic approach

- Liver and blood cleanse (blood cleanses benefit from the use of *yellow dock*, a herb that has been named" *the purifier of the body");*
- Immune system boosting.

Supplements:

- Probiotic supplementation, at least 10-12 billion germs a day;
- Antifungals: garlic, orally, as recommended.

Other measures:

- Topical antifungal substances: tea tree oil, myrrh or oregano oil applications as described above;
- Goldenseal compresses;
- Live yogurt is antifungal; apply topically to sooth itchy skin;
- Footbath with eucalyptus and/or lavender oil.

B. YEAST INFECTIONS

PYTIRIASIS VERSICOLOUR:

Etiology: yeast infection
Clinical aspect: brown white scaling macules that look lighter in the summer time (do not tan).
Diagnosis

- Clinical aspect;
- Microscopic and Wood lamp examinations.

Medical treatment: antifungals

Nutrition and holistic approach: as listed above, under *Athlete's foot*

C. SKIN CANDIDIASIS

Etiology: yeast infection by Candida Albicans
Clinical aspect: candidal paronychia (painful red swelling of the skin around the nails).
Medical treatment and **Nutritional approach**: as described above, under *Athlete's foot.*

◆PARASITIC SKIN INFECTIONS

SCABIES

Etiology: parasitic, transmissible skin infection, by a mite.

Clinical aspect:

- Superficial burrows, intense itching (especially at night, when the mite is more active), secondary infection (from scratching);
- Incubation lasts for one month followed by the initial sign, itching.

Diagnosis:

- Clinical aspect;
- Microscopic exam of the burrow with KOH will show presence of mites.

Medical treatment:
- Antiparasitic medication (Permethrin);
- Antihistaminic medication (due to the possibility of allergic reactions).

Nutrition and holistic approach:
- Liver and blood cleanse;
- Immune system boosting;
- Antiparasitic herbs: garlic;
- Local applications of tea tree oil or oregano grape oil;
- Topical lavender oil will help soothe the itching.

◆VIRAL SKIN INFECTIONS

A. HERPES SIMPLEX

Etiology: viral, Herpes simplex virus, transmitted by contact with erupted vesicles

Clinical aspect:
- Prodrome (initial phase, before the apparition of the eruption) with pain, itching, tingling;
- Chronic evolution with flare-ups caused by stress, infections, diseases, physical trauma, liver toxicity, improper diet (rich in refined sugar, saturated fat, stimulants, additives);
- *HSV 1 (Herpes Simplex Virus):* grouped, small vesicles on red base in herpetiform arrangement (crops) on skin (**cold sores**, on face and lips), rarely on mucous membranes;
- *HSV 2:* incubation (waiting time) of 2 to 20 days, vesicles present as described above, on mucous membranes (oral mucosa, vulvovaginitis or urethritis in males);
- Risk of transmission during the birth process.

Diagnosis:
- Clinical aspect;
- Tzank smear: microscopic exam that shows a special type of cells, multinucleated, giant epithelial cells;
- Viral culture.

Medical treatment:
- Compresses with antiseptic solutions;
- Acyclovir (antiviral).

Nutrition and holistic approach:
- Liver and blood cleanse;
- Immune system boosting;

- Identify allergic terrain (which may favor the development of flare-ups, as it overloads the immune system);
- Avoid food stimulants and allergens, alcohol, saturated fat, excessive refined carbohydrates;
- Restrict high arginine containing foods (arginine may promote the Herpes simplex virus growth): chocolate, nuts, peanuts;

<u>Supplements:</u>

- Vitamin C, 5-7 g/day (according to bowel tolerance) during flare-ups and at least 3 g/day in between flare-ups, for prevention;
- Bioflavonoid complex, to improve vitamin C absorption;
- Flax seed oil, two tablespoons/day;
- Lysine, 2 g/day, between meals (to decrease arginine levels).

<u>Other measures:</u>

- Antivirals: echinacea and goldenseal for flare-ups, not longer than 5-7 days; licorice and St. John's Wort in between flare-ups;
- Topically: vitamin E and zinc creams; applications of licorice in compresses (it is antiviral and also soothing);
- Bergamot oil, tea tree oil or St. John's Wort tincture applied at the onset may prevent the development of the eruption;
- Lavender oil in applications will help heal an erupted vesicle.

B. HERPES ZOSTER (SHINGLES)

Etiology*:* viral, (varicella zoster virus) which stayed dormant in the peripheral nervous system following childhood infection.
Risk factors*:* low immune system status, elderly population, stress, and concomitant disease process.

Clinical aspect:

- Prodrome: unilateral, "knife-like" pain and paresthesia ("pins and needles sensation") in a dermatome (territory served by a particular nerve);
- General symptoms: headache, mild fever, fatigue;
- Eruption after 3-5 days: small grouped vesicular eruptions; lesions last for days or weeks.

Diagnosis:

- Tzank smear;
- Clinical aspect;
- Viral culture.

Medical treatment:

- Topical applications of normal saline or betadine;
- Analgesic and antiviral medication

Nutrition and holistic approach

- Liver and blood cleanse;

- Eliminate high arginine containing foods;
- Use the same nutritional approach as for Herpes Simplex, with the addition of Quercetin, 500 mg three times a day, which seems to inhibit viral replication.

Other measures:

- Natural antiviral agents as described above;
- Avena sativa (oats) as a tea is very helpful; also, consider oats applications or oats bath;
- Topically: vitamin E and zinc cream, licorice, peppermint oil (if skin is not too sensitive).

C. WARTS

**common, contagious skin tumors caused by a human papillomavirus.*

They may appear single or in groups; can have various locations; the immune system's involvement is not proven.

Clinical aspect:

- Veruca plana: round, yellowish flat top, found mainly on the back of the hands;
- Venereal wart (sexually transmitted): pink, cauliflower like growth located on genitals;
- Plantar wart (verruca): flat wart on the sole of the foot.

Nutritional and holistic approach:

- Liver and digestive system cleanse;
- Identification and approach of allergic terrain;
- Immune system support;
- Vitamin C, 4g/day.

Other measures:

- Topically: aloe vera gel, myrrh, clove oil or tea tree oil;
- Fresh lemon juice or fresh garlic locally may help with softening and boosting of the immune system;
- Squeeze the fresh sap of a dandelion stalk and rub into the wart.

♦DERMATITIS (ECZEMA)

**superficial chronic inflammation of the skin characterized by itching, scaling, redness, papules and vesicles*

A. ALERGIC CONTACT DEMATITIS

Etiology:

- Inflammation of epidermis and dermis caused by Type 4 allergic reaction (cell mediated delayed hypersensitivity);
- Susceptibility to allergen is acquired and usually persists;
- Common allergens: poison ivy, latex, rubber, topical chemicals;

- Low zinc status (common in eczema cases);
- Altered EFA and prostaglandin metabolism.

Clinical aspect:
- Dry, itchy, scaling, red skin;
- Vesicles, papules, excoriations, lichenification (because of scratching);
- Lesions located at contact level, localized.

Diagnosis:
- Clinical aspect;
- Patch testing.

Medical treatment:
- Local and systemic corticosteroids;
- Avoidance of the etiologic factor.

Nutrition and holistic approach:
- Identify allergic terrain (even food sensitivities) as their presence will overload the immune system, which, in turn, will became more sensitive to **all** allergens;
- Liver and blood cleanse;
- Avoid the etiologic factor;
- Immune system boosting.

Supplementation:
- Vitamin A, 5000 IU daily;
- Vitamin E, 400 IU daily;
- Zinc, 50 mg daily during acute phase;
- EFA: flax seed oil two tablespoons daily.

Other measures:
Topically, zinc oxide applications, chamomile (if no ragweed allergy present) or licorice applications (either as creams or as teas); aloe vera gel; massage diluted oils of aspic or cedarwood into the area.

B. IRRITANT CONTACT DERMATITIS

Etiology: denaturation of keratin, modifications of the lipid layer of skin cell membranes, due to continuous exposure to irritants (soaps, dyes, detergents, oils).
Clinical aspect: as described above, localized, limited to contact area, various aspects (from only redness to scaling, vesicles, etc.).

Diagnosis: by clinical aspect and medical history will indicate contact with the irritant;

Medical treatment:
- Avoid exposure;
- Topical corticosteroids.

Nutrition and holistic approach:

- Avoid stressors, generally (coffee, alcohol, stimulants, additives, saturated fat, excess sugar consumption; whereas they are not etiologic factors, they may decrease the body's resistance to disease);
- Liver cleanse and support (a sluggish liver will not be able to detoxify chemical substances appropriately).

Supplementation:

- Multivitamin/multimineral formula;
- EFA's, zinc, vitamin A and vitamin C will increase the health status of the skin.

Other measures: topically, aloe vera gel and/or licorice (both are demulcents, soothing agents)

C. SEBORRHEIC DERMATITIS

**superficial greasy, reddish and yellow scaling papules located in areas rich in oil glands: scalp, face, eyebrows, behind ears, trunk, genital area; non-pruritic.*

Etiology*:* unknown; begins in infancy as "*cradle cap*";

Possible etiologies: genetic predisposition, stress, improper diet, fungal infections
Increased incidence in HIV cases;

Medical treatment:local antifungals and antiinflammatories.

Nutrition and holistic approach:

- General cleansing program: liver, blood, digestive tract;
- Identification and approach of allergies.

Supplementation:

- Vitamin B complex, 50mg/day, with additional Biotin (3 mg twice a day);
- Zinc , 30 mg/day;
- EFA's: flax seed oil, one tablespoon /day.

Other measures: topically, vitamin B6 ointment; local applications of olive oil.

D. ATOPIC DERMATITIS

Etiology:

- Subacute and chronic skin allergic reaction, caused by Type 1 hypersensitivity with Histamine release;
- *Risk factors*: increased family and personal medical history of allergies (may they be skin, asthma, hay fever; children of parents with an allergic terrain stand a high chance to develop allergies themselves, even so they may not develop the same allergy as the parents. For

example, an asthmatic mother may have a baby with eczema. The tendency to allergy counts here, not the type or the location of the allergic reaction);

- Zinc deficiency status;
- Affected EFA and prostaglandin metabolism (which will affect the strength of the cell membrane and also will affect the health of the immune system);
- Dysbiosis, Candidiasis: will create the conditions for Leaky gut and circulating allergens, which will overload the immune system, rendering it more reactive;
- Food sensitivities (by the mechanism described previously under *Dysbiosis, Candidiasis*).

Clinical aspect:

- Itching, vesicles, papules, excoriations, redness, lichenification, dryness (not all signs have to be present in order for eczema to be diagnosed); localized on face, scalp and extensor surfaces in infants and on the face, scalp, neck, flexural surfaces in childhood and adulthood;
- Secondary infection, due to scratching; also, the presence of local lesions decreases the skin resistance to infections (remember, the skin is part of our non specific defense system).

Medical treatment:

- Aveeno bath;
- Topical corticosteroids;
- Oral antihistaminic medication.

Nutritional and holistic approach:

*Dermatologic (skin) conditions treatment requires patience and faithful adherence to a particular diet and lifestyle approach

- Dietary approach: eliminate all major allergens and the foods the eczema client may be sensitive to; limit sugar and saturated fat consumption; eliminate stimulants and additives; increase fish consumption;
- Identify food allergies/sensitivities;
- Liver and blood cleanse;
- Dysbiosis and/or Candidiasis approach, if they are present;
- Immune system support and building; do not use immune system boosters as they may cause the immune system to further reactivity.

Supplementation:

- Vitamin A, 5000 IU daily;
- Vitamin E, 400 IU daily;
- Zinc, 50 mg daily;
- Vitamin C, 3grams/day, according to bowel tolerance; stabilizes mast cells membranes, inhibiting its degranulation and the release of histamine;
- Quercetin, 400 mg three times a day, before meals; stabilizes mast cells membranes;
- EFA's, flax seed oil, 1-2 tablespoons per day (for its anti-inflammatory effect and for the health of the cell membrane).

Other measures:

- Gingko Biloba has bioflavonoid effects; grape seed extract has the same effect; they also stabilize mast cell membranes;
- Green tea, for its antioxidant effect;
- Licorice, internally: has anti-inflammatory and anti allergic effects;
- Topically: licorice, aloe vera, calendula, and chamomile, either in bath or compresses;
- Burdock combines well with dandelion root in the treatment approach of eczema;
- Massage diluted chamomile, lavender and/or melissa oils into the affected area.

DISORDERS OF HAIR FOLLICLES AND SEBACEOUS GLANDS

A. ACNE VULGARIS/COMMON ACNE AND ACNE CONGLOBATA

**superficial, common skin condition of the hair follicles and oil glands characterized by the presence of white heads, black heads, pustules (presence of pus) and cysts.*

Types of acne:

1. **Acne vulgaris**: superficial lesions as mentioned above;
2. **Acne conglobata**: cystic acne (formation of cysts).

Etiology:

- Age: male teenagers seem to develop acne as a result of increased testosterone levels, which stimulates keratin production; keratin surplus may block skin pores. Also, testosterone increases sebum production;
- Infection: by a microorganism, Propionibacterium Acnes;
- Blood sugar irregularities: acne has been sometimes named" skin diabetes", as acne cases seem to have difficulties in metabolizing blood sugar properly.

Pathogenesis:

- Androgens (testosterone) stimulates sebum production, which is converted to free fatty acids by Propionibacterium acnes;
- Free fatty acids, in the presence of the skin bacteria create inflammation which causes hyperkeratinization (increased keratin) of the follicle lining with subsequent plugging.

Risk/exacerbating factors:

- Overuse of "junk food", excess sugar, saturated fat will overload the liver detoxification pathways, which in turn will allow toxins to circulate and increase the likelihood of flare ups ;
- Dysbiosis, Candidiasis: by creating the conditions for Leaky gut, increased circulatory toxins and /or allergens, which overload both the liver and the immune system;
- Drugs, medications (anabolic steroids, corticosteroids, oral contraceptives), chemical exposure act by overloading the liver;
- Face rubbing and touching will increase the possibility of infection and spread of infection.

Clinical aspect:

- Blackheads: dilated skin follicles with central plug of keratin;
- Whiteheads: inflammation by the skin bacteria;
- Pustules: when the inflammatory process results in pus formation;
- Cysts: formed by deep inflammatory collections that did not discharge to the surface of the skin;
- Sometimes scarring present;
- Lesions surrounded by redness;
- Location: face, shoulders, back.

Medical treatment varies according to the severity of the condition

- Local antiseptics;
- Antibiotic creams;
- General antibiotic treatment;
- Accutane (very high doses of vitamin A; average success rate, high liver toxicity potential; these clients have to undergo frequent laboratory investigations concerning the liver function).

Nutrition and holistic approach:

- Dietary advice: wholesome diet, rich in fruits and vegetables; avoid excessive sugar consumption and saturated fat; it seems that a high quality protein diet slows down the conversion of testosterone in its more active form, DHT (dihydrotestosterone);
- Liver and blood cleanse;
- Identify allergic terrain and take appropriate measures;
- Dysbiosis, candidiasis and /or Leaky gut approach, as described in the *Digestive system* chapter.

<u>Supplements:</u>

- Chromium, 200-400 mcg/day;
- Vitamin A, 10.000-20.000 IU/day, under careful monitoring, for short periods of time. High doses (higher than 5.000 IU/day) may result in birth defects if taken by pregnant women. Also, high doses of vitamin A should be avoided by cases with impaired liver function;
- Antioxidants: vitamin E ,400 IU/day and selenium, 200 mcg/day; selenium is very important in glutathione metabolism;
- EFA's: flax seed oil, 1-2 tablespoons/day;
- Zinc, 50 mg/day; firstly, zinc is important in testosterone metabolism; secondly, zinc decreases the testosterone conversion in DHT.

<u>Other measures:</u>

- Topically: tea tree oil and sulfur containing topical preparations;
- Facial steam with elderflower and calendula (marigold) may soothe and draw out the infection;
- Massage comfrey oil into old spots to reduce scarring;
- Exposure to sun helps.

B. ACNE ROSACEA

**chronic inflammation of the hair follicle and oil glands, characterized by facial flushing(due to capillary dilation), papules and pustules*; black heads are not present, as opposed to common acne

Etiology and precipitating factors:

- Excessive sebum production;
- Hypochlorhydria, which results in possible Leaky Gut syndrome and increased levels of circulating toxins; ultimately, the liver and immune system will be overloaded;
- Alcoholism, which increases vasodilatation;
- Exposure to heat and/or sun;
- Stress, which slows down the digestion, resulting in maldigestion, malabsorption and circulating allergens;
- Decreased pancreatic lipase: resulting in not sufficient lipid digestion.

Clinical aspect:

- Facial redness, of nose and cheeks;
- Papules, pustules of various sizes present;
- Mostly affecting middle age women.

Medical treatment:

- Topical and general antibiotics;
- Laser surgery for dilated vessels (telangiectasis).

Nutrition and holistic approach:

- Avoid risk and exacerbating factors, if possible;
- Avoidance of excessive sugar, caffeine, trans fatty acids, additives, saturated fat;
- Increase intake of fruits ,vegetables and fish;
- Identify allergic terrain and take appropriate measures;
- Liver and blood cleanse; dysbiosis, Leaky Gut approach, if necessary;
- Digestive enzymes, as prescribed;
- Hypochlorhydria approach;
- Vitamin B complex seems to be quite beneficial (with 40-50mg/day riboflavin);
- Probiotics, if they are on antibiotics.

♦SCALING PAPULAR DISEASES

PSORIASIS

**common chronic and recurrent disease characterized by clearly bordered red papules covered with silvery scales.*

Etiology and risk factors:

- Genetic defect at skin level, caused by rapid multiplication of skin cells;

- Incomplete protein digestion results in the possibility of apparition of toxic metabolites created by the action of the bowel bacteria on protein macromolecules (large protein molecules);
- Dysbiosis, Candidiasis, which create the conditions for increase toxin release;
- Improper liver function;
- Improper fatty acids metabolism;
- Stress, which impedes the digestion process on one side and slows down the liver's activity on the other side.

Clinical aspect:
- Red (erythematous) papules, covered with silvery scales, well contoured;
- Located on scalp, extensor surfaces, sites of trauma, pressure areas, nails;
- Koebner phenomenon: apparition of new lesions with new trauma;
- Auspitz sign: small bleeding upon removal of scales;
- There could be a pustular (pus forming) form and an arthritic form.

Medical treatment:
- Petroleum (as a lubricant);
- Corticosteroids;
- Vitamin D derivatives (inhibit hyperkeratinization).

Nutrition and holistic approach:
- Liver, blood, digestive system cleanse and support;
- Avoid excess sugar, fat, additives, and chemicals;
- Increase fish and fiber consumption;
- Food sensitivities identification and control (especially gluten).

Supplements:
- Multivitamin/multimineral formula;
- EFA's: flax seed oil or fish oils (compete with arachidonic acid-*which converts into inflammatory leukotrienes*- for the same binding sites);
- Vitamin A, 10.000-20.000 IU/day, in flare-ups; return to 5000IU/day for maintenance;
- Vitamin E, 400 IU/day;
- Selenium, 200mcg/day: supports glutathione metabolism.

Others:
- Sarsaparilla: promotes binding of bacterial gut toxins;
- Milk thistle: improves liver function, decreases cellular proliferation.
- Stress management;
- Ultraviolet exposure;
- Topically: licorice, chamomile (except cases who are allergic to ragweed; it has anti-inflammatory effects), capsaicin, (cayenne pepper extract) and vitamin D unguent;
- Gentle massage into the area bergamot essential oil or roman chamomile;

- Lavender and chamomile oil bath can relieve the tension that exacerbates the condition.

◆DISORDERS OF CORNIFICATION

CALLUSES and CORNS
**thickening of the skin due to repeated rubbing/pressure.*

Etiology:
- Mechanical trauma, pressure or friction;
- Aggravated by an acidic internal environment.

Location: mostly over bony prominences
1. Corns: more focal area of thickening; painful, conical, found over the toe joints and in between toes;
2. Callus: more diffuse thickening, superficial, found at the site of repeated trauma;

Medical treatment: topical acetylsalicylic acid.

Nutrition and holistic approach:
- Avoid etiologic factors;
- Increase the fruits and vegetables intake, to alkalinize the body.
- EFA's: flax seed oil, one tablespoon/day;
- Vitamin C, 2-3 grams/day.

Other measures:
- Topically, vitamin E applications help soften the callus;
- Also, the inner part of the banana peel seem to help with softening of the callus;
- Footbath with mustard seeds;
- Fresh lemon juice or vinegar may help softening the corns; fresh garlic compresses have the same effect.

◆BULLOUS DISEASES

PEMPHIGUS
**autoimmune disease, characterized by vesicles on red or normal skin base*

Etiology:

- Autoimmune, IgG produced against a skin's substance (desmoglein 3) that allows epidermal cells to separate from each other;
- Associated with Myasthenia gravis and malignancy.

Clinical aspect:

- Middle age onset (debut, beginning);
- May present with secondary (following) infection;
- Nikolsky sign: pressure on the skin induces apparition of lesion;
- Asboe-Hanson sign: vesicle/bulla (large vesicle) extends under finger pressure;
- Initially, mouth lesions, then skin lesions;
- First localized, and then generalized.

Medical treatment: immunosuppressive medication

Nutrition and holistic approach: tread carefully when approaching an autoimmune disease. Building the immune system is accepted, but boosting it is not (see under *Immune System*).

- Liver and blood cleanse;
- Immune system slow building;
- Adrenal support;
- Stress management.

◆BENIGN SKIN TUMOURS

SKIN TAGS: small, flesh colored pedunculated (having a neck) lesions, usually multiple. Medical treatment requires freezing or surgical removal. Nutritionally, it seems that they are a sign of abnormal blood sugar metabolism.

SEBORRHEIC KERATOSIS:
Pigmented superficial areas of thickened epidermis, occurring in old age, without a particular etiological involvement. Frequent locations are on trunk or temples. They may look like warts.

◆MALIGNANT TUMOURS

A. BASAL CELL CARCINOMA: common, decreased malignancy

Clinical aspect: shiny, dome-shaped nodules, central ulceration, pearly edge; slow spreading.

B. SQUAMOUS CELL CARCINOMA:

- Occur on sun-exposed areas;
- Fast growing, spreads to the lymph nodes;
- Scaly red papule, ulcerative lesions with raised border.

Diagnosis of the two above mentioned cancers:
- Clinical aspect; the most important detail when it comes to skin cancer, is **change;** a lesion that changes attributes (either color, dimension or shape) should be well checked and diagnosed;
- Biopsy.

Treatment*:* surgical

C. MALIGNANT MELANOMA: malignant tumour of melanocytes
- Sun exposure and family history are risk factors;
- Half of the cases develop from pigmented moles (well defined clusters of melanocytes, presenting as macules, papules or nodules).

Diagnosis:
- Clinical aspect: change in symmetry, colour, dimensions (increase in size) and /or border;
- Biopsy.

Medical treatment: surgical removal

Nutrition approach for skin cancers: *see **Cancer approach** in Neoplasia chapter*

HAIR CONDITIONS

ALOPECIA
**hair loss*

Types of alopecia:

- **ALOPECIA AREATA**: patch of baldness; multiple possible etiologies: family history, immunologic conditions, stress; hypothyroidism;
- **FEMALE PATTERN ALOPECIA**: common, thinning of hair frontal and lateral mostly;
- **MALE PATTERN ALOPECIA**: very common, family history, lateral hair loss followed by vertex (top of head) hair loss;
- **TINEA CAPITIS**: fungal infection; patches of hair broken off close to scalp, itching; diagnosis by KOH skin scraping;
- **TOXIC ALOPECIA**: patchy or complete hair loss caused by febrile illnesses, hypothyroidism, infectious diseases, after pregnancy, drugs, radiation, vitamin A overdose.

Nutrition and holistic approach will depend on the etiologic factor
- General body systems support;
- Address cause, if possible (stress management, antifungals, etc.);
- Protein malnutrition could be a cause for hair loss.

Supplements:

- EFA's: flax seed oil, one tablespoon/day;
- Vitamin B complex, 50mg twice a day;
- Biotin ,50mg three times daily (very important for hair growth);
- Vitamin, C 3grams/day;
- Vitamin, E 400 IU/day.

Other measures:

- Horsetail hair wash;
- Sage tea and nettle tea, both as local applications and internally;
- Massage scalp with oils of fenugreek or ginger;
- Lavender, rosemary, sage and/or cedarwood oils can be used for gentle massage;
- Gingko Biloba increases circulation;
- Avoid foods containing raw eggs (contains avidin, a protein that binds Biotin and inhibits its absorption);
- Massage scalp to increase circulation;
- Use milder hair products and avoid as much as possible chemical treatment of hair.

NAIL CONDITIONS

ONYCHOLYSIS: detachment of the nail from its bed; caused by trauma, psoriasis, thyrotoxicosis (high thyroid function) or fungal infections
PARONYCHIA: infection of the soft tissue around the nail, caused by minor injuries followed by inflammation
THICKENING OF NAILS: suggest either Psoriasis or fungal infection

Nutritional approach:

For fungal or bacterial infections:

- Immune system building;
- Garlic, internally;
- Probiotic supplementation;
- Topically, tea tree oil;
- Supplement with zinc if white spots are present on nails (sign of zinc deficiency)

CHAPTER 15

THE RESPIRATORY SYSTEM

One of my students was saying a few months ago when she heard how the respiratory system works: "Wow, we have one great exhaust system!"
So very true...the respiratory system takes care of the gases exchange and of the acid-base balance, by means of carbon dioxide. Also, this is a system not so difficult to assess: you either breathe well ...or not so well. You have either normally coloured lips, or bluish lips. You either cough...or not.
Without further ado, allow us to present the respiratory system: your exhaust system.

IMPORTANT NUTRIENTS FOR THE RESPIRATORY SYSTEM

Nutrient	Role
Vitamin A and beta carotenes	Protection of respiratory mucus membranes
Vitamin B complex	Vital for energy production
Vitamin C	Antioxidant, collagen formation, stabilizes the membrane of mast cells, thus rendering it useful in allergies and asthma
Quercetin	Stabilizes mast cells; indicated for prevention and treatment of asthma
Coenzyme Q10	Increases cellular oxygenation
Germanium	Increases cellular oxygenation
Magnesium	Relaxation of smooth muscle tonus
Cysteine	It seems that it can help breaking down excessive mucus, thus used in respiratory tract conditions

Table 15.1-Important nutrients for the respiratory system

Common symptoms/signs: runny nose, sneezing, cough (dry cough usually signifies irritation of the mucus membranes, whereas productive, wet cough signifies presence of secretions in the respiratory tree), shortness of breath (dyspnea).

ASSESSMENT

MEDICAL	NUTRITIONAL
1. Clinical aspect: based on the signs and symptoms listed above;	1. Dietary and supplemental analysis: to assess if the building blocks necessary for the development and maintenance of the respiratory tract are provided;
2. Physical examination: will assess presence of secretions in the respiratory tree(by listening with the stethoscope) and possible presence of pneumonia, pleurisy, etc.;	2. Digestive system status, as a malfunctioning digestive system may result in malnutrition and overloaded liver function (see preceding chapters);

MEDICAL	NUTRITIONAL
3. Sputum analysis, to assess presence of infectious agents;	3. Liver status assessment, as a sluggish liver will not be able to process the necessary nutrients for the respiratory system; also, improper detoxification may result in increased levels of circulating toxins affecting the health of the respiratory system (especially asthma cases are susceptible to this aspect);
4. Imaging techniques: X-ray, ultrasound, CT scan, MRI, to assess presence of various conditions of the respiratory tract: pneumonia, cancer, etc.;	4. Immune system status, as an impaired immune system will not be able to properly eliminate allergens, therefore creating the terrain for allergic reactions;
5. Spirometry; assesses the breathing capacity of the lungs;	5. Identification of food allergies, as they pose a threat for the immune system.

Table 15.2-Assessment of the respiratory system

PULMONARY DISORDERS

♦ ALLERGIC CONDITIONS

A. ASTHMA

**condition characterized by spasm of the bronchial tree and shortness of breath*

Classification:

1. EXTRINSIC (ATOPIC/ALLERGIC) ASTHMA: allergic condition, characterized by increased levels of IgE (cross reference *Immune System*).

Etiology:

- Various allergens (dust, pollen, house pets, etc.);
- Food allergies, as they weaken the immune system's status, rendering it more susceptible to various allergens' action;
- Early introduction of solid food in an infant's diet, as the digestive system is not quite developed yet and it may allow the conditions for the development of Leaky Gut, with the obvious consequence of overloading the immune system; (cross reference *Leaky gut/Digestive system*); the same mechanisms apply to the presence of low stomach acid, which results in insufficient protein digestion;
- Maldigestion and malabsorption weaken the immune system by not providing the necessary nutrients for the building of immune system's elements;
- Various vaccinations have been quoted as weakening the immune system's status;
- Stress/low adrenal gland function, as stress may slow down the digestion, with the consequence listed under previous paragraph.

2. INTRINSIC ASTHMA: is associated with cold air exposure, exercise, infections, stress, toxins (risk factors enclosed in the definition).

Pathogenesis:

- In allergic asthma, exposure to allergen will stimulate the increase in IgE, which, in turn will attach to the mast cells (which contain Histamine); their attachment will result in mast cells degranulation (their cell membrane breaks down, releasing the histamine granules that are contained inside the cell); histamine release has the following consequences:

    1. Bronchoconstriction: the smooth muscles of the bronchioles goes into spasm; the calibre of the bronchiole will diminish;
    2. Increased blood vessels permeability, which creates edema;
    3. Increased mucus secretion.

    All these events will render the bronchioles calibre smaller than normal, which impedes on air circulation; the clinical manifestation will be dyspnea (shortness of breath).

- In intrinsic asthma, exposure to cold or increased exercise; a common cold; toxin exposure; all these factors will elicit an inflammatory reaction with very similar consequences as the ones listed above. Some authors quote the involvement of mast cells as well in intrinsic asthma as in extrinsic asthma, whereas some authors quote the fact that the mast cells are not that involved in the pathogenesis of intrinsic asthma, but other cells and chemicals (macrophages, leukocytes; kinins, leukotrienes, inflammatory prostaglandins). Nevertheless, the pathological response of the body is very similar.

Clinical aspect: common to the two asthma forms:

- Beginning of a dry, irritating, tickling cough associated or not with chest tightness;
- Shortness of breath, laboured breathing;
- Wheezing (sound on exhalation) present.

In certain situations, the asthma episode may turn into an **asthma attack**, when all the previously described signs and symptoms are very severe.

> **Note:** an asthma attack **IS A MEDICAL EMERGENCY!!!**
> Seek medical attention immediately!!!

Evolution: usually asthma sufferers are healthy between attacks; in time though, in some cases, progressive obstruction of the airways is maintained, and the person has troubles recovering between arracks. This form of asthma may progress into COPD (*see below*).

Nutrition and holistic approach:

- If possible, avoid the precipitating factors: avoid smoke, dusty rooms, always wipe the dust with a wet cloth, turn mattresses often and clean them, etc.;

- Identify and approach food allergies;
- Identify and approach possible etiologic factors: malabsorption, low stomach acid, etc.;
- When having an asthma episode, some sources say that hot fluids help (heat will relax smooth muscle tonus); increased fluid intake may help coughing out the mucus;

> **Note:** when having a cold or an asthma episode, avoid orange juice, as it is mucus forming; milk and dairy products may have the same effect.

- For prevention, increase intake of alkaline foods and reduce the intake of saturated fat and animal products, as they feed into the inflammatory pathway, giving raise to pro-inflammatory prostaglandins and other inflammatory substances;
- Immune system support; building, not boosting, as this is an allergic condition and boosting may increase the reactivity of an overloaded immune system;
- Increase general intake of onions, garlic and flax seeds; fish oils are anti-inflammatory as well;
- Avoid excessive salt consumption; it seems that it is associated with increased bronchial reactivity.

Supplements:

- Vitamin C with bioflavonoids, 2-4 g/day, or up to bowel tolerance, as it is antioxidant and it stabilizes the cell membranes of mast cells, rendering them less susceptible to degranulation;
- Quercetin, 500 mg three times a day, as it stabilizes mast cells as well;
- Magnesium, 400-600 mg/day, as it relaxes the smooth muscle tonus;
- Vitamin E, 400 IU/day, as an antioxidant;
- Fish oil supplements, as prescribed;
- Vitamin A, 5000 IU/day, as an antioxidant and protective agent of the respiratory mucosa.

Others:

- Echinacea, astragalus, are immune system herbs (cross reference *Immune System*);
- Elecampane, mullein, thyme, chamomile and peppermint are helpful;
- Essential oils of chamomile and/or lavender in a steam inhalation/vaporizer or bath may help.

B. HAYFEVER/ALLERGIC RHINITIS

**allergic reaction to pollens*

Etiology and predisposing factors: ragweed, tree and grass pollen (spring hayfever is usually due to flower and tree pollens and the end summer form is usually due to grass pollen).
Pathogenesis: allergic reaction type I (Immediate hypersensitivity reaction) characterized by mast cell degranulation with effects limited to the nasal passages; increased mucus production; no bronchial constriction.

Clinical aspect:

- Runny nose, sneezing, increased lacrimation (tear secretion);
- Redness and discomfort of mucus membranes;

- Itchy nose and eyes;
- Sometimes, throat itchiness and irritation may be present.

Nutrition and holistic approach: very similar to the one described previously in asthma, as in diet, general measures and supplements.

♦ COPD (CHRONIC OBSTRUCTIVE PULMONARY DISORDER)

**disease characterized by progressive airflow obstruction*

Forms:

1. ASTHMA ,has been described previously

2. CHRONIC BRONCHITIS

**inflammation of mucosal lining of lower respiratory tract*, characterized by excessive mucus production due to chronic irritation of bronchial lining.

Etiology: chronic smoking associated or not with chronic, damp atmosphere.

Clinical aspect: Cough (dry at first, then increased productivity) and sputum for more than three months a year, for a period of at least two years; diagnosis requires the timing of the clinical appearance and will also include performed spirometry.

3. EMPHYSEMA

**permanent dilatation of bronchioles and enlargement of air space*; loss of elasticity; lungs are chronically hyper inflated, not enough oxygen circulating to the body systems and increased concentration of carbon dioxide.

Pathogenesis: chronic irritation of lungs.

Etiology:

- Chronic smoking or environmental chemical exposure;
- Chronic bronchitis;
- Asthma;
- Genetic link.

Clinical aspect:

- Shortness of breath, heavy weight sensation on the chest;
- Dry, rattling cough;
- Enlarged thorax ("barrel chest");
- Cyanosis (blue-ish color of mucus membranes).

Note: emphysema is an irreversible condition

Nutrition and holistic approach:

- Avoid etiologic and predisposing risk factors;
- Avoid inflammatory and mucus forming foods (as described under *Asthma*);
- Increase intake of antioxidant rich foods;
- Immune system building;

Food therapy:

- Carrot and parsley juice is a good cleansing combination;
- Parsnip juice has been known to help those suffering from COPD;
- Chilli peppers may thin the mucus;
- Garlic is a natural antibiotic, consume liberally.

Supplements:

- Vitamin C with bioflavonoids, 2-4 g/day;
- Vitamin E, 400 IU/day ,as it increases tissue elasticity;
- Vitamin A, 10000-15000 IU/day (with the necessary precautions regarding the liver status and a possible pregnancy);
- Green food supplements, as prescribed, for renewal and rejuvenation;
- NAC (N-acetyl cysteine), as prescribed, as it is a mucolytic agent (breaks down mucus).

Others:

- Horsetail, agrimony, mullein, lobelia, chamomile and peppermint are helpful;
- Eucalyptus oil steam or bath inhalation may open up airway passages; other helpful oils are cedarwood or peppermint.

♦ COMMON COLD

**upper respiratory tract infection*

Etiology: infectious, by various viral strains, transmitted either by air or by direct contact (for routes of transmission and stages of disease, cross reference *Infectious diseases*).

Clinical aspect:

- Fever, sometimes chills (which is more suggestive of a flu virus);
- Sneezing, runny nose, headache;
- Coughing, sore throat.

Nutrition and holistic approach:

- First of all, rest; whereas you need to be nourished, there is no need for heavy meals (as a fair amount of energy goes into digestion); have plenty of teas and fluids, diluted fruit

juice (except orange, which is mucus forming) and soups; (according to Chinese medicine, soups are healing foods);
- Lemon juice and honey help with recovery;
- Fresh garlic and onion, liberally;
- Mustard poultice on the chest or a mustard foot bath will help relieve congestion;
- Ginger helps relieve the sore throat.

Supplements:
- Vitamin C with bioflavonoids, up to bowel tolerance, 500-1000 mg every few hours;
- Vitamin A , 5000-10000 IU/day (with necessary precautions);
- Zinc, 30-45 mg/day; zinc lozenges as prescribed soothe the sore throat;
- Garlic supplements, as prescribed.

Others:
- Cinnamon and thyme are quite useful for congestion;
- Take echinacea at the very first sign of cold, this is when you benefit most from it; you can take it for 5-7 days at the most;
- Peppermint, ginseng, mullein are helpful;
- Essential oils of tea tree, lemon and lavender, either in a burner or in the bath help relieve the cough and congestion.

♦ PNEUMONIA
**acute infection of the lung tissue*

A. BACTERIAL PNEUMONIA
**bacterial infection of the lower respiratory passages including alveoli*

Etiology: infectious (by the pneumococcus bacteria).

Risk factors:
- Preceding upper respiratory infection;
- Immunocompromised, with low immune system status;
- Alcoholism, smoking;
- Underlying chronic lung disease (asthma, emphysema);
- Age extremes (very young and very old), as their immune system status usually is not optimal.

Pathogenesis: the alveoli of a certain part of the lung are destroyed by infection and that segment is practically solid and non-workable on a temporary basis.

Clinical aspect*:*
- Onset may be slow, insidious, with fever, fatigue, headache, dry cough initially;
- Cough (of purulent or blood-tinged sputum);
- Fever (chills may be present);

- Dyspnea, rapid breathing;
- Chest pain;
- Pleurisy may or may not be present.

Diagnosis*:* respiratory exam, radiology (consolidation), leukocytosis (increased number of white blood cells), sputum culture, blood cultures.

> **Note**: acute bacterial pneumonia **IS A MEDICAL EMERGENCY!!!**

Nutrition and holistic approach:

- Decrease intake of pro-inflammatory foods;
- Increased intake of fluids (teas, diluted fruit juices, soups) and alkaline forming foods;
- Follow the general suggestions under *Common cold.*

<u>Supplements:</u>

- Vitamin C and bioflavonoids, one gram every few hours up to bowel tolerance;
- Vitamin A, 10000-20000 IU/day (take all necessary precautions);
- Vitamin E, 400 IU/day;
- Zinc , 30-45 mg/day;
- Garlic supplements, as prescribed;
- Probiotics, as prescribed, as your clients will be on antibiotic therapy for pneumonia;
- Vitamin B complex, 50 mg /day, as it is very important for energy production.

<u>Others:</u>

- Ginseng is a good tonic; elderflower will promote sweating and healing; chamomile, mullein, thyme, cinnamon, plantain, marshmallow are helpful;
- Steam or bath inhalation of tea tree and eucalyptus oil help decrease the infection, respectively, congestion.

B. VIRAL PNEUMONIA (INTERSTITIAL PNEUMONIA)

**viral infection of the lower respiratory passages including alveoli*

Etiology: various viruses.

Risk factors*:* malnutrition, immunocompromised, exposure to infected people, elderly.

Clinical aspect*:* headache, fever, myalgia (muscle pain), cough, rash, no consolidation/solidification.

Diagnosis*:* leukocytosis, x-ray shows diffuse lesions (as opposed to the bacterial one, where a part of the lung was not functional), negative sputum culture (no bacteria present).

Nutrition and holistic approach: cross reference *Bacterial pneumonia.*

♦ ACUTE BRONCHITIS

**infection of upper respiratory passages*, usually by viruses, characterized by increased phlegm production;

Risk factors:

- More common in winter;
- May be preceded by viral upper respiratory tract infections;
- Malnutrition, smoking.

Clinical aspect: sneezing, runny nose, fatigue, myalgia, fever, productive cough, pharyngitis, dyspnea.
Diagnosis: clinical exam, no consolidation on radiological examination.

Nutrition and holistic approach: see under *Pneumonia.*

♦ PNEUMOCONIOSES (DUST DISEASE)

**lung disease due to chronic inhalation of dust*

Types:
*1. **Silicosis**:* metal mining, pottery, sandstone or granite cutting, sandblasting; usually asymptomatic in the beginning, then cough, dyspnea, sputum, worsening of symptoms as the disease progresses;
***2. Asbestosis*:** mining, insulation application, asbestos removal; gradual onset of dyspnea on exertion, productive cough, wheezing, pleural infection (pleurisy);
3. Coal: black lung disease; symptoms similar to emphysema.

Nutrition and holistic treatment: these are very chronic diseases in nature and unfortunately, in quite a few cases, debilitating; our approach will be supportive, providing dietary and lifestyle advice according to the individual's status.

♦ LUNG CANCER

*highly lethal cancer of the bronchial epithelium

Risk factors: smoking, exposure to radiation, chemicals, heavy metals (cross reference also the chapter *Neoplasia*).
Clinical aspect: cough (often with blood tinged sputum), local chest pain, local wheezing, weight loss and weakness, pleural effusion (pleurisy).
Evaluation: chest films, biopsy.

Nutrition and holistic approach: see chapter *Neoplasia.*

CHAPTER 16

CARDIOVASCULAR DISORDERS

Think of your blood as the medium that carries everything throughout the body: nutrients, wastes, respiratory gases such as oxygen and carbon dioxide. Any need for thyroid hormone? The blood will carry it away from the thyroid gland to all cells and tissues that need it. Did we eat too much meat? Have we become too acidic? The pH of your blood will dictate certain changes that will allow your body to fall back in balance (homeostasis).

Of course, in order for your blood to circulate, we need a healthy heart, which is, simply, just a very special pump, and hopefully elastic and healthy blood vessels. Unfortunately, this being the study of pathology, we will mostly discuss, in the following, the unhealthy.

IMPORTANT NUTRIENTS FOR THE CARDIOVASCULAR SYSTEM

Nutrient	Role
Vitamin E	Inhibits platelet aggregation
Bioflavonoids	Increase vitamin C absorption and control capillary fragility
Vitamins C and K	Blood thinners
Vitamin B_1	Increases heart muscle tone, therefore useful in congestive heart failure
Folic acid (along with vitamin B_6)	Decreases homocysteine* levels
Vitamin B_6	Improves fat absorption; indicated in atherosclerosis
Antioxidants (vitamins C, E and A) and selenium	Counteract free radical damage, thus being indicated for atherosclerosis prevention
Coenzyme Q10:	Increases tissue oxygenation
Lysine	Lowers high levels of triglycerides, therefore indicated in hyperlipidemia
Taurine	Found in heart muscle; component of bile, which is needed in fat digestion; indicated in CHF, hypertension
Carnitine	Involved in fat metabolism; indicated in atherosclerosis
Choline	Indicated in atherosclerosis (as component of lecithin)
Inositol	Involved in fat and cholesterol metabolism; indicated in atherosclerosis
Calcium/magnesium	Vital in muscle contraction; magnesium relaxes the smooth muscle; indicated in hypertension
Potassium	Regulates the heart rhythm; indicated in prevention of CV diseases
Methionine	Assists in the fat break down
EFA	Reduce blood pressure, lower lipid levels and reduce the risk of blood clots formation

Table 16.1- Important nutrients for the cardiovascular system

Homocysteine: intermediate compound in the conversion of methionine to cysteine; elevated levels have been linked with increased risk for cardiovascular disorders (homocysteine is harmful by directly damaging the artery wall and by interfering with collagen fibers formation).

NUTRITIONAL ABNORMALITIES OF THE CARDIOVASCULAR SYSTEM

Cause	Nutritional abnormality
Decreased vitamin C and bioflavonoids level	Bleeding
Decreased calcium and magnesium levels; vitamin B_1 deficiency	Heart palpitations
Decreased levels of vitamin B_1 and magnesium	Tachycardia
Decreased EFA status; decreased levels of calcium and magnesium	Hypertension
Sodium and water imbalance; adrenal fatigue	Hypotension

Table 16.2-Nutritional abnormalities of the cardiovascular system

Common symptoms/signs:

- Pallor (pale skin and mucus membranes);
- Cyanosis (blue colour of the mucus membranes);
- Shortness of breath;
- Tachycardia (fast heart beat);
- Bradycardia (low heart rhythm);
- Heart palpitations;
- Chest pain;
- Claudication (leg pain due to lack of oxygen supply to the leg muscles).

ASSESSMENT OF THE CARDIO-VASCULAR FUNCTION

MEDICAL ASSESSMENT	NUTRITIONAL ASSESSMENT
1. Clinical aspect: based on symptoms/signs; 2. Physical examination: will include heart assessment from the heart sounds point of view; manually palpated pulse; also measures heart dimensions; 3. Laboratory testing: of cholesterol, LDL, HDL, lipoprotein (a), fibrinogen (coagulation factor), homocysteine; 4. X-ray: to asses heart's dimensions; 5. Phonocardiogram: to assess heart sounds; 6. EKG (Electrocardiogram): registers the electrical activity of the heart;	1. Nutritional status assessment based on the symptoms/signs mentioned above; 2. Liver function, as liver is responsible for lipid metabolism and transport; 3. Digestive system assessment: to identify possible causes of malnutrition/maldigestion, which will greatly impede the cardiovascular health, by nutrient depletion; 4. Free radical status assessment (as in exposure assessment and antioxidant status); 5. Immune system assessment, as a weak immune system will not be able to deal with circulating toxins and harmful substances, rendering the possibility of free radical damage;

MEDICAL ASSESSMENT	NUTRITIONAL ASSESSMENT
7. Echocardiogram: assessment of the strength of heart contraction (ejection fraction); assessment of heart chambers; 8. Stress testing: assessment of cardiac activity upon stress/exercise; 9. Doppler studies (echogram of the blood vessels): to assess the health of the blood vessels and eventual presence of obstacles in the vascular tree; 10. Angiography: introduces a contrast substance intravenously, then an X – ray is being taken that allows the view of all blood vessels already filled with the contrast substance.	6. Stress levels assessment, as stress is a leading risk factor of cardiovascular diseases; 7. Adrenal gland assessment, as the adrenal gland is the one that reacts in stressful situations; 8. Chronic diseases presence; which constitutes a risk factor in themselves, because of the stress level that accompanies them; 9. Presence of diabetes: refer to *Diabetes* and the role of glycosylation in the debut of cardiovascular disease; 10. Assessment of physical activity level, as physical inactivity is a risk factor for cardiovascular disease.

Table 16.3-Assessment of the cardiovascular function

CARDIOVASCULAR CONDITIONS

As we live in this fast paced, chemically enriched society, being continuously exposed to damage from the free radicals, increased stress levels, unclean air, no wonder that our cardio-vascular system is taking quite a beating. Following, we will explain the basic mechanism that underlines the pathology of the cardiovascular system and is responsible for the development of such dramatic situations as stroke or heart attacks and the risk factors that allow for these pathological changes.

ATHEROSCLEROSIS

means "hardening of the arterial wall";* the end result is the development of a **plaque that gradually obstructs the artery, diminishing the blood supply to the area that the artery supplies and consequently, depriving the tissue of oxygen; the blockage does not elicit symptoms up until it occupies almost ninety percent of the arterial lumen (the cavity or channel within a tubular organ, like the artery);

Most affected areas are:

- The heart (resulting in CAD-*Coronary Artery Disease*),
- The brain (resulting in *stroke*)
- The legs (resulting in *Peripheral vascular disease*).

Etiology:

- Dietary and lifestyle factors: high saturated fat, high refined sugar intake, deep fried, too much meat, too many additives, too many chemicals, too many stimulants, too little exercise*, too much environmental toxic exposure**, too much stress (it does look like the description of your next door neighbour's day to day life, doesn't it?);
- Obesity;
- Diabetes, high blood pressure;
- Family history of cardio vascular disease;
- Abnormal lipid metabolism.

**Exercise*: improves the oxygen supply to the heart (by increasing the number of mitochondria in the cells, therefore increasing the oxygen holding capacity), decreases obesity, and reduces high blood pressure;
***Smoking*: the chemicals contained in tobacco can affect the artery wall directly or they can modify the LDL molecule, which in turn damages the artery; consider second hand smoke as a risk factor as well.

Other risk factors:

- **Low antioxidant status:** fats are easily damaged by free radicals; this leads to a process called *lipid peroxidation* (creation of toxic fat derivatives by the action of free radicals); lipid peroxides easily damage the artery walls; antioxidants will block their formation;
- **Low vitamin E status:** vitamin E incorporates easily into the LDL molecule and prevents against free radical damage; doses between 400 IU and 800 IU are most beneficial; use the doses on the higher range if you are exposed to toxins;
- **Low vitamin C status:** vitamin C is the antioxidant in the fluid environment of the body (being water soluble); it can also regenerate oxidized vitamin E; strengthens the collagen structure of the arteries; inhibits platelet aggregation (in the beginning of plaque formation, platelets clump together, as explained below, under *Pathogenesis*);
- **Low levels of EFA:** increased intake of EFA lower levels of LDL molecules, inhibits platelet aggregation and lowers blood pressure;
- **Low levels of magnesium:** magnesium improves energy production within the heart, increases dilation of the coronary arteries (the arteries that supply the heart muscle itself), inhibits platelet aggregation;
- **Increased platelet aggregation:** platelets have a tendency to become "sticky" and adhere to the arterial wall easier, increasing the risk for plaque formation, if the dietary saturated fat intake is increased as opposed to increased intake of EFA; vitamin C and garlic have the effect of decreasing platelet "stickiness";
- **Increased fibrinogen:** fibrinogen is a clotting factor that helps platelets aggregate and increases blood viscosity (renders the blood thicker in consistency); exercise, vitamin B3, EFA and garlic help decrease fibrinogen levels;
- **Increased homocysteine levels:** which poses a risk for cardiovascular disease; vitamin B6 and folic acid are the treatment of choice.

Pathogenesis of atherosclerosis

1. **Weakening of the glucoseaminoglycan (GAG) layer** that protects the endothelial cells; allows for damage by free radicals, immune, physical, mechanical, viral, chemical and drug factors;
2. **Site of injury becomes permeable** to lipoproteins, which increases the affinity for cholesterol; monocytes and trombocytes adhere to damaged area as well;
3. **Smooth muscle cells** from the middle layer of the arterial muscular wall will migrate into the inner layer, where they undergo proliferation, increasing plaque formation;
4. **Fibrous cap forms** (scar tissue, collagen, elastin) over the inner layer of the arterial muscular wall; fat and cholesterol accumulate;
5. The plaque continues to grow until it blocks the artery (totally or partially).

Clinical aspects: atherosclerosis manifests in the development of coronary artery disease, peripheral artery disease (both will be approached below) and stroke (which has been presented within the *Neurology* chapter).

Nutrition and holistic approach: just general measures will be presented here, as the specific approach will be described along with the specific disease:

- Identify and approach the etiologic factors of atherosclerosis: dietary and lifestyle factors, obesity, hyperlipidemia, etc.;
- Employ a diet rich in fiber, low in saturated fat, rich in EFA and antioxidants;
- Use onions, ginger and garlic as much as possible;
- Cold water fish, pecans (which are a good source of protein and of EFA) are highly recommended;
- Barley water may help prevent heart disease by promoting the normal functioning of the heart

Supplements:

- Good multivitamin and mineral formula;
- Bromelain may help diminishing the size of arterial plaques;
- Beta carotene may prevent lipid peroxidation (25000 UI/day);
- Niacin helps reduce high levels of Lipoprotein (a); see recommendations under *Hypercholesterolemia*;
- Vitamin B6, 50-100 mg/day and folic acid, 400 mcg/day are the choice for high levels of homocysteine;
- Chromium, 400 mcg/day;
- Vitamin C , 2-3 g/day, or up to bowel tolerance;
- Vitamin E, 400-800 IU/day;
- Helpful: L-carnitine 1-1.5 g/day.

Other measures:

- Hawthorne berries and lime flowers are both very helpful in supporting the health of the arteries;
- Lavender oil supports the heart's activity; it can be used in a bath or in a vaporizer;

- Alfalfa juice contains magnesium and it has a relaxant effect on the blood vessels;
- Cayenne pepper may lower cholesterol levels; so does gugulipid.

♦SYNDROME X

a condition characterized by blood sugar instability and insulin resistance, associated with hyperlipidemia, high blood pressure and obesity; possible angina associated symptoms

Etiology:

- Increased intake of refined carbohydrates, leading to blood sugar imbalances;
- Genetic predisposition.

Pathogenesis:

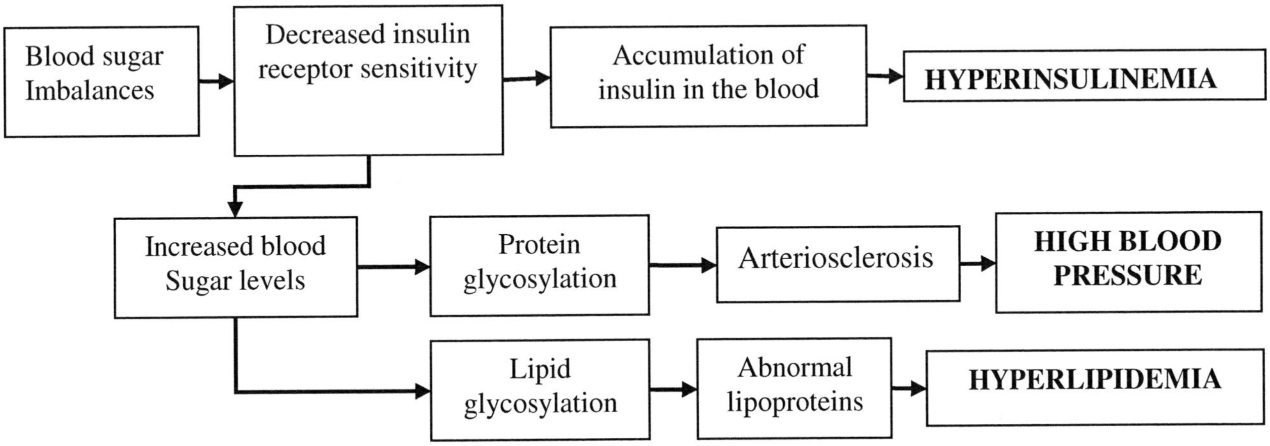

Diagram 16.1-Pathogenesis of Syndrome X

Diagnosis:

- Blood sugar imbalances with a tendency towards hyperglycemia;
- Decreased sensitivity of the insulin receptors;
- Hyperinsulinemia;
- Hyperlipidemia;
- High blood pressure;
- Obesity.

Nutrition and holistic approach:

Please, follow the suggestions under *Atherosclerosis*

♦ CORONARY ARTERY DISEASE (CAD)

blockage of one or more of the branches of the coronary artery* (which supplies the heart muscle- ***myocardium*- with blood);
*it is an image of the discrepancy between the *oxygen supply* (which is low, because of the blockage) and *oxygen demand* (which is high, as the heart muscle needs high amounts of oxygen and nutrients).

Etiology: atherosclerosis; any of the etiologies and/or the risk factors presented under *Atherosclerosis* could constitute a cause for CAD

TYPES OF CAD:

A. ANGINA

**chronic evolution of CAD;*

Clinical aspect:

- **<u>Chest pain</u>** (lack of oxygen of the myocardial tissue manifests as pain).
  <u>Location</u>: precordial (the area above the heart), retrosternal (behind the breast bone), radiating either in between the shoulder blades and/or in the left arm;
  <u>Character</u>: claw-like, gripping, squeezing, pressure;
  <u>Duration</u>: short, up to 10-15 minutes per episode.
  <u>Aggravating factors</u>: (anything that would increase the need for more oxygen): physical effort, stress/emotion, after eating, cold days;
  <u>Relieving factors</u>: rest.
- **Dyspnea** (shortness of breath): sometimes, it may be the only manifestation of lack of myocardial oxygen
- **Other symptoms:** nausea, sweating (pale, clammy skin), anxiety

Diagnosis:

- Clinical aspect;
- Laboratory testing: may identify the etiologic factor: hyperlipidemia, high homocysteine, diabetes, etc.;
- Stress test (see under assessment);
- Electrocardiogram, which will show a characteristic wave pattern.

Medical treatment: will employ various drugs and, if the blockage is significant, cardiac surgery. The procedures used are either *bypass surgery* (which simply "skips" the blocked segment by constructing an alternative pathway from the vein of the leg) or *balloon angioplasty* (which means introducing a small balloon inside the artery and thus expanding its diameter).

Nutrition and holistic approach:

> **ATTENTION:** Angina may precede a heart attack! It is important that a doctor would seriously evaluate this person; our approach will be **supportive only**!

- Therapeutic approach will depend upon the cause;
- Generally, avoid precipitating factors of the angina attack;
- Decrease further degradation of the artery by focusing on a diet low in saturated fat and refined carbohydrates and rich in fiber, nuts, grains, onion, garlic, fish and EFA's;
- Apply an exercise protocol evaluated by a specialist and according to the severity of the angina;
- Avoid stimulants and high salt intake (as it may increase the blood pressure).

Supplements:
Use the supplement list provided under *Atherosclerosis,* to which we may add:

- Good multivitamin and mineral formula;
- Coenzyme Q 10, 150-200 mg/day, as it increases tissue oxygenation;
- L-carnitine, 1.5 g/day, in divided doses, as it transports fatty acids into cells to be used for energy purposes;
- Magnesium, 400-600 mg/day, as magnesium deficiency induces coronary artery spasm.

Other measures:

- Hawthorne supports the health of the heart, by increasing the blood flow to the heart muscle;
- Calming, relaxing herbs are: chamomile, lavender, lemon balm; use as teas or in a bath;
- Lime flowers are heart and circulatory system tonics;
- Chelation therapy is very useful (see appendix H)

> ***Note****: there are many forms of angina; for example,* ***Variant angina*** *(Prinzmetal's angina) is unrelated to exercise and it manifests in the night time;* ***Unstable angina*** *can manifest in any circumstances, even at rest, thus the denomination of "unstable" and it poses a higher risk for an acute event. The type of angina described in details above is* ***Stable angina.***

B. MYOCARDIAL INFARCTION (HEART ATTACK)
[*]***acute*** *coronary insufficiency*; the myocardium area that is being nourished by the blocked artery will die (necrosis) because of sudden interruption of the blood flow.

> **Note: MYOCARDIAL INFARCTION IS A MEDICAL EMERGENCY!!!**

Clinical aspect: very similar to the picture of angina, but the duration changes to over **30 minutes.**

- In a case like this, due to the dying of a part of the heart muscle, markers of necrosis (named cardiac enzymes) can be measured in the blood stream; also, the electrocardiogram shows a characteristic pattern. Unfortunately, once dead, the affected heart muscle will not regain normal function, so the heart will shunt the blood away from the necrosis area through collateral vessels.
- The most important aspect here is **prevention**. Once exposed to an acute cardiac event, you would like to take measures so it does not ever happen again.
- All dietary, nutritional and lifestyle suggestions described above, under *Angina*, are quite useful.

♦ HEART ARRHYTHMIAS

**modifications of the normal cardiac rhythm;*

- Normally, the heart beats regularly, rhythmically, 60-80 beats /minute, as dictated by the sinoatrial node (a special mixture between the muscular and nervous tissue that is capable to automatically set the heart rhythm). From the sinoatrial node, the electrical involuntary impulse that allows the heart to contract will be transmitted to the atrio-ventricular node, then to the wall between the ventricles (Purkinje fibers). Lastly, the electrical impulse will reflect on ventricles walls, bilaterally.
- Exercise and emotional states (sympathetic responses) will physiologically increase the heart rhythm.

Etiology:

- Stimulants intake;
- Conditions that affect the heart structures; therefore, the normal electrical conduction between one node and the other will be impeded (lack of oxygen to the part of the heart muscle where the node is located, for example);
- Infections, hypoxia (low oxygen), acidosis, metabolic imbalances (of calcium, magnesium or potassium);
- Organic conditions: hyper or hypothyroid, anemia;
- Anxiety, panic attacks;
- Allergies.

Types of arrhythmias:

1. **Tachycardia:** abnormally rapid heart rate (more than 100 beats/minute); presents with palpitations, dizziness, dyspnea, chest discomfort, possible fainting;
2. **Bradycardia**: abnormally slow heart rate (less than 60 beats/minute); often asymptomatic; presents with dizziness, fatigue, dyspnea;
3. **Irregular heart rhythm:** presents with palpitations, discomfort, and anxiety.

There are many aspects that apply to medically diagnosed arrhythmias: some of them are linked to disease conditions of the ventricles; some of them are linked with disease conditions of the atrias. These cases will be on antiarrhythmic medication. The diagnosis is based on the presence of the clinical picture and on cardiac and general investigations (laboratory, x-rays, echogram, etc.).

Our approach will be **supportive** only:

- Avoid stimulants, decrease intake of saturated fat and refined carbohydrates;
- Employ a healthy, wholesome diet;
- Identify and approach sources of stress on the body: liver toxicity, allergies, malabsorption, allergic terrain, etc.;
- Good multivitamin and mineral complex.

Following, we will present the classical picture of well-known **palpitations**. When there is no medical reason to explain the presence of palpitations, their etiology usually refers to *stress* or *exertion.* Sometimes lack of sleep or overuse of stimulants (like coffee or alcohol, smoking) may be responsible for their apparition.

They are not accompanied by any of the symptoms presented above (dizziness, fainting, etc.) and do not present with abnormal laboratory results and/or with abnormal investigations results.
Palpitations are perceived like " *a skipped beat"*, which is actually a premature heart beat followed by a compensatory pause.

Nutrition and holistic approach:
*will be applied **ONLY** after making sure that there is no organic condition responsible for the apparition of palpitations:

- Identify all causes of stress on the body and address them appropriately (as listed above);
- Eliminate stimulants and antinutrients (excess saturated fat, refined carbohydrates, chemicals) and apply a healthy diet and lifestyle
- Good multivitamin and mineral formula;
- Antioxidant complex, as prescribed;
- Flax seed oil, one tablespoon/day;
- Lime flowers and valerian are helpful when palpitations are brought in by stress or lack of sleep;
- Essential oils of lavender, mandarin, melissa and rosemary are soothing and calming and can be used either in a bath or in the vaporizer.

♦ VALVULAR HEART DISEASE

**any disease condition that applies to the heart valves*

Almost **all** of heart valves could be affected by disease.

Types of valvular disease:

1. Prolapse

*it applies to the mitral valve and the condition is called **Mitral Valve Prolapse** (MVP); it is the bulging of the mitral valve leaflets into the left atrium during the heart's contraction;

Etiology:

- Multifactorial;
- It can be idiopathic;
- Thyroid diseases (Graves');
- Rheumatic heart disease;
- Anxiety;
- Magnesium deficiency.

Clinical aspect: usually asymptomatic; sometimes fatigue, dizziness, orthostatic hypotension (see adrenal fatigue for explanation)

Diagnosis: by heart auscultation (with the stethoscope);

Nutrition and holistic approach:
- General dietary and lifestyle recommendations;
- Multivitamin and mineral formula;
- Magnesium, 400-600 mg/day.

> **Note:** keep in mind that these cases will have to undergo prophylactic (preventive) antibiotic therapy when they visit their dentist, as this condition may predispose to cardiac infections; do add *probiotics* to their protocol before, during and after the antibiotic treatment.

2. Regurgitation (Insufficiency, Incompetence)

******allows for retrograde flow (backwards) from one heart chamber into the other;* the valve does not close properly and the blood keeps being re-pumped; it can affect any of the heart valves

Etiology:
- Rheumatic fever (acute inflammatory complication of an infection with a germ called Streptococcus);
- Infective endocarditis (inflammation and infection of the endocardium);
- Abnormal wear and tear of the papillary muscles (muscles in the walls of the ventricles);
- Coronary Artery Disease;
- Congenital malformations.

3. Stenosis

**blood flow obstruction because of narrowed valve orifice;* the valve is stiff and the heart has to work more in order to pump the blood; any heart valve can be affected by stenosis

Etiology:
- Endocarditis;
- Rheumatic heart disease;
- Congenital malformations.

The last two types of conditions are serious and more than likely to be on various medication protocols. Our approach would be the general supportive one outlined under *General therapeutic approach to disease.*

♦ CONGESTIVE HEART FAILURE

> **Note: THIS IS A MEDICAL EMERGENCY** presented here for information purposes only

*insufficient function of the heart (decompensation) leading to systemic hypoxia (generalized lack of oxygen)

Etiology:

- Atherosclerosis;
- Valvular disease;
- Cardiac infections (endocarditis, pericarditis);
- Lung diseases;
- Coronary artery disease.

Clinical aspect:

- **LHF (Left Heart Failure):**
  - "The pink puffer", will exhibit symptoms related to lung circulation and oxygen depletion (the left side of the heart receives oxygenated blood from lungs);
  - Dyspnea (shortness of breath);
  - Orthopnea (can not breath properly in a lying down position, has to sit up);
  - Pulmonary rales (upon lung auscultation with a stethoscope, the presence of sounds that show secretions accumulation in the lung tissue);
- **RHF (Right Heart Failure):**
  - " The blue bloater" will exhibit symptoms related to venous overload, as the right side of the heart receives venous blood from the whole body, via vena cava;
  - Dilated jugular (neck) veins;
  - Liver enlargement;
  - Edema;
  - Ascites (fluid accumulation in the abdominal cavity);

♦ BLOOD PRESSURE ABNORMALITIES

Blood pressure is the pressure of the blood against the interior walls of the arteries; it usually refers to the pressure in the large arteries close to the heart

Blood pressure is measured *only in the arteries*. As the blood is strongly pumped from the left ventricle into the aorta, it circulates as a pulse wave, based on the elasticity of the arterial walls, in an *expand-release* motion.

Our blood pressure can increase physiologically when we are under sympathetic stimulation (exercise, emotions, etc). We can have the elasticity of our arteries checked when the blood pressure is measured. During one minute, the heart will contract and relax rhythmically 60 to 80 times. Every time another pulse wave will stretch the arterial wall.

Blood pressure

- **SYSTOLIC:** the higher one; measures the pressure of the blood at the time of the ventricular contraction (how well the arteries stretch);
- **DIASTOLIC:** the lower one; measures the pressure of the blood when the ventricles relax between contractions (how well the arteries bounce back);

Diagram 16.2- Blood pressure presentation

If the arterial wall is not elastic (presence of *atherosclerotic plaques*), the blood will have to push harder against the arterial wall in order to stretch it, which will increase the blood pressure. Also, any factor that creates *vasoconstriction* (narrowing of blood vessels) may lead to higher blood pressure levels. Some examples are: smoking and stress.

What happens when our *blood volume* is increased (too much water circulating via the blood)? If the kidney function is normal, the entire water surplus will be eliminated via urination. If, for one reason or another, the kidneys are not able to eliminate the excess water, then high blood pressure may develop, because of increased blood volume (heart has to pump stronger).

On the other hand, what happens when we forget to drink water? We may become dehydrated, which means that the blood volume will decrease. Your body needs to balance this situation. Therefore, a kidney enzyme called renin will be released. **Renin** release will stimulate the release of a vasoconstrictor substance called **angiotensin**, which, in turn will stimulate the adrenal cortex to release **aldosterone** (this hormone works by retaining sodium ions at kidney levels; but, wherever sodium goes, water will follow, thus sodium absorption will result into water absorption and ultimately, blood volume increase).

A. HIGH BLOOD PRESSURE (HYPERTENSION)

**elevated blood pressure levels;*

Normal values:

Blood pressure

- **Systolic:** between 90-140 mmHg
- **Diastolic:** between 60-90 mmHg

Therefore, a blood pressure of 120/88 mmHg is normal; so is BP: 135/70 mmHg; but a blood pressure of 144/94 mm Hg is higher than normal; also, a blood pressure of 88/56 mm Hg is lower than normal.

Etiology:

1. **Primary Hypertension:**

- Unknown etiology;
- Heredity;
- Increased sodium intake (which affects the blood volume, increasing it);
- Obesity;
- Stress;
- Nicotine consumption;
- Increased peripheral vascular resistance by either an atherosclerotic plaque or increased blood volume and/or consistency (viscosity).

2. **Secondary Hypertension**

- Renal diseases (because of impaired water and/or sodium reabsorption);
- Adrenal gland disorders (because of increased aldosterone release; its effect is an increase in blood volume, with subsequent high blood pressure).

HIGH BLOOD PRESSURE CLASSIFICATION:

CLASSIFICATION	SYSTOLIC VALUES	DIASTOLIC VALUES
Borderline	120-160	90-94
Mild	140-160	95-104
Moderate	140-180	105-114
Severe	160+	115+

Table 16.4 –High blood pressure classification

Clinical aspect:

- Relates to the cause;
- Mild hypertension does not exhibit any symptoms;
- High levels of blood pressure may result in dizziness, headache, visual impairment;
- Unfortunately, in some cases the high blood pressure is identified after the development of complications: heart attack, stroke, kidney damage, ocular damage

In order to diagnose Hypertension, **three measurements** are to be made and at least two of them should show higher levels. Even so, if the blood pressure levels are not too high, the initial recommendations will be dietary and lifestyle changes. Unfortunatelly, if a case is suggested to take blood pressure medication, there are some risks for side effects

Nutrition and holistic approach:

- Avoid intake of saturated fat, salt, refined carbohydrates and food additives;
- Avoid alcohol, smoking, coffee;
- Exercise!

- Increase intake of fiber rich fruits and vegetables (high in potassium, which is beneficial for the blood pressure levels) and fish;
- Avoid aspartame use (it may increase blood pressure by creating lesions in the arterial wall);
- Approach obesity, liver cleanse and digestive system status;
- As high blood pressure has been linked to calcium and/or magnesium deficiency, increase intake of calcium and magnesium rich foods, like green leafy vegetables and nuts and seeds.

Food therapy:

- Asparagus may help reduce blood pressure levels, as it acts as a diuretic;
- Avocados, tomatoes, cabbage, bananas, oranges and raisins are high in potassium and low in sodium;
- Eat garlic liberally as it reduces the cholesterol levels;
- Celery intake has been linked with lowering blood pressure levels;

Supplements:

- Good quality multivitamin and mineral formula;
- Flax seed oil, one tablespoon/day or Evening Primrose Oil ,500 mg three times/day;
- Calcium and magnesium, 800-1200 mg/day to 400-600 mg/day, as they relax the smooth muscle of blood vessels;
- Coenzyme Q 10, 100 mg twice a day, as it increases tissue oxygenation;
- Vitamin C, 1-2 g/day, with bioflavonoids;
- Vitamin E, 400 IU/day.

Other measures:

- Hawthorne reduces blood pressure levels and improves heart functionality;
- Mistletoe is indicated in cases with decreased arterial elasticity;
- Horseradish is a diuretic; so is parsley;
- Oats are calming and reduce cholesterol levels;
- Apples can also reduce cholesterol levels;
- Valerian, chamomile and rosemary are soothing and relaxing;
- Essential oils of lavender and marjoram may help;
- Avoid using licorice in its usual form, as it increases water retention; use instead DGL (deglycyrrhizinated licorice), which does not have this effect ,

B. HYPOTENSION (LOW BLOOD PRESSURE)

[*]*decreased blood pressure levels*

Etiology:

- Normal, in athletes;
- Idiopathic;
- Physical inactivity, dehydration (by lowering blood volume);
- Diseases processes: anemia, excessive vomiting, burns, hemorrhage;
- Adrenal fatigue: insufficient production of stress hormones;
- Malnutrition.

Clinical aspect:

- Fatigue, dizziness, " space-out " feeling (not enough blood reaching the brain vessels);
- Fatigue, coldness of extremities;
- Tachycardia (as the heart is trying to pump more blood).

Orthostatic hypotension: abrupt fall in blood pressure levels upon brusque (sudden) standing up.

Nutrition and holistic approach:

- Will rely upon etiologic factors identification;
- Adrenal fatigue protocol, if applicable;
- Eat small, nutritious meals 4-5 times/day;
- Vitamin B5 deficiency increases salt excretion, which may lower blood volume; consume wheat germ and nuts, to supply vitamin B5;
- Licorice is very helpful in cases with adrenal fatigue, by increasing water retention, consequently, increasing blood volume.

Supplements:

- Good multivitamin and mineral formula;
- Vitamin C with bioflavonoids 2-3 g/day;
- Flax seed oil, one tablespoon/day;
- Vitamin B complex, 50-100 mg/day.

Other measures:

- Ginger, ginseng and rosemary have beneficial effects;
- Essential oils of black pepper, lemon, sage or rosemary are helpful in massages or baths.

♦ ANEURYSMS

**dilation of one segment of an artery due to a defect/weakness in the muscular arterial wall*; they can have different shapes and sizes

- Occur at major branching point of arteries and in subarachnoid space (between the meninges of the brain);
- Unfortunately, they run the risk of rupture, which leads into hemorrhages; depending on the size and /or location of the aneurysm the consequences could be dramatic.

Risk factors: collagen disorders, family history, hypertension, smoking, atherosclerosis, physical stress at times of onset.

THIS IS A MEDICAL EMERGENCY!!!

Clinical aspect:
- Depends on location:
  - It may present with severe headache, if the location is intracranial, or
  - Abdominal pain and pulsation feeling, if the aneurysm affects the abdominal aorta.

♦ PERIPHERAL VASCULAR DISORDERS
group of disorders affecting the blood vessels of the extremities

A. PERIPHERAL ARTERIAL OCCLUSION
occlusion of the arterial blood supply to the extremities

Etiology:
- Atherosclerosis;
- Thrombosis (thrombus is a stationary blood clot; it is attached to the inner wall of a blood vessel, creating obstruction);
- Embolism (an embolus is a "traveling" obstacle; it can dislodge from a blood clot, it can also be an air bubble or a piece of fat; as it travels via the blood, it can lodge itself in an artery, blocking it and cutting the blood supply to the area served by that particular blood vessel).

Clinical aspect: depends on the obstacle's location, the extent of obstruction and whether there are collateral vessels that can supply the affected tissue.

Acute occlusion: it happens fast; sudden onset of severe pain (the tissue that lacks oxygen supply will react through pain – remember the chest pain in myocardial infarction?), coldness, numbness and pallor; the pulses below the level of obstruction are difficult to be felt.

Chronic occlusion: is more frequent, it develops in an insidious (slowly progressive) way and it manifests as *intermittent claudication* (pain, ache or cramp in the lower leg upon walking or physical effort, which is when the leg muscles will need more oxygen; if the arterial supply is diminished, then the muscle will react by pain); relieved by rest.

Medical treatment for chronic obstruction (**the acute one is a medical emergency**) involves mild controlled exercises, prevention (stop smoking), and vasodilators.

Nutrition and holistic approach (applied to the chronic obstruction)
- Identify and approach therapeutically the etiological factors involved (mostly applicable to atherosclerosis): preexistent hypertension, hyperlipidemia;
- Avoid all factors that could lead to vasoconstriction (smoking, for example);
- Avoid all saturated fats, trans fatty acids, excessive refined carbohydrates;
- Focus on a diet rich in fruits and vegetables, fish, nuts, grains and legumes.

<u>Supplements and other measures</u>: please refer to *Atherosclerosis* treatment.

B. RAYNAUD'S DISEASE AND PHENOMENON

**spasm of arterioles (smaller arteries) in the fingers and, rarely, in the toes;* more common in women and it usually starts in early adulthood.

Etiology:

RAYNAUD'S DISEASE: idiopathic; cold exposure is the main trigger; emotion, embarrassment (when the sympathetic nervous system is activated and results in vasoconstriction) could prove to be aggravating factors;

RAYNAUD'S PHENOMENON: secondary to connective tissue disorders (scleroderma), obstructive arterial disease, trauma, drug intoxication.

Clinical aspect:

- Sudden onset with arteriolar spasm,
    - resulting in *pallor* (white color; the fingers only, not the whole hand);
    - then, if the spasm persists, in *cyanosis* (blue coloration, due to lack of oxygen);
    - followed by *redness* (because of reflex vasodilation, as blood vessels can not stay contracted for too long a time; this is a homeostatic mechanism);

  Sometimes the clinical aspect is only biphasic (cyanosis and redness, no pallor);

- While the attack persists, the person will experience pain, numbness and tingling in the affected area, followed by burning, when the circulation is reinstated;
- The attacks last for only minutes, usually; normally, there are no pathologic modifications of the tissues, but if the disease persists for a long period of time and the attacks occur often, complications may develop (ulcers, gangrene(*decay and death of tissue due to lack of blood supply)*.

Nutrition and holistic approach for Raynaud's disease:

- Identify food allergies and approach them, as it is suggested that they may aggravate the disease (the mechanism is not clear yet; possibly the general overload that allergies put on the immune system and ultimately, on the liver);
- Liver cleanse and support, as all nutritional factors that are needed for support are metabolized by the liver, and also all toxic factors that may affect the health of the arteries and ultimately, aggravate the disease, have to be detoxified by the liver;
- Avoid all saturated fat, trans fatty acids, refined carbohydrates, smoking, emotional upset, exposure to cold, as they all may contribute to smaller vessel caliber, which may predispose to the disease;
- Increase intake of fish, fish oils and liver friendly foods; also germanium containing foods (onions, garlic, shiitake mushrooms) as it increases tissue oxygenation.

<u>Supplements</u>

- Good multivitamin and mineral formula;

- Vitamin E, 400 IU/day, as it helps relieve the numbness;
- Evening primrose oil, 500 mg three times/day, as it improves circulation and it has healing effect on the blood vessels;
- Coenzyme Q10, 50 mg/day, as it increases tissue oxygenation;
- Vitamin B complex ,50 mg/day with additional B3, 50 mg/day;
- Magnesium, 400-600 mg/day, as it relaxes the smooth muscles of the blood vessels;
- Vitamin C with bioflavonoids, 1-2 g/day, as it is supportive for the health of the blood vessels, by increasing their strength.

<u>Other measures:</u>

- Massage hands and feet with mustard and sesame seed oil, to improve circulation;
- Fresh ginger and cayenne improve circulation;
- Gingko biloba increases circulation to extremities;
- Essential oils of black pepper, lemon or rosemary can be massaged into the area.

Raynaud's phenomenon approach is based on the etiology. All the above-mentioned measures can be supportive.

C. VARICOSE VEINS

******swollen, weakened veins;* commonly found on legs; other locations: rectum (where they present as hemorrhoids), and scrotum (varicocele).

Pathogenesis:

Normally, the venous flow, as it returns to the right heart, is being controlled by the *muscle pump* (as you move, the skeletal muscles contract and press against the veins, forcing open the venous valves located from place to place along the vein's trajectory and the blood is pushed forward). When the venous valves become weak, the blood has a tendency to pool locally and accumulates, creating reverse flow (thus, the bulging veins) instead of returning to the heart. The excess fluid pressure will allow water to migrate into the tissues, creating edema. In time, impaired venous circulation will create local modifications like skin thinness, easy bruising and possibly, later on, leg ulcers.

Etiology:

- Occupational (because of gravitation): individuals who spend a long time standing or perform heavy lifting;
- Obesity (which creates an overload on the circulatory system and decreaseds venous elasticity);
- Age: due to loss of muscle mass and increased vascular fragility (vessels have a tendency to rupture);
- Pregnancy (increased abdominal pressure), also ascites (water accumulation in the abdominal cavity);
- Venous valves damage by inflammation;
- Nutritional imbalances: lack of vitamin C (collagen formation) and bioflavonoids (improve vascular fragility).

Clinical aspect:

- Sore, tender, enlarged veins;

- Leg swelling and aching; feeling of heaviness and tiredness present;
- Bruising and discoloration;
- Later, in severe cases, leg ulcers;
- Complications: deep vein thrombosis, as the pooling of blood creates the conditions of clots formation.

Medical treatment involves compression support, sclerosing therapy (injections of substances that may fibrose the vein wall) and surgery.

Nutrition and holistic approach:

- Avoid prolonged standing up, or, if you have to, walk and move as much as possible;
- Identify and approach obesity, constipation (which strains the rectal veins), liver overload (as circulating toxins may affect the vascular wall; also, proper liver function ensures proper blood flow);
- To avoid vascular problems, generally, avoid saturated fat and trans fatty acids;
- Increased fiber intake;
- Regular exercise improves the function of the muscle pump;
- Increase intake of garlic and onion, as they help break down fibrin (a substance involved in clots and scars formation);
- Either pineapple or bromelain help break down fibrin, as well;
- Raw beetroot has tonic and strengthening effects;
- Mustard poultices applied locally may improve circulation.

Supplements:

- Vitamin E, 400 IU/day, to improve circulation;
- Vitamin C, 2-3 g/day;
- Bioflavonoids complex (especially rutin and hesperidin), as prescribed, as they improve the venous wall tone;
- Vitamin B complex, 50 mg/day, as it is needed to strengthen the blood vessels (vitamins B are strongly involved in the energy producing pathways).

Other measures:

- Dandelion root supports liver's health;
- Gingko improves circulation;
- Horse chestnut, witch hazel, yarrow: repair and strengthen the veins walls;
- Calendula applications (as a compress, or in a bath);
- Rosemary oil in a light carrier oil, as a massage;
- Bilberry helps strengthen capillaries;
- Keep your legs in an elevated position, to improve the circulation.

D. BRUISING

**also called ecchymosis; broken blood vessels release the blood into the interstitial tissue;* the array of colours that the bruise goes through is due to haemoglobin modification and absorption.

Etiology: trauma, in most of the cases; sometimes is due to diseases as leukemia or hemophilia.

Clinical aspect:

- Presence of the bruise;
- Pain on pressure or upon moving the involved area;
- Possible local swelling.

Nutrition and holistic approach: **(will apply to trauma only)**

- Cabbage leaves, cut and in small pieces and warmed up can be applied as a compress; roasted onions compress has a healing effect as well;
- Vinegar compress (heat it lightly) will help with the bruising;
- Witch hazel or yarrow compresses are healing;
- Arnica is very helpful;
- Increased intake of vitamin C and bioflavonoids.

E. THROMBOSIS

**the formation or presence of a thrombus (blood clot);* when it affects the superficial veins it is called Thrombophlebitis; when it affects the deep veins it is called Deep Vein Thrombosis
*Phlebitis means venous inflammation

Etiology:

- Varicose veins; inflammation;
- Trauma;
- Prolonged bed rest or immobilization;
- BCP (Birth Control Pills) use.

Clinical aspect:

- Acute superficial thrombophlebitis arrives with local inflammatory signs: a long, red, swollen cord can be seen and palpated; local pain; it will require antibiotic and anti-inflammatory treatment;
- Chronic DVT (Deep Vein Thrombosis) exhibits local heaviness, tenderness, pain, swelling, skin discoloration and presence of superficial veins; a doctor can diagnose it by eliciting pain in the calf.

Nutrition and holistic approach (applied to chronic conditions)

- Liver cleanse (see above, under *Varicose veins*);
- Increase intake of EFA's, fiber, vitamins E and C rich foods;

- Supplement with a good formula of multivitamins and minerals, evening primrose oil, 500 mg three times/day; vitamin C and bioflavonoids ,1-2 g/day and vitamin E ,400 IU/day;
- White willow is anti-inflammatory;
- Witch hazel, yarrow and horse chestnut relieve blood stagnation and help strengthen the venous walls;
- Garlic is a natural blood thinner.

CHAPTER 17

HEMATOLOGY* AND ONCOLOGY

At any given moment, your Red Blood Cells (RBC) travel throughout your entire body, transporting oxygen (which we cannot do without); your White Blood Cells (WBC) are fighting infections and allergies, and your thrombocytes (platelets) are involved in coagulation. Sometimes, though, things go amiss, and normal cells become abnormal and multiply, creating life-threatening situations. Let us begin by reviewing the blood constituents and what is involved in coagulation.

**Hematology is the study of blood, blood forming elements, their physiology and pathology*

BLOOD CONSTITUENTS

PLASMA (the fluid compartment of the blood)	CELLULAR COMPARTMENT		
➢ Water ➢ Electrolytes ➢ Proteins ➢ Nutrients ➢ Wastes ➢ Gases ➢ Hormones	RBC	➢ Contain Hemoglobin (iron binding protein) ➢ Oxygen transport	
	WBC	Neutrophils	Involved in acute infections
		Basophils*	Contain Histamine
		Eosinophils	Involved in allergies and parasitic infections
		Lymphocytes	Cells of the Immune System
		Monocytes**	Involved in chronic infections and "later phase" fight against pathogens
	Platelets (Thrombocytes)	➢ Blood clotting	

Table 17.1- Blood constituents

* In tissues, become *mast cells*, involved in allergies;
** In tissues, become *macrophages.*

BLOOD CELLS FORMATION (HEMATOPOIESIS)

Everything starts with a mother cell, or stem cell, called **Hemocytoblast**, which we find in the red bone marrow (located in children in the long parts of long bones, and in adults in our breast bone and other limited locations).

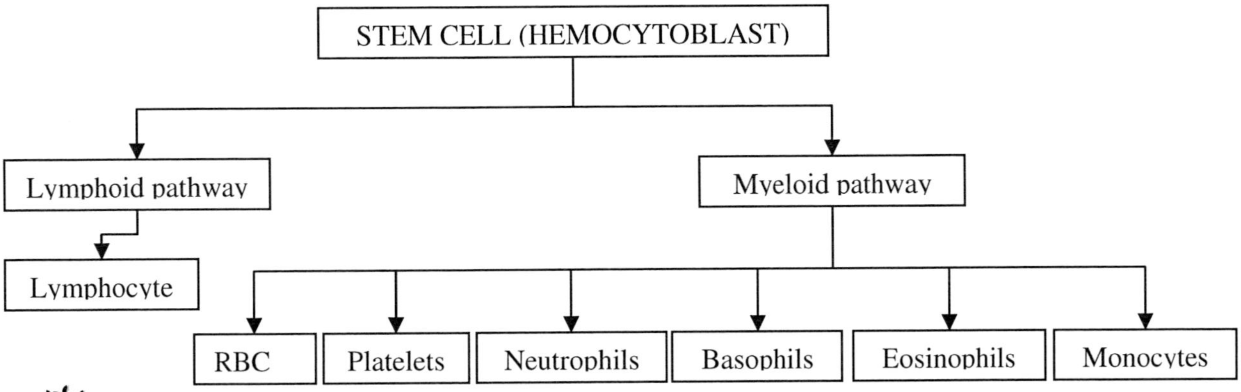

Diagram 17.1- Blood cells formation

Erythropoietin: glycoprotein secreted by the kidney that stimulates the stem cells of the bone marrow to produce more RBC; its secretion is dependent upon oxygen levels in the blood.
If we look at the above diagram we can see that practically all blood cells sprout from one cell. This is why, if the cause of a blood condition is not clear (for example, anemia) your doctor may decide that a *bone marrow biopsy* is necessary to see if the problem resides in the periphery (blood stream) or in the bone marrow.

HEMOSTASIS (STOPPAGE OF BLOOD)

- will occur when the blood vessel is traumatized and repair mechanisms are activated

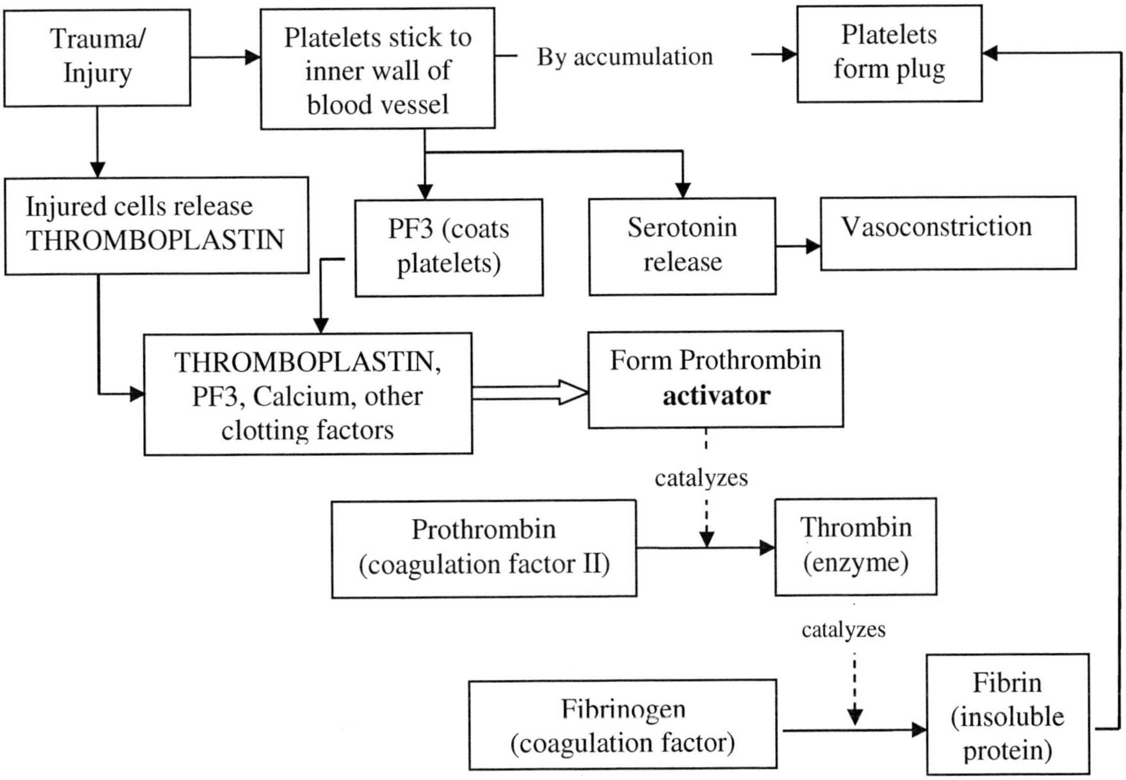

Diagram 17.2-Hemostasis

There are 13 coagulation factors. Any disorder or lack of any of them can lead to coagulation problems (like in Hemophilia, hereditary disease which lacks factors VIII, IX or XI).

IMPORTANT NUTRIENTS FOR THE BLOOD

Nutrient	Role
Vitamin B_{12} and folic acid	New blood cells formation
Vitamins B_1 and B_2	Assist in blood cells formation
Bioflavonoids	Control capillary fragility
Vitamin K	Production of prothrombin
Vitamin C	Blood thinner
Vitamin B_6	Promotes RBC formation
Calcium	Important in blood clotting
Iron	Oxygen transport
Copper	Important in RBC formation
Germanium	Carries Oxygen into the cells
Taurine	Important in WBC formation

Table 17.2 –Important nutrients for the blood

Common signs/symptoms: pallor (white coloration of skin and mucous membranes), cyanosis (blue coloration of mucous membranes), weakness, fatigue, dizziness, tachycardia, tachypnea (increased respiratory rhythm);

ASSESSMENT

Medical assessment	Nutritional assessment
1. Clinical aspect: based on signs / symptoms described above. 2. Physical examination: of skin, mucous membranes, lymph nodes; possible bleeding sites 3. Laboratory analysis: shows the whole cellular spectrum of blood, the number of cells, the shape, the color 4. Bone marrow biopsy: analyses microscopically the morphology (structure) of the blood stem cell	1. Signs and symptoms as mentioned above 2. Hydrochloric acid assessment: as hypochlorhydria does not allow for iron ionization, which decreases its absorption 3. Type of diet: a vegan diet without proper supplementation may result in vitamin B12 deficiency, which in turn leads to pernicious anemia 4. Liver function assessment, as the liver is responsible for the clotting factors production 5. Nutrient intake assessment, as lack of vital nutrients leads to anemia cases 6. Free radical status assessment, as free radicals can lead to oncologic etiology of disease

Medical assessment	Nutritional assessment
5. Imaging techniques, to asses the bleeding presence and location	7. Digestive system status assessment, as the nutrient absorption depends on the health of the digestive system 8. Immune system status assessment, as the immune system is responsible for destroying pathogens and abnormal cells

Table 17.3- Assessment of blood and blood elements

♦ ANEMIAS

[*]*group of disorders with multifactorial etiology that are characterized by low oxygen capacity in the blood stream due to lack of hemoglobin.*

MAJOR TYPES OF ANEMIA

TYPES OF ANEMIA	SUBTYPES	PATHOGENESIS	ETIOLOGY
ANEMIA CAUSED BY BLOOD LOSS	Acute post hemorrhagic anemia.	Loss of RBC number.	Rapid massive hemorrhage (trauma, rupture of a large blood vessel).
	Chronic blood loss.		Prolonged, moderate blood loss (peptic ulcer, gynecological problems).
	Iron deficiency anemia.	Iron deficiency[*] will result in not enough hemoglobin production[**], which lowers its capacity to transport oxygen.	➢ Deficient intake. ➢ Deficient absorption, either by deficient hydrochloric acid (which ionizes iron, making it fit for intestinal absorption), or diseases of the intestine, which, ultimately, interfere with iron absorption. ➢ Blood loss.
ANEMIAS CAUSED BY DEFICIENT ERYTHRO POIESIS (blood cells formation)	Anemia of chronic diseases.	Shorter RBC survival. Decreased marrow responsiveness (will not produce blood cells fast enough). Kidney conditions (impaired erythropoietin synthesis).	Cancer, chronic infections, leukemia.

TYPES OF ANEMIA	SUBTYPES	PATHOGENESIS	ETIOLOGY
	Aplastic anemia.	Loss of RBC precursors, either a bone marrow problem or a defect in the stem cell.	➢ *Idiopathic (in adolescents and young adults).* ➢ Chemicals, radiation, drugs (antineoplastics, antibiotics, NSAID).
	Vitamin B12 and folic acid deficiency anemia (Pernicious /megaloblastic anemia).	Both vitamin B12 and folic acid are required for RBC formation.	➢ Deficitary intake. ➢ Absorption deficit (lack of intrinsic factor, required for vitamin B12 absorption and/or intestinal problems). ➢ Increased requirement (pregnancy, lactation, increased metabolism).
ANEMIAS CAUSED BY EXCESSIVE HEMOLYSIS (destruction of red blood cells)	Anemia caused by immunologic abnormalities.	Autoimmune hemolysis by presence of antibodies that react with RBC.	➢ SLE, lymphoma, chronic leukemia. ➢ Interaction with various drugs (penicillin, cephalosporines).
	Anemia caused by mechanical injuries (Traumatic hemolytic anemia).	When RBC are exposed to excessive turbulence, abnormally shaped fragments of RBC may appear in the blood stream; they will not have the same oxygen carrying capacity that the normal RBC do.	➢ Within the heart, because of valvular disease; may cause turbulence (which, in turn, may break down RBC's). ➢ In arterioles, because of malignant hypertension (very high levels). ➢ In defects of coagulation (usually coagulation factors deficit).
ANEMIAS CAUSED BY EXCESSIVE HEMOLYSIS (destruction of red blood cells)	Anemias caused by defective hemoglobin synthesis: ➢ *Sickle cell disease.* ➢ Thalassemias.	These are called "hemoglobinopathies". Abnormally shaped or abnormally microstructural hemoglobin (defect of one or more protein chains) will not be able to carry enough oxygen.	➢ Genetic defects of shape or lack of /abnormality of the protein chains that are making up the globin part of the hemoglobin.

Table 17.4-Major types of anemias

**The most important storage form for iron is* Ferritin*; when a possible anemia is investigated, it is advisable that Ferritin levels are measured along with hemoglobin levels, (hemoglobin may still be normal, but if the reserve is low, it means that anemia is already on its way and this client will require supplementation)*

*** The absorbed iron, transported via a transporting protein called **transferrin** will enter the RBC; iron will then be transferred onto the mitochondria and the iron will attach to a molecule named protoporphyrin, forming a structure named heme; heme will attach a protein (globulin) in order to become hemoglobin; so, as you can see, if there is not enough iron, there will not be enough hemoglobin; if there is not enough hemoglobin, then the oxygen carrier capacity will diminish, hence anemia*

The above table presents the most common anemias encountered in the medical practice. Following, we will describe the most approachable anemias from a nutrition point of view: Iron deficiency anemia and Pernicious anemia (with a few notes on the clinical aspect of hemolytic anemia).

Clinical picture

General/common symptoms and signs for all anemias	Iron deficiency anemia	Pernicious / Megaloblastic anemia	Hemolytic anemia
• Pale skin and mucus membranes • Fatigue, dizziness, headaches •Tachycardia (because the heart tries to pump more blood in the circulation as to satisfy the oxygen needs of cells) • Tachypnea (fast respiratory rate), because the body is trying to get in as much oxygen as possible)	• All common signs/symptoms	• Restlessness • Tingling and numbness of the legs • Tongue burning • Loss of appetite • Depression, mental confusion	• Possibility of yellow tinge of skin and mucus membranes, because of increased hemoglobin destruction • Possible splenomegaly (enlarged spleen), because the spleen is the organ that has to filter all worn out or destroyed RBC

Table 17.5- Clinical aspect of anemias

Nutrition and holistic approach:

- The nutritional approach will very much depend on the cause of the condition (it is very important that the anemia is properly diagnosed as in etiology, as the therapeutic approach is different according to cause);
- Assessment of stomach acid level, liver status and digestive system status, as all of these may be predisposing factors of anemia;
- Avoid all body stressors (allergies, toxicity presence, etc), as they may pose a burden and further overload the detoxification/absorption pathways.

A. Iron deficiency anemia:

- Increase intake of iron rich foods: liver, green leafy vegetables, raw leeks (they contain vitamin C as well, which is important for iron absorption), parsley, spinach, dried beans, dried apricots, oats, pumpkin seed;
- Nutritional yeast helps the body absorb iron;
- Iron absorption is inhibited by coffee or tea intake; avoid them;
- Stinging nettle, carrot, beet, dandelion and alfalfa are rich in iron.

Supplements:

- Iron, 20-30 mg/day, according to the severity of the condition (keep in mind that these clients may already be on iron supplementation; your approach will be supportive);
- Vitamin C, 1-2 g/day, as it enhances iron absorption;
- Calcium, zinc and vitamin E may impede iron absorption, so they should be taken at a different time of the day.

B. Vitamin B 12 and folic acid anemia

- Increase intake of brewer's yeast, dried beans, green leafy vegetables, grains; if you are a vegan, it is suggested you take vitamin B_{12} supplementation;

Supplements:

- Vitamin B_{12},1000 mcg/day;
- Folic acid, 1-1.2 mcg/day.

♦LEUKEMIAS

malignant neoplasms of the blood forming organs, resulting in excessive proliferation and defects of certain white blood cells

Etiology: uncertain; genetic factors; exposure to radiation and/or toxic substances

TYPES OF LEUKEMIA

A. ACUTE:

- More common in children;
- Sudden onset;
- Fatigue, weight loss, fever, night sweats, anemia, weakness, easy bleeding and bruising; liver, lymph nodes and spleen may increase in size; increased susceptibility to infection.

B. CHRONIC:

- Affects adults mostly;
- Similar symptoms as the one listed above, but milder;
- Slow onset of tiredness and weakness;
- Progressive spleen enlargement with eventual pain and distension feeling in the upper left quadrant of the abdomen.

Medical treatment will employ chemotherapy and/or radiation. For more details on interactions with supplementation, please refer to *Neoplasia* chapter.

Nutrition and holistic treatment: will be supportive. A clear medical diagnosis has to be established, as different types of leukemia may require different approaches. Generally, please refer to and employ the approach outlined in *Neoplasia* chapter.

♦LYMPHOMAS

**neoplasms of the lymphoid tissue*

A. HODGKIN'S DISEASE

a form of malignant lymphoma affecting mostly the lymph nodes and the bone marrow

Etiology: unknown, but factors involved are:

- Genetic;
- Infectious;
- Environmental;
- Occupational toxicity.

Clinical aspect: anorexia (appetite loss), weakness, fatigue, and weight loss, night sweats; painless, progressive enlargement of lymph nodes and spleen.

Diagnosis is based on the clinical picture and the presence of characteristic cells called Reed-Sternberg (large, having two nucleus)

B. NON-HODGKIN'S LYMPHOMA

malignant proliferation of lymphoid cells of the lymph nodes, bone marrow, spleen, gastro-intestinal tract and liver

Presents with peripheral lymphadenopathy; later, the lymph nodes may become matted; edema of face and neck because of local compression;

Nutrition and holistic approach: cross reference to *Neoplasia.*

TERMINOLOGY IN HEMATOLOGY

TERM	DEFINITION/DESCRIPTION
Polycythemia vera	Idiopathic chronic increase in haemoglobin concentration and RBC mass
Thrombocythemia	Increased number of platelets
Hemophilia	Hereditary bleeding disorder due to clotting factors deficiency
Thrombocytopenia	Decreased platelets number
Purpura	Bleeding disorder characterized by increased bruising because of increased vascular fragility
Leukopenia	Decreased number of circulating WBC
Neutropenia	Decreased number of circulating neutrophils (leading to increased susceptibility to infection)
Eosinophilia	Increased number of eosinophils

Table 17.6-Terminology in haematology

CHAPTER 18

THE URINARY SYSTEM

You cannot help but be amazed how perfectly we were created. In the following chapter we will approach a system that filters the blood, eliminates the water-soluble waste, and keeps the blood balanced from the point of view of water and electrolytes balance and from the acid-balance point of view. And, as all other systems, it has a language of its own, which we will present in the following paragraphs.

IMPORTANT NUTRIENTS FOR THE URINARY SYSTEM

Nutrient	Role
Vitamin A	Protection of all mucus membranes
Vitamin B complex	Energy pathways
Vitamin C	Antioxidant, collagen formation
Coenzyme Q10	Increases cellular oxygenation
Germanium	Increases cellular oxygenation
Magnesium with vitamin B_6	Help reduce calcium kidney stones
Potassium	Deficiency has been associated with proteinuria
Valine	Maintains proper nitrogen balance in the body, thus lessening the work of the kidneys

Table 18.1-Important nutrients for the urinary system

Common signs/symptoms: increased urinary frequency, burning on urination, nocturia (urination in the nighttime), urinary colic (pain; will be described under *Kidney stones*), incontinence (incapacity of holding urine).

ASSESSMENT

MEDICAL	NUTRITIONAL
1. Clinical aspect, as per signs and symptoms listed above;	1. Dietary and supplemental analysis: to assess if the building blocks necessary for the development and maintenance of the urinary tract are provided;
2. Physical examination, to assess presence of lesions, trauma, kidney stones;	2. Digestive system status, as a malfunctioning digestive system may result in malnutrition and overloaded liver function (see preceding chapters);

MEDICAL	NUTRITIONAL
3. Blood work: will assess certain markers, like **creatinine,** which should be filtered out by the kidneys; if found in a certain amount in blood, this leads to the conclusion that the kidneys could not eliminate it, therefore it accumulated in the blood stream;	3. Liver status assessment, as a sluggish liver will not be able to process the necessary nutrients for the urinary system; also, improper detoxification may result in increased levels of circulating toxins affecting the health of the urinary system ;
4. Urine analysis: assesses pH, gross presence of blood, glucose or WBC, etc, in urine;	4. Immune system status, as an impaired immune system will not be able to properly eliminate infectious agents, therefore creating the terrain for infections;
5. Urine microscopy and urine culture: identifies the microorganism that may be causing the disease;	5. Identification of food allergies, as they could elicit cystitis (see below, under *Cystitis*);
6. Diagnosis imaging: X-ray, ultrasound, CT scan, MRI: assesses presence of stones, tumors, malformations, etc.	

Table 18.2- Assessment of the urinary system

URINARY SYSTEM DISEASES

♦ URINARY TRACT INFECTIONS (CYSTITIS)

**inflammation of the urinary bladder and /or of urethra*

Etiology:

- Infectious: various microorganisms, frequently E. Coli (usually bacteria goes up from urethra; also urethra is close to the anus and vagina, allowing for microorganisms in those areas to gain access to the urinary system);
- Irritation: barrier contraception, sexual intercourse, chemical irritants like soap, detergent, etc.;
- Poor hygiene;
- Food allergies (the theory states that some of the food allergies may target the urinary bladder's mucosa, which swells up because of the allergic reaction, and by doing so, decreases the capacity of the urinary bladder, therefore, resulting in the frequent urination and no burning characteristic for the food allergies reactions);
- Pregnancy;
- Malformations of the urinary tract, that may slow down the flow of urine, therefore creating urine stagnation, which in turn allows for invasion by bacteria;
- Excessive antibiotic use, which may destroy the local flora, especially the one in the vagina; this decreases the local protective capacity, allowing for bacterial growth;

Clinical aspect:

- Burning pain on urination;
- Increased urinary frequency (but not the quantity);
- Cloudy, foul smelling urine, low abdominal pain.

Diagnosis: by urine analysis.

Nutrition and holistic approach:

- Increased water intake, to keep the urinary system well flushed; watermelon and celery juice help with flushing;
- Unsweetened cranberry juice contains a substance that decreases the bacterial adherence to the urinary mucosa;
- If fruit juices are used, dilute them (sugar allows for bacterial growth);
- Carrot juice is known to flush out acid waste;
- Avoid sugar intake (which depress the immune system) and acid forming foods(which increase the irritation);
- Increase intake of alkaline forming foods.

Supplements:

- Vitamin C with bioflavonoids, 4-6 g/day, in divided doses ,and up to bowel tolerance, as it supports the urine system and acidifies the urine (bacteria has troubles living in an acidic environment); some authors quote urine alkalinization, as it seems that clinical results may support this theory;
- Vitamin A, 20000 - 30000 IU/day, for the protection of the mucus membranes; return gradually to 5000 IU/day, after a few days;
- Zinc, 30 mg /day, for immune system support;
- Probiotics, as prescribed, to restore normal flora in the pelvic area;
- Garlic supplements, as prescribed, as a natural antibiotic.

Other measures:

- Uva ursi(bearberry) is very helpful; buchu and cornsilk help as well;
- Goldenseal has antimicrobial properties; use on a short term basis; it can be added to sitz bath (see *sitz bath* under *Hemorrhoids*).

♦ URINARY CALCULI (KIDNEY STONES)

**formation of stone deposits at the kidney and ureter level;*

Etiology:

- Dehydration, which allows for mineral accumulation;
- Infections, which disturb the local balance, creating the terrain for mineral deposits;
- Conditions that allow for urine stagnation (allow depositing of minerals);

- Metabolic disturbances (hyperparathyroidism, destructive bone disease, oxaluria); all these diseases allow for accumulation/lack of excretion of various minerals;
- Increased refined carbohydrate intake will increase calcium excretion from the body with an increase of calcium levels in the urine;
- Increased dietary phosphorus (meat, pop) will increase calcium excretion;
- Increased urinary oxalate (from consuming foods like almonds, cashews, kale, rhubarb, spinach, cocoa) may elicit oxalic acid stones formation.

Definition: "Gravel" means small kidney stones

Pathogenesis: due to the causes listed above, the minerals accumulate in the kidneys and the stone begins to grow by new deposits attached to the core accumulation.

Stone composition: calcium salts, uric acid, non-calcium crystals (magnesium, oxalate).

Clinical aspect:

- If there is gravel, the symptoms are usually discomfort and cloudy urine; a person usually knows that they are eliminating gravel;
- A kidney stone of a certain dimension will elicit what is called a **"urinary colic".**

Note: Urinary colic: develops when the stone dislodges and it travels downwards throughout the urinary system:

- Excruciate, intermittent, radiating pain, originating in flank (back);
- nausea, vomiting, abdominal distension;
- possible blood in urine, as the passing of the stone creates lesions;;

If superimposed infection: fever, chills, urinary frequency increased.

Diagnosis: by ultrasound

Nutrition and holistic approach:

- Decreased calcium intake will not solve the problem; accepted literature says that the approach stands with metabolic abnormalities which have to be corrected, not with decreased calcium intake;
- Increased water intake, as a general measure for flushing out purposes;
- Avoid urine stagnation (incomplete urination, etc.);
- Determining the type of stone is important, as the dietary approach is different for each stone; this could be achieved by stone analysis, or, if this aspect is not possible, by laboratory investigations which will determine which metabolic abnormality stays at the base of the problem;
- It seems that a vitamin A deficiency allows for stone constituents to deposit;

- Increase your sources of plant protein as opposed to meat protein (phosphorus increases calcium excretion; also it may increase uric acid deposition);
- Avoid consumption of oxalic acid foods (as outlined in the etiology) and increase vitamin B_6 intake, as it helps eliminate oxalic acid;
- Fresh lemon juice in warm/hot water is believed that it can break down kidney stones;
- Increase intake of green leafy vegetables, rich in vitamin K which promotes the production of a protein responsible for inhibition of oxalate stones;
- Avoid alcohol intake, as it increases calcium excretion, on one hand and it increases uric acid precipitation, on the other hand;
- Avoid cysteine rich foods if you have a history of kidney stones, as it seems to result in stone formation in susceptible individuals.

Supplements:
- Magnesium, 500 mg/day, as magnesium deficiency increases the likelihood for developing kidney stones;
- Vitamin B_6, 50 mg/day, for oxalic acid control;
- Vitamin A, 5000-10000 IU/day, for protection of mucosa; return to maintenance doses or use beta carotenes upon elimination of stone; attention to vitamin A intake if the liver is damaged or if a woman is pregnant;
- It seems that calcium supplementation prevents the formation of oxalic acid stones.

Others:
- Parsley, gravel root, stone root and celery seeds may help dissolve kidney stones;
- Cornsilk or yarrow help during an attack;
- Aloe vera, slippery elm and marshmallow root are demulcents, soothing the inflamed mucus membranes.

♦ KIDNEY INFLAMMATIONS

A. PYELONEPHRITIS
**inflammation of the kidney*

Etiology:
- Infectious, often from repeated cystitis;
- Urine stagnation, as by malformations or kidney stones;
- Dehydration;
- Chronic use of drugs with kidney elimination.

Clinical aspect:
- Low back pain, pain on urination;
- Increased urinary frequency;
- Cloudy, smelling urine; sometimes blood may be present as well;
- Severe infections may present with nausea and vomiting.

B. GLOMERULONEPHRITIS

**bilateral infection at glomerular level* (the units that are filtering the blood)

Etiology:

- Infectious;
- Autoimmune, by circulating immune complexes.

Clinical aspect:

- As it follows an infectious process (usually a strep throat), symptoms will include fever, headaches, fatigue, low back pain;
- Edema (periorbitar-*around the eyes*- and around the ankles);
- Cloudy, reddish urine.

Note: chronic aspects of these diseases may develop insidiously, slowly, resulting in gross abnormalities of the kidney function: hematuria (blood in urine), proteinuria (proteins in urine), edema, hypertension, uremia (accumulation of urea from the protein breakdown; it is a toxic product for the body, in high quantities); the end result could be kidney failure

These conditions require **immediate medical attention;** our approach will be supportive:

Nutrition and holistic approach:

- Employ a low protein diet, to prevent urea accumulation;
- Increase intake of healthy, alkaline, simple foods and avoid any dietary stressors which may overload the kidneys excretion and elimination mechanisms (fat, sugar, salt, alcohol, additives, etc.);
- Garlic is a natural antibiotic;
- Parsley juice in water encourages kidney function.

<u>Supplements:</u>

- Vitamin A, 10000-20000 IU/day, taking the necessary precautions listed under *Kidney stones;*
- Vitamin E, 400 IU/day, is an antioxidant and prevents scarring;
- Vitamin B_6, 100 mg/day, helps decreasing levels of urea;
- Vitamin C, 1-2 grams a day, for immune support and to strengthen the vessel wall.

<u>Other measures:</u>

- Horsetail, dandelion leaves, bearberry, fennel and alfalfa; they all help in various combinations; consult a herbalist.

CHAPTER 19

GYNECOLOGY

Medical dictionaries define Gynecology as *"the branch of medicine that deals with diseases of the genital* tract in women"*. We, alternative medicine practitioners, come along and would now like to add to the definition. How about "gynecology is the branch of medicine that deals with diseases of the genital tract in women caused by imbalances of the digestive tract and/or toxic environmental exposure"? Or, how about "the liver is at the root of many etiologies of the female genital tract"? Or "an apple a day keeps the harmful estrogen away"?

Allow me to explain all these claims in the following chapter and let us start by presenting the list with the most important nutrients for the female genital system.

**genital: pertaining to reproductive organs*

IMPORTANT NUTRIENTS FOR THE FEMALE REPRODUCTIVE SYSTEM

Nutrient	Role
Vitamin A	Protects the mucus membranes of the genital tract
Vitamin B_3	Sex hormones synthesis
Vitamin B_6	Sodium balance; acts as a mild diuretic, therefore is indicated in PMS
Folic acid and vitamin B_{12}	Necessary for formation of red blood cells (thus, indicated in cases that present with increased bleeding)
Folic acid	Indicated in cases with cervical dysplasia
Vitamin C	Antioxidant, cancer prevention; reduces bleeding by strengthening the blood vessel wall
Vitamin E	Antioxidant, cancer prevention; indicated in cases of infertility
Bioflavonoids	Increase blood vessels wall strength; indicated in cases with bleeding
Magnesium	Relaxation of smooth muscle
Iron	Hemoglobin production; indicated in cases with bleeding
Vitamin B complex	Involve in regulation of estrogen metabolism (the liver does not inactivate estrogen properly when there is a B complex deficiency)
EFA	Anti-inflammatory

Table 19.1-Important nutrients for the female reproductive system

Common symptoms/signs: low abdominal pain (it may be central or sided), bleeding between periods and of irregular nature (metrorrhagia), increased menstrual bleeding, (menorrhagia), dysmenorrhea (painful menstruation), dyspareunia (painful intercourse), various discharges;

ASSESSMENT

MEDICAL	NUTRITIONAL
1. Clinical appearance, as listed above; 2. Physical examination (genital exam): which detects masses, bleeding origin, cervix aspect, etc.; 3. Laboratory tests: hormones levels, blood work assessing anemia, infection, etc; 4. PAP smear: shows cellular abnormalities, if any at cervix levels and can also assess the presence of infections; 5. Transvaginal ultrasound assesses the aspect of uterus, fallopian tubes and vagina; 6. Biopsy: to assess the aspect and function of the endometrium (the lining of the uterus);	1. Presence of symptoms/signs as listed above; 2. Dietary and environmental analysis, to assess the estrogen exposure and also the potential liver stressors; 3. Digestive system status assessment, as maldigestion impedes nutrient absorption; (necessary for hormones synthesis) and also it may allow bowel toxins to travel freely, overloading the liver; 4. Liver function assessment, as an overloaded liver will greatly impede on the hormones degradations and detoxification;

Table 19.2- Assessment of the female reproductive system

REPRODUCTIVE ENDOCRINOLOGY

GLAND	HORMONE	ACTION
Hypothalamus	Gonadotropin releasing hormone	Acts on the pituitary gland to release **FSH** and **LH**
Anterior Pituitary gland	FSH (Follicle-stimulating hormone)	Stimulates the production of ova (cells of the reproductive system);
	LH (Luteinizing hormone)	Stimulates the ovaries to produce estrogen and progesterone;
Ovaries	Estrogen*	Regulation of menstrual cycle; health of the organs of the reproductive system;
	Progesterone*	

Table 19.3- Reproductive endocrinology

*Estrogen and progesterone are both derived from the cholesterol molecule

THE MENSTRUAL CYCLE

	Follicular phase (proliferative) ***Days 1-14***(includes the menstrual bleeding)	**Ovulatory phase** ***Day 14***[*]	**Luteal phase** (secretory) ***Days 14-28***
Pituitary hormones	Slight increase of FSH	LH peak	LH and FSH levels decline
Ovarian cycle	One follicle starts undergoing maturation	Ovulation: oocyte release	Formation of corpus luteum
Ovarian hormones	Estrogen levels increase	High estrogen starts declining and progesterone starts increasing	Increased progesterone levels
Endometrium	Increases in thickness due to increased blood supply and glands	Endometrium continues to become thick	Continuous increase of blood supply and endometrial glands

Table 19.4- The menstrual cycle

[*]The ovulatory phase varies from one person to the other

> **Note:** the menstrual cycle may vary from one person to the other, as in number of days; there are cycles as short as 23 days and as long as 30-35 days; even though the length is different, the events that make up the cycle are developing as described above

Comments:

- The first part of the menstrual cycle is dominated by increased estrogen levels, whereas the second part of the cycle is dominated by increased progesterone levels (secreted by the corpus luteum, which is what was left of the ovarian follicle after the ovum was released);
- The endometrium grows and becomes velvety as the body prepares for the implantation of an embryo (stage of development up to nine weeks);
- If fertilization (the combination of the male and the female cell) does not occur, the thick endometrium will be sloughing off after day 28 as menses (bleeding).

THE HORMONAL BALANCE

For us to be healthy, the estrogen and progesterone should be in balance. Unfortunately, it seems that lately the estrogen has a tendency to greatly increase in our bodies, unopposed by progesterone, which creates a situation called ***Estrogen dominance***. Let us take a look at these two hormones and in which way their imbalance can affect us.

A. ESTROGEN:

- Has a steroid base;
- It is being produced by ovaries at puberty;
- It increases in the first half of the menstrual cycle and declines in the second half.

Types of Estrogen:

1. **Estradiol** (E2; 10-20%): produced by ovaries; the strongest type of estrogen; linked to increased risk for breast cancer;
2. **Estrone** (E1; 10-20%): the type of estrogen that our fat cells produce, especially after menopause; linked to breast cancer risk, as well, but in a lesser extent than estradiol; estradiol and estrone may be converted into each other;
3. **Estriol** (E3; 60-80%): produced by ovaries; has a protective effect, except when supplemented in high amounts; the liver can convert estradiol and estrone into estriol.

Roles of Estrogen:

- Prepares the body for ovulation;
- Responsible for the development of sex characteristics (breast and hips enlargement, etc.);
- Generally, promotes growth and cell division;
- Aids in the use of glucose by the brain and also increases blood flow to the brain;
- Maintains the elasticity, thickness and lubrication of vulva, vagina and urethra;
- Part of the hormonal balance that affects libido and sexual activity (along with testosterone);
- Incorporation of calcium in bone depends on estrogen;
- Seems that it may increase HDL and decrease LDL; increases anti-oxidant activity in the blood, protecting against high blood pressure (this is why hormone replacement therapy used to be recommended in menopausal women for prevention of cardio-vascular disease; of course, there are other way of accomplishing cardio-vascular health- see *Chapter 16*);
- Affects the texture of hair and skin (as in increased elasticity and lubrication);
- Involved in water balance (an estrogen excess may lead to water retention).

> **Note**: Estrogen receptors are located in brain, bone and heart (beta receptors) and in uterus and breasts (alpha receptors); it seems that the soy isoflavones prefer the beta-receptors

Sources of Estrogen:

1. **Endogenous source** (our bodies produce it)

- Ovaries;
- Placenta, during pregnancy (mostly estriol);
- Fat tissue;
- Adrenal gland cortex (produces androgens, which are precursors for the estrogen).

Other endogenous sources:

- Liver breaks down estrogen for elimination; we excrete estrogen via urine and feces; urinary estrogen is completely eliminated, whereas the estrogen in our gut may be recycled, increasing the endogenous estrogen pool; thus, impaired liver function may lead into improper estrogen breakdown, which will make it available to the body;
- Intestinal health: constipation will slow down transit time allowing the estrogen bound to feces to be reabsorbed and recycled; gut bacteria produces an enzyme (*beta-glucuronidase*) that splits the estrogen from its carrier in the intestines, making it more available for recycling;
- Candida may produce chemicals that resemble the estrogen.

2. **Xenoestrogens:** environmental chemicals that mimic the structure of the estrogen molecule; they have a tendency to accumulate in the fat tissue; some examples are: pesticides, plastics (it is said that you should not be squishing your plastic water bottle out of shape, as the distortion may allow xenoestrogens molecules to leach in the water; also, be aware of foods that are packaged in plastic, especially when they are fatty, as the fat absorbs toxins), chlorine, detergents, solvents, hormones fed animals;

3. **Synthetic estrogens**: provided by Hormone Replacement Therapy (HRT), birth control pills (BCP), fertility drugs;

4. **Phytoestrogens**: estrogen-like molecules found in plants; they act as weak estrogen molecules and have a protective effect on the body, as they may displace the xenoestrogens from their sites and also they may displace the excessive body estrogen from their receptor, but they are too weak to stimulate cell division.

Classification of phytoestrogens:

Class of Phytoestrogens	Sub-class	Comments	Sources
Steroids		Found in many plants at a very low level	Pomegranate and apple seeds
Saponins		Found in many plants at very low levels	
Terpenoids			Black cohosh and licorice
Phenolic	Flavones	They have a chemical structure that is similar to steroid hormones. They are abundant in the human diet	Most red and yellow colored fruits and vegetables
	Isoflavones		Legumes, chickpeas, lentils, red clover, soy
	Lignans		Flax seed, rye, millet, buckwheat, sunflower seeds; most cereals
	Flavonols		Citrus fruits, onion, apples, red wine
	Coumestans		Young sprouting legumes

Table 19.5- Sources of phytoestrogens

Estrogenic herbs: angelica, black cohosh (the commercial preparation is *Remifemin*), red clover (the commercial preparation is *Promensil*), hops, thyme, turmeric, and yellow dock.

Notes on soy: lately there has been a lot of talk about soy and how much should we have; Soy is a powerful phytoestrogen so a high intake will result in excessive estrogen activity. Some sources are quoting that three ounces of soy three times a week is more than enough. Please, do not forget that a diet high in fruits, vegetables, seeds and grains provides a good intake of phytoestrogens. The panel is still out on the soy story; my belief is that the secret is in moderation. Do not discard it, but do not live on it. Of course, every person is different and you will do well to work individual assessments.

B. PROGESTERONE

- Has a steroid base (progesterone formation precedes estrogen formation);
- Released at puberty, dominates the second half of the menstrual cycle;
- There is only one type of progesterone.

Roles of Progesterone:

- Precursor of estrogen and testosterone;
- Maintains endometrial health;
- Balances estrogen excess;
- By balancing estrogen, helps protect against breast cancer;
- Promotes the survival of embryo and fetus during pregnancy;
- Protects against fibrocystic breast disease;
- Protects against endometrial cancer;
- May help sex drive;
- Normalizes blood clotting;
- Promotes fat burning for energy;
- Aides thyroid metabolism;
- Helps keep blood sugar levels regular;
- Natural diuretic, as it normalizes water balance;
- Natural antidepressant.

Sources of Progesterone:

1. **Endogenous source:**

    - Ovaries;
    - Testes, adrenal cortex and placenta (smaller quantities).

2. **Plant source**: Mexican wild yam contains a substance *–diosgenin-* which is extracted and converted in a laboratory to bio-identical natural progesterone, then is incorporated into a cream (mostly known as Natural Progesterone cream); it has good absorption and good results; the percentage form (3, 7 or 10%) applies to wild yam cream without added natural progesterone; it doesn't have progesterone in it (you need a laboratory for that, as mentioned above), but women have been using it for many years with various clinical results; the number of grams/ounce form has added natural progesterone to it; (dosages vary greatly from 2 mg/ounce to 400 mg/ounce); consult your naturopath for the appropriate dosage;

3. **Herbs:** Sarsaparilla, blue cohosh, blood root, fenugreek, yucca and Chaste tree.

ESTROGEN DOMINANCE APPROACH

- Avoid the exposure to xenoestrogens;
- Increase intake of phytoestrogens (a balanced diet, with increased intake of fruits, vegetables, grains and legumes should be more than enough);
- Ensure digestive system health and optimal transit time (see under *The Digestive system*);
- Ensure liver health (see under *Liver*);
- Obesity approach, if necessary;
- Increase exercise levels;
- Increase the melatonin levels (melatonin is secreted by the pineal gland between one and three am, in conditions of darkness; melatonin decreases the number of estrogen receptors; bananas and St. John's wort may increase melatonin levels);
- Folic acid decreases the effects of estrogen in the body;
- Iodine helps minimizing the effects of estrogen on the breast tissue;
- Increased intake of flax seed oil, which decreases the effects of estrogen on the breast tissue; Evening Primrose Oil should be avoided, as it has the opposite effect.

Besides all the information we accumulated so far, there are some factors to be considered, when it comes to *increased exposure to estrogen:*

- **The number of years** while a woman has menstrual cycles: the younger the onset age and the later the menopause age, the more menstrual cycles a woman has; every cycle is accompanied by increased estrogen levels, so this factor should be taken into consideration when we assess the estrogen exposure;
- **The length of menstrual cycles**: the shorter the cycle (less than 26-28 days), the more cycles a woman has, which increases her risk to exposure;
- **The number of live births**: the more you have, the lower the risk (as the hormones secreted during pregnancy are estriol, which is protective, and progesterone);
- **The woman's age when she has her first born**: the younger you are when you have your first child, the lower the risk; it seems that the breast cells fully mature and are less vulnerable to estrogen exposure once a woman goes through her first full pregnancy;
- **The number of months spent breastfeeding**: the longer the breast feeding time, the lower the risk, as it seems that the longer we nurse, the more we metabolize fat and toxins from the body;
- **Number of bowel movements**: the more we have, the lower the risk, as every bowel movement eliminates more estrogen.

PATHOLOGY OF THE REPRODUCTIVE TRACT

♦MENSTRUAL ABNORMALITIES AND ABNORMAL UTERINE BLEEDING

A. PREMENSTRUAL SYNDROME (PMS)

**cyclic occurrence of specific physical , emotional and behavioural changes experienced every month between ovulation and menstruation.*

Etiology: multifactorial, see below under presentation

- Possible common denominator: high estrogens to progesterone ratio (except PMS-D);
- Low liver function (impedes estrogen degradation) associated or not with low thyroid function (which slows down the body's metabolism, therefore affecting both the digestive system and the liver).

PMS PRESENTATION

SUBGROUP	SYMPTOMS	MECHANISM
PMS-A (anxiety)	Anxiety, irritability, mood swings, emotional instability, panic attack	High estrogen- progesterone ratio; high estrogen decreases serotonin levels in mid cycle;
PMS-C (craving)	Increased appetite, headache, fatigue, palpitations, craving for sweets and salt	Altered carbohydrates metabolism Altered prostaglandin metabolism;
PMS-D (depression)	Depression, crying, forgetfulness, confusion, insomnia	Low neurotransmitters levels It seems that these cases actually present with low estrogen levels;
PMS-H (Hyper hydration)	Fluid retention, weight gain, breast tenderness, abdominal bloating	Excess aldosterone, as a result of increased estrogen and decreased magnesium.

Table 19.6-PMS presentation

Note: every time when you see a PMS case, question the liver function; my experience showed that just on a mild liver cleanse alone, these cases were getting much better, as the internal balance starts restoring

Nutrition and holistic approach:

- Employ the estrogen dominance approach listed above;
- Greatly increase the intake of fruits and vegetables (vegetarians excrete higher amounts of estrogen than the meat eaters), and reduce sources of arachidonic acid;
- Fresh apples, celery and grapes will diminish the bloating if eaten during the week before the apparition of menses;

- Barley water, which is rich in vitamins B ease the PMS symptoms;
- Eat oats for their calming effect.

Supplements:

- Vitamin B_6, 50 mg twice a day, as it is needed for the conversion of tryptophan into serotonin and supports progesterone synthesis;
- Vitamin E, 400 IU/day, as it helps stabilize hormonal imbalances and reduces breast tenderness;
- Evening Primrose oil, 500 mg three times/day, as it supports the prostaglandin E1 synthesis;
- Magnesium, 400-600 mg/day, as it is involved in vitamin B_6 metabolism; also, stabilizes moods and provides relaxation of the smooth muscle of the genital tract;

Note: Cravings for chocolate may be actually a cry of the body for more magnesium!

- Zinc, 30 mg/day, as it involved in hormones production.

Other measures:

- Natural progesterone cream, as prescribed, as it balances out estrogen levels;
- Chaste berry helps with hormone balancing ;yarrow and lady's mantle relieve cramps; corn silk and burdock help relieve bloating; chamomile and peppermint help relieve nausea;
- St John's wort, oats, lemon balm and passion flower relieve symptoms of PMS A and D;
- Essential oils of geranium and rosemary in the bath may help symptoms of water retention and irritability;
- Light abdominal massage with lavender oil may be very helpful.

B. DYSMENORRHEA

**painful menstruation;* usually the cramping occurs in the lower abdomen and it is worse on the first day of flow

Onset: usually within two years of menarche (first menstrual period), with peak between 15-24 years.

Types:

1. Primary: pain occurs in the absence of a physical abnormality or pelvic disease; tends to decrease with age and it will usually disappear after childbirth.
   Causes:
   - Psychological factors: stress about adolescence, anxiety, depression, etc.;
   - Physical factors:
     - Cervical stenosis (the cervix orifice is small and enlarges with childbirth);
     - Increased release of prostaglandins, which causes muscle contraction, and thus, pain.

2. Secondary: pain due to a disease process; starts later in life and increases in intensity; chronic dysmenorrhea with a history of infertility suggests either endometriosis or PID (Pelvic Inflammatory Disease)

Causes:

- Endometriosis: this pain is worse with menses, not only related to menses;
- PID: physical examination will lead to diagnosis;
- IUD (Intrauterine device);
- Uterine malformations/anomalies;
- Ovarian cysts: the pain is unilateral, though;
- Uterine fibroids.

Clinical aspect:

- Various intensity of low abdominal pain;
- Nausea and vomiting, which is a common reaction to pain;
- Diarrhea, as the movements of the large intestine and those of the uterus are linked (you may have loose bowel movements with uterus movements);
- Low back pain, because of water retention and increased tissue swelling, pressing on nerves;
- Headache, dizziness.

Note: dysmenorrhea could be so intense that many women are incapacitated for a few days every month!

Nutrition and holistic approach:

- Avoid all dietary liver stressors, alcohol, increased sugar, additives; reduce salt intake as it promotes water retention;
- Avoid all saturated fat, as it increases the arachidonic acid within the body with increased prostaglandins E_2 release, which are pro-inflammatory and pain-prone;
- Increase intake of fish, nuts, fruits and vegetables;
- Smoking and obesity are risk factors for dysmenorrhea;
- Foods that help reduce inflammatory prostaglandins levels: spinach, beans, millet, alfalfa and mangoes.

<u>Supplements:</u>

- Vitamin B_3, 50 mg twice a day, as it reduces the menstrual cramps;
- Vitamin C and bioflavonoids, 1-3 g/day, as it supports vitamin B_3 effect and improves vessels health;
- Calcium and magnesium, 800-1000 mg/day to 400-500 mg/day, for relaxation of smooth muscle;
- Vitamin E, 400 –800 IU/day, as it seems to relieve somehow spastic dysmenorrhea;
- Evening Primrose Oil, 500 mg three times/day, as it is anti-inflammatory;
- Bromelain, 500 mg twice a day, as an anti-inflammatory.

<u>Other measures:</u>

- Crampbark is useful for menstrual cramps; peppermint may help ease the pain;
- Ginger seems to have a calming effect on the smooth muscle;
- Oats and valerian, also lemon balm are calming;
- Cypress and lavender essential oils has antispasmodic properties and can be massaged into the abdomen or used in a bath;

- Exercise, stress management, relaxation techniques.

C. AMENORRHEA

**absence of menstrual bleeding*

> **Note:** *Physiological amenorrhea* means that this is a normal occurrence: before puberty, during pregnancy, during lactation, after menopause.

1. **Primary amenorrhea**: no vaginal bleeding occurred by the time of expected beginning
   - Genetic defect;
   - Congenital absence of vagina.

2. **Secondary amenorrhea**: no bleeding for three months in a woman who had regular cycles or no bleeding for six months in a woman who had irregular cycles; we will list the most well known causes here, followed by individual therapeutic approaches from a nutritional and holistic point of view

2a. Ovarian failure (the ovary does not respond to pituitary stimulation)
- Diet focused on fruits and vegetables, mostly greens, fish, nuts, seeds, grains, legumes (especially soy);
- Black cohosh, for its estrogenic effects;
- Natural hormone replacement (see your naturopath; the holistic approach does not replace the prescribed treatment that your clients are on):
  - a combination named Tri Est, that contains a combination of estrone, estradiol and estriol provides estrogen;
  - Natural progesterone cream, that provides progesterone;
  - Multivitamin and mineral formula.

2b. Hypoestrogen states (associated with weight loss, stress, anorexia)
- Make sure that your clients have the appropriate caloric intake;
- Increased intake of fruits and vegetables, soy, flax, fish;
- Multivitamin and mineral formula;
- Black cohosh (see above);
- Natural hormone replacement (see above).

2c. Anovulatory amenorrhea (there is no ovulation; usually the estrogen levels are normal, but the progesterone levels are low; polycystic ovary is an example):
- Employ a low carbohydrate and high protein diet, as these cases may result in obesity;
- Increase intake of fish, legumes, nuts and grains;
- Chaste tree, as it balances the pituitary gland and it is progesteronic;
- Natural progesterone cream, as prescribed.

> *Transient amenorrhea*: weight changes, travel, extreme stress, excessive exercise
> - Address the cause

♦GYNECOLOGIC INFLAMMATIONS AND INFECTIONS

A. VAGINITIS

**Infections/inflammations of the vagina*

Types:

1. Hormonal: menopause and women whose ovaries have been removed;
2. Irritant: allergies to different chemical substances (condoms, spermicidal substances, soaps, detergents) or to sanitary napkins, abrasions, hot tubs;
3. Infectious (the most frequent cause of vaginitis).

In the following we will approach the infectious vaginitis:

A1. Bacterial vaginosis

Etiology: different agents; decreased levels of normal local flora (lactobacilli) and increased levels of microorganisms like Gardnerella and other bacteria.

Risk factors and comments:

- Not clear if sexual transmission is involved, so the treatment of partners is not mandatory; in severe cases that occur often, it is recommended;
- Complications: PID, by migration into the upper genital tract.

Clinical aspect:

- Thin, frothy, smelly discharge (fishy);
- Mild itching/burning of vulva;
- No signs of inflammation;
- Visualization under the microscope of special cells, "clue cells".

Nutrition and holistic approach:

- Systemic immune system boosting, as we are dealing with an infectious condition;
- Decrease saturated fat, excessive sugar, alcohol, smoking, coffee;
- Increased intake of fruits and vegetables, nuts, legumes and water;
- Probiotics, as prescribed ;
- Insert one lactobacillus capsule into vagina in the morning;
- Vitamin E locally, one capsule introduced inside vagina, for a few days;
- Goldenseal is antimicrobial; garlic is a natural antibiotic.

A2. Candida vaginitis

Etiology: Candida albicans

Risk factors and comments:

- Recurrent candida vaginitis are usually present in women with a low immune status;

- Excessive sugar in the diet, antibiotic use, various drugs (hormones, radiotherapy, chemotherapy), pregnancy, nylon pantyhose and underwear and tight clothes may constitute risk factors;
- Sexual contact may be a source for re-infection;
- Some authors say that the re-infection may be possible from the gastro-intestinal tract via rectum and that recurrent vaginal infections are a sign that there is systemic candidiasis.

Clinical aspect:

- Intense local itching;
- Vaginal discharge looks like "cottage cheese", classically;
- Irritation, vulvar burning;
- Symptoms become worse the week preceding menses;
- Microscopic examination of vaginal discharge establishes the diagnosis.

Nutrition and holistic approach:

- See dietary advice above, under *Bacterial vaginosis*;
- Probiotics, as prescribed;
- Boric acid powder capsule, introduced intravaginally, as prescribed;
- Local acidophilus capsules may be introduced intravaginally;
- Douches with tea tree oil or apple cider vinegar;
- Garlic, as a natural antibiotic.

A3. Trichomonas vaginitis

Etiology: Trichomonas vaginalis

Risk factors and comments:

- Multiple sexual partners;
- Sexually transmitted diseases acquired previously;
- Co-existence with other infections;
- Transmitted sexually.

Clinical aspect:

- Vaginal and vulvar itching and irritation;
- Discharge is frothy and yellow green;
- Painful intercourse;
- Vaginal redness present;
- Diagnosis by microscope visualization;

Nutrition and holistic approach:

- Immune system boosting;
- Dietary factors recommendations as above;
- Tea tree oil washes and douches;

- Probiotics, as prescribed.

B. PID (PELVIC INFLAMMATORY DISEASE)
**infections and inflammations of the uterus (endometritis), the ovaries and/or the fallopian tubes (salpingitis);* the etiology is infectious.

Risk factors:
- Multiple sexual partners;
- Genital tract infections (like bacterial vaginosis);
- IUD use;
- Recent abortion or recurrent PID.

Clinical aspect:

1. **Acute**: fever and chills, dyspareunia, discharge, vaginal bleeding, severe abdominal pain and possible low back pain

THIS IS A MEDICAL EMERGENCY!!!

2. **Chronic:** fatigue, low abdominal and back pain, nausea, pain on urination, irregular spotting;

Nutrition and holistic approach will apply to the ***chronic*** aspect, as the acute one is a medical emergency:
- Immune system boosting, as an infection is present;
- Avoid all dietary and lifestyle stressors of the immune system;
- Focus on a healthy, wholesome, balanced and natural diet; increased bioflavonoids rich foods;
- Probiotics, as prescribed;
- Garlic is a natural antibiotic; eat liberally or use it in supplementation, as prescribed;
- Red clover is a blood cleanser; if pain present, crampbark may help;
- Aloe vera and slippery elm soothe irritated membranes.

♦ENDOMETRIOSIS
**endometrial tissue migration outside of the uterus;* usually located in the pelvic cavity, along abdominal organs, on the pelvic floor and on the ovaries

Etiology: much discussed, but still in theory form:
- Weak immune system with a tendency towards autoimmunity (do assess food sensitivity in this context);
- Retrograde bleeding from vagina into the fallopian tubes and then in the pelvic cavity (the "Retrograde menstruation theory");
- Embryonic defect;
- Environmental toxins exposure;
- Emotional aspect.

Clinical aspect:

- Pelvic pain, severe, may be cyclic or constant;
- Dyspareunia;
- Dysmenorrhea;
- Pain with bowel movement;
- Pain with urination;
- Pain on movement.

Diagnosis: these cases undergo multiple diagnosis procedures, starting with physical examination, ultrasound, which is not very helpful, and ultimately, laparascopy (the surgical opening of the abdomino-pelvic cavity) which proves the presence of endometriosis, often as "*chocolate cysts*" (dark cysts with blood).

> **Note**: endometriosis is one of the main causes of infertility

Nutrition and holistic approach:

- Employ all measures under estrogen dominance, as it seems that endometriosis is one of the conditions that mirrors it;
- Increase fish and nuts intake for their anti-inflammatory effect;
- Seafoods and sea vegetables are rich in iodine, which seems to protect against endometriosis.

Supplements:

- Vitamin C, 2-4 g/day, as it improves the vessel wall health;
- Beta carotenes, 25000-50000 IU/day, as they are vitamin A precursors and support the health of the mucus membranes;
- Vitamin E, 400 IU/day, as it inhibits the arachidonic acid formation;
- Evening Primrose Oil, 500 mg three times a day or flax seed oil, 1-2 tablespoons/day, for their anti-inflammatory effects;
- Vitamin B complex, 50 mg/day, as it benefits hormone balancing and supports the liver;
- Bromelain and papain, as they are anti-inflammatory and break down scar tissue (being enzymes);

Other measures:

- Cramp bark diminishes the pain; Chaste tree helps balancing hormones;
- Valerian is relaxing and antispasmodic; so is motherwort;
- Shepherd's purse may help diminish the bleeding; dandelion root is a very good liver detoxifier;
- Natural progesterone cream, as prescribed;
- Castor oil packs may help diminish the pain.

♦OVARIAN CYSTS

**closed sacs, usually filled with fluid*; they are not uncommon and more often than not they are discovered during a routine examination; the etiology is not very clear; some authors quote hormonal imbalances, other quote pelvic congestion (from exposure of extremities to cold; wearing high heels may also compromise pelvic circulation), and it seems that most of them agree on a sluggish liver theory (as the liver would create imbalances by not properly dispose of hormones).

Classification:

1. Single cysts;
2. Multiple cysts.

Pathogenesis: it seems that ovarian cysts develop from an ovarian follicle that neither released an ovum, nor degenerated; instead it accumulated fluid and increased in size
(They may range in size from very small to the size of a grapefruit!);

Clinical aspect:

- Depending on their size and location, cysts may range from painful to very painful; pain varies in intensity and it is usually present above the hip bone or unilaterally, in the lower abdomen; sudden moves will elicit pain;
- Pain during intercourse;
- Irregular bleeding;
- If a cyst develops a stem that attaches it to the ovary, it is possible that sometimes the cyst stem will torsion, resulting in high levels of pain.

> **Note:** Polycystic ovary syndrome is a condition characterized by the presence of a few cysts, usually unilaterally, irregular menses or amenorrhea, mild obesity and increased tendency to develop excessive hair; the estrogen levels seem to be elevated;

Nutrition and holistic approach:

- Liver detoxification, cleanse and support, as outlined in the *Liver* chapter, from a dietary and supplemental point of view;
- Vegan diet seems to help, as it will decrease the estrogen burden on the liver;
- Avoid all fried foods, smoking, coffee, alcohol, excess sugar.

Supplements:

- Vitamin E, 400 IU/day, seems to be helpful in preventing and reducing cysts;
- Evening Primrose oil, 500 mg three times/day, for its anti-inflammatory properties;
- Vitamin A, 5000 IU/day or beta carotenes, 25000 IU/day, for the protective effect on the lining of the ovary.

Other measures:

- Dandelion root is very good for liver cleansing; yellow dock is a body purifier;
- Licorice is soothing for the mucus membranes;
- Castor oil packs on liver and on the affected ovary may relieve symptoms.

♦UTERINE FIBROIDS (MYOMAS)

**benign tumors developing in the uterus muscle (myometrium);* they occur frequently and , depending on the location and size, they may range from asymptomatic (no symptoms) to various clinical pictures, as described below; they are the most common cause of a pelvic tumor; according to size and bleeding level, they may require surgery; rapid growth of a fibroid when pregnant, due to estrogen stimulation; they decline after menopause, due to declining levels of estrogen; they could be single or multiple.

Etiology and risk factors:

- Fibroids seem to be due to estrogen dominance;
- High fat diet, obesity, will increase the risk;
- Coffee intake will increase the risk also (coffee contains methylxanthines, which contribute to growth);
- High stress levels;
- Pregnancy;
- High estrogen intake (from any source; fibroids have a high number of estrogen receptors).

Clinical aspect:

- A pelvic mass may be palpated (felt) on physical examination, by your doctor;
- Bleeding (high bleeding with menses and in between); could lead to anemia;
- Pain, when present, depends on the location of the fibroid;
- There could be increased pain with menses and pain with the intercourse; also, there may be a pressure-sensation against rectum, on bowel movements.

Types of fibroids:

- Cervical: within the walls of the cervix;
- Prolapsed: coming through cervix;
- Pedunculated: it has a stalk;
- Intramural: within the uterus wall;
- Submucosal: protrude into the uterine cavity and they are the cause of most of the bleeding.

Medical diagnosis:

- Clinical signs and symptoms;
- Physical examination;
- Ultrasound, CT scan.

Complications:

- Anemia, by continuous bleeding;
- Obstruction, by large fibroids pressing against ureters.

Medical treatment will employ hormonal medication and /or surgery; if the fibroid is large and complicated, hysterectomy (uterus removal) will be performed

Nutrition and holistic approach:

- Estrogen dominance approach, as outlined above;
- Obesity approach, if necessary;
- Increase intake of vitamin K containing foods, to approach the bleeding;
- Increased intake of EFA's for their anti-inflammatory and antispasmodic properties;
- Increased intake of iron rich foods, to prevent anemia.

Supplements:

- Vitamin C with bioflavonoids, 1-2 g/day, as it enhances iron absorption and strengthens the vessels walls;
- Vitamin B complex, 100 mg/day, as it assists in liver function and the health of red blood cells;
- Evening Primrose oil, 500 mg three times/day;
- Lipotropic factors (choline, inositol, etc), as prescribed, as they help liver remove fat, and by doing so, improving its function;
- Green food supplements, as they provide minerals and vitamin K;
- Vitamin A, 5000 IU/day, as it supports the health of mucus membranes;
- Vitamin E, 400 IU/day, as it helps the liver detoxify estrogen.

Others:

- Cinnamon bark and beets seems to help regulate the bleeding;
- Natural progesterone cream, as prescribed;
- White ash is helpful when uterus is enlarged due to fibroids presence;
- Shephard's purse is an anti-hemorrhagic;
- Essential oils of geranium, rose or cypress, gently massaged into the abdomen or in a bath are helpful;
- Do see your naturopath or herbalist, as there are many helpful herbal combinations.

♦MENOPAUSE

**cessation of menstruation due to decreasing ovarian function;* it usually happens around the age of fifty, but it can occur much earlier than that; we will not discuss here the menopause due to removal of ovaries or of uterus, though our approach will be very similar.

Climacteric/perimenopause: the years around menopause, characterized by multiple changes that lead into the menopausal picture; the duration could span from 2 to ten years!—it is due to changeable hormonal levels.

Hormonal changes of perimenopause:

- Menstrual cycles begin to vary (some are short, some are very long);
- Estrogen levels will vary for a while, going up and down, which explains the erratic cycles;
- Progesterone levels seem to decline before estrogen levels;
- Eventually, estrogen levels will decline so that no menstrual cycle occurs.

Clinical aspect:

- Hot flashes and palpitations: related to a decline in ovarian function; their physiology is not very well understood; it seems that the body responds to a sudden and transient resetting of the body's set point, in the hypothalamus; obvious triggers are stress, spicy foods, hot drinks, warm environment;
- Sleep disruption and insomnia: difficulty falling asleep and staying asleep;
- Anxiety and depression: estrogen levels do have a positive effect on mood;
- Memory loss and changes in cognition: it seems that they are due to estrogen decline, as well;
- Irregular bleeding, due to decreased ovarian function;
- Osteoporosis, as estrogen is responsible for incorporation of calcium in the bone;
- Vaginal dryness and thinning of walls and similar changes in the urethra: due to loss of estrogen. This results in dry and possibly bleeding vulva and vagina, easy trauma after sex, an increased likelihood of bladder infections and of prolapse (uterus or vagina slip forward due to lack of strength and elasticity of the structures that keep them in place);
- Decreased sexual response; this has a dual aspect; one is due to the hormonal changes the other one may be due to the discomfort elicited by vaginal dryness;
- Increased hair growth on face and body, due to increased levels of androgens and decreased estrogen levels.

Medical treatment employs HRT (Hormone Replacement Therapy) using **Premarin**, which is estrogen derived from the urine of pregnant mares; unfortunately, it is not metabolized by the liver in the same way the natural estrogen is and has a tendency to accumulate and exhibit multiple side effects:

- Breast tenderness, headaches, leg cramps;
- Blood clots, high blood pressure, fluid retention;
- Increased risk of endometrial and breast cancer.

Nutrition and holistic approach: we would like to add here that we do not suggest that clients should not take what their doctor prescribes; there are cases where the benefits will outweigh the risk. What we do here is to present a mild, preventive and supportive approach for women who go through menopause:

- Dietary changes as early as possible in life are very important: focus on a diet rich in fruits and vegetables, grains, legumes and fish; avoid as much as possible the dietary and lifestyle stressors listed under *Liver;*
- Do increase your calcium intake early in life and employ exercise, to prevent osteoporosis.

<u>Supplements:</u>

- Calcium and magnesium, 1000 mg/day to 500 mg/day, for osteoporosis prevention and also for calming effects;
- Vitamin E, 400 IU/day, as it helps diminish hot flashes and vaginal dryness;
- Flax seed oil, one tablespoon/day;
- Vitamin C with bioflavonoids, 1-3 g/day will help with collagen formation and diminish vessel wall weakness; helps relieve the hot flashes;
- Vitamin B complex, 100 mg/day is important for liver function and energy production;

- Natural hormone therapy, as prescribed (see your naturopath).

Other measures:
- Vitamin E oil capsule placed inside vagina may relieve the dryness;
- Valerian, hops, oats, lemon balm help with the anxiety and tension;
- Ginseng helps with alertness; gingko increases blood flow to brain;
- Chaste berry, angelica, black cohosh help regulate female hormones.

Note: our advice is to see a naturopath or a herbalist, as there are many helpful herbs; also, lately, commercial preparations indicated for menopause are becoming more and more popular.

♦GYNECOLOGIC CANCER

This will be a presentation of the most known gynecological cancers in a very summary form. The nutrition and holistic approach will follow the principles outlined in the chapter *Neoplasms.*

TYPE OF CANCER	PRESENTATION/COMMENTS
VAGINAL CANCER	Presents with vaginal bleeding and the lesion will be seen on vaginal exam; the biopsy confirms the diagnosis;
CERVICAL CANCER	
1. Cervical dysplasia:	Cellular abnormality proven by PAP smear; it may be a pre-cancerous lesion; Do suggest to your clients to see a naturopath, as cervical dysplasia benefits greatly from nutritional and natural therapy treatments.
2. Cervical carcinoma	Presents with abnormal uterine bleeding accompanied or not by vaginal discharge, the lesion may be seen, PAP smear is positive.
ENDOMETRIAL CANCER	Bleeding with menses and in between, estrogen dominance picture, diagnosis by endometrial biopsy;
OVARIAN CANCER	Leading cause of death due to cancer in women; few early symptoms, so difficult to assess; the bleeding irregularities are not remarkable; often, the first sign is abdominal swelling, which is not an early sign.

Table 19.7- Gynecologic cancer

Rule of thumb: upon any of the gynecological signs or symptoms presenting, do insist that your client will have a serious check-up

♦ BREAST DISORDERS

A. FIBROCYSTIC BREAST DISEASE (FBD)

**development of cysts in the breast tissues that are responsible for cyclic and usually bilateral changes;* they are an image of estrogen dominance; they are not considered pre-cancerous lesions, but the risk for developing breast cancer seems to be increased in cases with FBD (probably because it is difficult to assess a change in the lumps when they are multiple).

Etiology:

- All factors leading to estrogen dominance could be responsible;
- Increased caffeine intake may increase the risk because of the presence of methylxanthine, which promotes growth.

Clinical aspect:

- Painful breasts, usually bilaterally, because of the swelling of the cysts due to increased estrogen levels (higher in the first half of the cycle); breast tenderness decreases while on menses and appears the following month (cyclic pattern);
- The cysts are palpable (you can feel them), painful, soft, they move with the tissue underneath.

Nutrition and holistic approach:

- Apply the estrogen dominance protocol including the liver cleanse and support.

Supplements:

- Flax seed oil, 1-2 tablespoons a day (usually evening primrose oil is recommended, but use caution; if there is silent breast cancer, then evening primrose oil may accelerate its growth);
- Vitamin E, 400 IU/day, reduces pain and size of lumps; also vitamin A, 5000 IU /day;
- Vitamin C with bioflavonoids, 1-2 g/day;
- Vitamin B complex, 100 mg/day ;
- Lipotropic formula, as prescribed.

Other measures:

- Castor oil packs on breasts are soothing;
- Make sure you wear a well fitted bra as lymphatic drainage may be impeded by a constrictive bra;
- Marigold, marshmallow, nettles and yellow dock are helpful;
- Essential oils of geranium, juniper, lavender or rosemary are helpful.

B. BREAST CANCER

In most of the cases, it is an image of *estrogen dominance.*

Risk factors:

- Female, early onset of menstruation, late menopause, never breast fed, delayed child birth (see information under *Increased estrogen exposure*);
- Obesity, alcohol use, impaired liver and digestive system status;
- Family history;

- Chemical exposure, artificial hormone therapy.

Clinical appearance:
- Unilateral lump that changes shape and consistency, but not from one menses to the other; usually, the lump is not so soft;
- Lump does not move with the underlying tissue, non painful, possible bleeding/discharge from nipple;
- Skin dimpling, retracted nipple (these sign appear late in the evolution of the disease);
- Enlarged axillary (armpit) lymph nodes.

Nutrition and holistic approach:
- Employ *estrogen dominance approach* as presented;
- Apply the protocol outlined in the *Neoplasia* chapter.

The above-mentioned protocols are to be applied from a diet and supplements point of view.

Others:
- Essential oil of lavender encourages death of breast cancer cells;
- Green tea and shark cartilage may interfere with formation of new blood vessels (angiogenesis) that feed the tumor.

♦INFERTILITY
**inability to conceive over 12-18 months when regular and unprotected sex is present*

Causes:
- Genetic disorders, local trauma, cancer, chronic diseases, family history, medication, chemical and /or environmental exposure, history of PID, sexual transmitted disorders, endocrine diseases.
-

Lifestyle habits that can increase the risk for infertility

HABITS	EFFECTS ON WOMEN	EFFECTS ON MEN
Alcohol	Decreases estrogen and progesterone levels	Damages the liver and increases the estrogen levels
Smoking	Damages the liver	Damages the liver and it is toxic to the sperm, decreasing its motility
Stress	• Inhibits pituitary gland • Decreases levels of sex hormones • Damages the liver	
Eating habits	Anorexia/bulimia affect ovulation Obesity: creates conditions for estrogen dominance	

HABITS	EFFECTS ON WOMEN	EFFECTS ON MEN
Over exercise	May interfere with ovulation	May be associated with steroid use, which is associated with male infertility;
Personal hygiene	Repeated infections decrease mucus quality	Suggest they not wear tight underwear and sit too much, as it changes the local scrotal temperature (sperm cells need a lower temperature than the body temperature);
Sexual habits	• Lubricants may decrease mucus and survival time of sperm • Long abstinence or too frequent intercourse (for ability to conceive, it is being recommended to ejaculate at least once a month and to have intercourse every other day during the fertile period, as intercourse every day may decrease the amount of sperm per ejaculate).	

Table 19.8- Lifestyle factors that increase the risk of infertility

Nutrition and holistic approach: will apply to the cause of infertility; following you will find general considerations and suggestions:

- DETOXIFICATION! It is very important, as the body will need two **healthy** cells in order to create a new life; a toxic liver may definitely be in the way of conceiving (**if all medical causes have been assessed already**); do employ a sustained liver detoxification and abstain from conceiving while detoxifying, as circulating toxins may affect the cells of the new life; my son arrived following seven years of marriage after I did a two weeks fruit and vegetable detoxification program (and I thought that all that nausea was due to the detox program!);
- Diet and lifestyle counseling: encourage avoidance of dietary and lifestyle stressors and ensure that they focus on a healthy, natural, antioxidant and EFA rich diet.

<u>Supplements:</u>

- Vitamin E, 800 IU/day, as it regulates the cervical mucus production and is very important for sex hormones production;
- Vitamin B_6, 50 mg twice a day, for six months, as it seems to balance progesterone levels;
- Good multivitamin and mineral formula;
- Vitamin C with bioflavonoids, 1-2 g/day.

<u>Other measures:</u>

- Stress management is very important.

Note: In these cases, patience is the key; in the absence of medical causes, cleansing, detoxification and supplements can make a great improvement.

CHAPTER 20

THE MALE REPRODUCTIVE SYSTEM

No other system receives less attention from the health care practitioners than the male reproductive system. Men do not go to the doctor, and that's a given, even when they feel like there is no reason to live any more. They are even less than likely to go to have a check-up when it comes to the reproductive system. But they will probably tell somebody they love and trust that something is wrong. When you have a male client with a health problem pertaining to the reproductive system, please keep in mind how difficult it must have been for them to come and see you and how relieved they may feel when they hear that you can help them ...quite a bit. Here is how:

IMPORTANT NUTRIENTS FOR THE MALE REPRODUCTIVE SYSTEM

Nutrient	Role
Vitamin A	Protection of all mucus membranes
Vitamin C	Antioxidant, collagen formation
Vitamin B complex	Important for the energy pathways
Vitamin E	Deficiency may lead to infertility
Coenzyme Q10	Increases cellular oxygenation
Germanium	Increases cellular oxygenation
Magnesium	Relaxation of smooth muscle tonus
Molybdenum	Deficiency has been associated with erectile dysfunction
Selenium, with zinc and vitamin E	May help in prostate hypertrophy
Vanadium	Low levels have been associated with decreased reproductive function
Zinc	Vital for testosterone production and prostate health
Arginine	One of the components of the seminal fluid; indicated in infertility cases
Glycine	Maintains prostate health

Table 20.1- Important nutrients for the male reproductive system

Common symptoms/signs:

- Bladder urinary outlet obstruction: increased urinary frequency, nocturia (urination in the nighttime), interrupted flow
- Difficulty achieving or maintaining an errection;difficulty ejaculating;
- Burning and discomfort at urethra level
- Rarely, blood in urine, as a sign of prostate cancer.

ASSESSMENT

MEDICAL	NUTRITIONAL
1. Clinical examination, based on the signs and symptoms listed above	1. Dietary and supplemental analysis: to assess if the building blocks necessary for the development and maintance of the reproductive tract are provided
2. Physical examination: of possible malformations; of the size and aspect of the prostate gland (last one performed by rectal exam)	2. Digestive system status, as a malfunctioning digestive system may result in malnutrition and overloaded liver function (see preceding chapters)
3. PSA(Prostate specific antigen), which is a prostate cancer marker when elevated (just mild elevated values are not indicative of cancer; BPH is accompanied by low levels of PSA in a number of cases)	3. Liver status assessment, as a sluggish liver will not be able to process the necessary nutrients for the reproductive system; also, improper detoxification may result in increased levels of circulating toxins affecting the health of the reproductive system (especially infertility cases are susceptible to this aspect)
4. Ultrasound: for identification of possible prostate cancer	4. Immune system status, as an impaired immune system will not be able to properly eliminate abnormal cells, which may result in cancer formation
5. Biopsy, see under 4. above	
6. Sperm analysis, to assess its viability	

Table 20.2-Assessment of the male reproductive system

PATHOLOGY OF THE MALE REPRODUCTIVE SYSTEM

◆PROSTATE CONDITIONS

A. ACUTE BACTERIAL PROSTATITIS

**inflammation of the prostate gland, caused by retrograde infection*

Etiology: infectious; STD (sexually transmitted disease) related; usually preceded by a urinary tract infection that allowed germs to travel upwards and infect the prostate tissue

Clinical picture: fever, chills, pain, dysuria (pain/burning on urination), abdominal pain. It could progress towards chronic infection and/or urethral blockage.

Nutrition and holistic approach:

- increase water, antioxidant rich foods, fiber and essential fatty acids intake
- immune system boosting

Supplements:
- Vitamin C , 2-4 g/day, or up to bowel tolerance
- Vitamin A , 5000 IU/day
- Vitamin E , 400 IU/day
- Evening primrose oil, 500 mg three times/day
- Zinc, 25-40 mg/day
- Vitamin B complex , 50-100 mg/day

Others:
- Alfalfa, burdock, bearberry, goldenseal, garlic, Oregon grape, echinacea, marshmallow, slippery elm are all helpful

B. BENIGN PROSTATE HYPERTROPHY (BPH)
**enlarged, non tender/inflamed prostate*

Etiology:
- Hormonal changes associated with the age; it seems that there is an increased testosterone levels in the prostate gland and also increased conversion of testosterone into DHT (dehydrotestosterone), a potent form of testosterone; this conversion is catalyzed by an enzyme (5 alpha reductase); it also seems that increased estrogen levels in a male body slows down the elimination of DHT from the prostate gland, therefore creating the conditions for BPH ;
- Increased intake of saturated fat and alcohol, as the liver burden increases and the metabolism of hormones may be affected;
- Low zinc (very important in testosterone production) and low essential fatty acids status (allows for presence of inflammatory markers);
- Toxic exposure increases the activity of 5 alpha reductase

Clinical aspect:
- Urinary frequency and urgency (they seem the need to urinate "right now");
- Nocturia;
- Hesitancy and intermittency;
- Reduced force of urine.

All of the above are symptoms characteristic to the "*urinary outlet obstruction*", which means that the urethra is being pressed upon by the progressively increased size of the prostate gland

Diagnosis: by prostate exam and PSA levels (in almost half of the cases PSA levels are present but low, which does not signify the presence of cancer).

Nutrition and holistic approach:
- Avoid toxic exposure, alcohol, saturated fat intake;
- Increase intake of phytoestrogens (to encourage elimination of DHT from the prostate), antioxidant rich foods, essential fatty acids;
- Pumpkin seeds are rich in zinc; increase their intake;

- Higher good quality protein diet decreases the activity of 5 alpha reductase, diminishing testosterone conversion.

Supplements:

- Flax seed oil, one tablespoon/day;
- Zinc, 50 mg/day;
- Vitamin B complex , 50 mg/day; increases zinc absorption;
- Vitamin C with bioflavonoids, 1-2 g/day.

Others:

- Saw palmetto inhibits the testosterone conversion into DHT;
- Stinging nettle, horsetail, and watergrass are helpful;
- Flower pollen extract and Pygeum africanum seem to help the condition.

C. PROSTATE CANCER

**cancer of the prostate gland*

Etiology: cross reference *Neoplasia* chapter

Clinical aspect:

- Blood in urine;
- Painful urination, pain in lower back, pelvis and upper tights;
- PSA present and high.

Nutrition and holistic approach: cross reference *Neoplasia* chapter; Saw palmetto can be used as well

♦ERECTILE DYSFUNCTION

**inability to attain/maintain an erection.*

Etiology (any cause that affects the pelvic circulation)

1. Organic:
    - Vascular insufficiency (atherosclerosis, pelvic trauma);
    - Drugs, alcohol, tobacco use;
    - Endocrine disorders (diabetes, hypothyroidism);
    - Neurological disorders (multiple sclerosis).
2. Psychological/stress (as stress has vasoconstricting, narrowing effect)
    - Lack of desire;
    - Depression;
    - Fear of failure.

Nutrition and holistic approach:

- Stress and/or couple counselling, if appropriate;
- Decrease alcohol intake (whereas enhances the sexual desire, it hinders performance); smoking is a vasoconstrictor;
- Increase intake of fresh fruits of vegetables, fish oils, nuts and niacin rich foods(peanuts, yeast, wheat germ, avocado; niacin is a vasodilator);
- Erectile dysfunction may be affected by magnesium deficiency; increase intake of magnesium rich foods;
- Sesame seeds may enhance sexual vigour;
- Coriander is an aphrodisiac.

Supplements:

- Vitamin B complex, 50 mg/day;
- Zinc, 30-45 mg/day;
- Vitamin, A 5000 IU/day;
- Vitamin, C 1-2 g/day, as it strengthens the vascular wall;
- Vitamin E, 400 IU/day, is very important for the health of the reproductive system;
- Flax seed oil ,one tablespoon/day;
- Coenzyme Q10 and germanium, as they increase cell oxygenation;
- Arginine 250 mg/day; this aminoacid increases sperm count, sperm motility and male reproductive hormones production.

Others:

- Clove, ginger, cinnamon and cardamom are aphrodisiacs;
- Ginseng is a male tonic; gingko increases circulation;
- Potency wood (muira puama) is helpful; damiana is an aphrodisiac.

◆INFERTILITY

**inability to conceive a child after 6-12 months of unprotected sex in the absence of female causes.*

For "*Lifestyle habits that can increase the risk of infertility*", cross reference the *Gynecology* chapter

Etiology:

- Deficient sperm production/reduced sperm motility;
- Ductal obstruction (malformations, strictures);
- Ejaculatory dysfunctions;
- Inflammation/disorder of accessory glands;
- Hypothalamo-pityitary-axis disorders (affects FSH and LH);
- Free radical damage(affect sperm quality);

- Zinc deficiency(sperm production depends on testosterone levels, which depend on zinc levels).

Sperm-damaging factors:

- Increased scrotal temperature (sperm is produced at a lower temperature than the body's temperature; anything that increases scrotal temperature may affect sperm formation);
- Infections;
- Increased estrogen levels (will imbalance testosterone levels);
- Heavy metals (may affect the sperm quality).

Nutrition and holistic approach:

- Identify and approach appropriately etiologic factors and sperm damaging factors;
- EFA rich foods stimulate sex hormones production;
- Increase intake of pumpkin seeds.

Supplements:

- Vitamin B complex , 50 mg/day;
- Zinc , 30-45 mg/day;
- Flax seed oil ,one tablespoon/day;
- Vitamin E, 400 IU/day;
- Vitamin C with bioflavonoids, 1-2 g/day.

Others:

- Damiana and saw palmetto are the herbs of choice;
- Oats, lemon balm, chamomile are calming;
- Essential oil of rose may increase sperm count.

CHAPTER 21

SPECIAL SUBJECTS

♦CHRONIC FATIGUE SYNDROME

*long standing marked fatigue in the absence of physical or psychological causes

Etiology: multifactorial

- Unknown;
- Persistent viral infections (various agents have been nominated);
- Stress/low adrenal function;
- Weak/non-optimal immune system ;
- Pre-existing physical condition: cardio-vascular diseases, multiple sclerosis, diabetes, cancer, etc;
- Depression;
- Impaired liver function.

Clinical aspect

- New beginning of fatigue(they were all right before all these started)causing half reduction in activity for at least six months and exclusion of other causes of fatigue (these cases are thoroughly investigated, because the condition may mimic anything, from cancer to degenerative diseases); all clinical examinations, laboratory and imaging investigations will not find any cause of another disease; this is a diagnosis " *by exclusion*";
- Mild fever, sore throat, painful lymph nodes;
- Muscle weakness, muscle pain, joint pain;
- Prolonged fatigue after exercise/housework/any physical activity (usually they need more than a day of rest after doing even a mild activity; these cases learn a lot about their strength; they will plan their activities carefully);
- Headaches, poor memory and concentration;
- Sleep imbalances: insomnia or hypersomnia;
- Neurological problems: "pins and needles", difficulty performing certain fine tasks, etc.

Nutrition and holistic approach:

- Do your best to identify anything that could create an imbalance in the body, as this will add to an already overwhelmed organism: allergies, low stomach acid, candida, sluggish liver, malnutrition, etc; approach them carefully, as in these cases their balance is fragile: liver detoxification should be approached slowly, but sustained, adrenal gland support should be the center of your attention, etc;

Note: it is difficult to assess how a CFS case will progress/or regress; suffice to say that I have seen multiple cases that were **very much** improved by the dietary and nutritional measures.

- Carefully assess their nutritional status and take the appropriate measures (I have seen great results with intravenous vitamin and mineral therapy);
- Increase intake of oats, as they are calming; also increase intake of tryptophan rich foods;
- Avoid hypoglycemia;
- Remove , as much as possible, all dietary and lifestyle stressors; suggest they decrease their exposure to a polluted environment;
- Encourage an alkaline, healthy diet; increased water intake; increase intake of vitamin and mineral rich foods.

Supplements:

- Vitamin A, 5000IU/day; vitamin E, 400 IU/day; vitamin C with bioflavonoids, 1-3 g/day;
- Multivitamin and mineral formula;
- Flax seed oil, one tablespoon/day;
- Green food supplements, as prescribed;
- Vitamin B complex , 100 mg/day;
- Calcium and magnesium, 800-1000 mg/day to 400-500 mg/day;
- Digestive enzymes and probiotics, according to the condition.

Others:

- Licorice, ginseng, as they support the adrenal function;
- Chamomile, lemon balm and passion flower are calming;
- Essential oils of bergamot, rose and neroli are soothing.

CHAPTER 22

PSYCHIATRIC DISORDERS

Psychiatry is defined as the branch of medicine dealing with the study, diagnosis and treatment of mental illnesses. What is the mind? It is defined as the psyche; the brain function by which we are aware of what surrounds us, and by which we experience feelings, emotions and desires.

We can approach a client from a medical point of view, from a nutritional point of view; or from an herbalist's point of view…but sometimes signs and symptoms of a disease are just physical images of a psychiatric disorder. Does she lose weight? Maybe she is on a diet, maybe she is anorexic. Does she become irritable? Maybe she is hypoglycemic, but maybe she is anxious…does she become easily depressed? Maybe it is her thyroid; maybe it is a deep sense of loss…

Allow us to present, in the following chapter, an array of psychiatric disorders and their nutritional approaches.

IMPORTANT NUTRIENTS FOR BRAIN FUNCTION

Nutrient	Role
Thiamin (vitamin B_1)	Supports cognitive activity and brain function;
Riboflavin (vitamin B_2)	Needed for tryptophan metabolism;
Niacin (vitamin B_3)	Helpful in cases with Schizophrenia; memory enhancer;
Pantothenic acid (vitamin B_5)	"The anti stress vitamin"; neurotransmitter synthesis; helpful for depression and anxiety;
Pyridoxine (vitamin B_6)	Needed for normal brain function, as it is involved in sodium potassium balance, red blood cells formation and nucleic acids synthesis;
Vitamin B_{12}	Acetylcholine synthesis; aides in memory and learning;
Biotin	Important in fatty acids production, thus important for the brain cell membrane;
Choline	Part of acetylcholine; indicated in Parkinson disease;
Folic acid	Helpful for depression and anxiety; it is considered a "brain food";
Inositol	Has a calming effect; important in lecithin synthesis;
PABA	Indicated in depression;
Vitamin C	Required for anti-stress hormones synthesis; strong antioxidant;
Coenzyme Q10	Increases oxygen uptake in the cells;
Calcium	Transmission of nerve impulse; it has calming effects;
Germanium	Increases cellular oxygenation;

Nutrient	Role
Magnesium	Deficiency leads to irritability and nervousness;
Glutamine	"Brain fuel"; in the brain tissue, glutamine turns into glutamic acid, vital for brain function;
Phenylalanine	Precursor of dopamine and norepinephrine;
Taurine	Has protective effects on the brain; used in anxiety treatment;
Tryptophan	Precursor for serotonin;
EFA	Essential for the brain cells membranes;

Table 22.1-Important nutrients for brain function

ASSESSMENT OF MENTAL STATUS

MEDICAL ASSESSMENT	NUTRITIONAL ASSESSMENT
1. Level of consciousness: refers to alertness and the person's state of awareness of the environment; 2. Attention: ability to focus or concentrate over time on one task and activity; 3. Memory: capacity of storing information • Short term memory: memory over an interval of minutes, hours or days • Long term memory: refers to intervals of years; 4. Orientation: depends on both memory and attention, in relation to time, space and other people; 5. Perception: awareness of the objects in the environment and their qualities and interrelationships; 6. Thought process: refers to sequence, logic, coherence and relevance of a person's thought as it leads to selected goals; describes how people think Thought content: refers to what people think about; 7. Affect and mood 8. Language, speech difficulties/impairment	1. Liver function: an overloaded liver will allow for exacerbations of psychiatric diseases, via toxicity; 2. Digestive system status, as malnutrition will deplete the CNS of its nutrients; 3. Heavy Metal Toxicity testing, as heavy metals with brain affinity may interfere with various brain functions; 4. Hypoglycemia status assessment, hypoglycemia will increase irritability and will allow for increased frequency of panic attacks, depression and disorientation; 5. Free radical status assessment, free radicals have been involved in some psychiatric disorders etiology; 6. Adrenal gland function assessment, as low adrenal function may result in anxiety and depression exacerbations.

Table 22.2-Assessment of the mental function

Common symptoms are described below:

Abnormalities of thought content:

1. Compulsions: repetitive behaviors or mental acts that a person feels the absolute need to perform in order to produce or prevent something that may happen in the future, although expectations of such an outcome are utterly unrealistic;

2. Obsessions: recurrent, uncontrollable thoughts, images or drives that a person considers unacceptable fearful or not belonging to him/her;

3. Phobias: persistent, irrational fears accompanied by a strong desire to do everything in their power to avoid the particular stimulus;

4. Anxieties: apprehension, feelings of intense fear, tension, uneasiness that may be focused (phobia) or generalized (a sense of not so clear dread or impending doom);

5. Delusions: false, difficult to change personal beliefs that are not shared by any other person in the nearby vicinity (family, social group, etc); the culture may consider those beliefs to be completely unrealistic or fantasies.

Abnormalities of perception:

1. Illusions: misinterpretation of real external stimuli;

2. Hallucinations: subjective sensory perceptions in the absence of relevant external stimuli: visual, auditory, olfactory, gustatory, tactile or somatic.

Physical disorders that have psychiatric/psychological symptoms:

- HIV, burn sequelae, cancer, CFS, congenital anomalies, fibromyalgia, impotence, irritable bowel syndrome, pain, sleep disorders, stroke, terminal illness, transplantation issues (they may present with depression, anxiety, panic attacks).

Psychiatric or psychological disorders that have physical symptoms:

- ADHD, alcohol and drug abuse, anxiety, bipolar disorder, depression, eating disorder, schizophrenia (they may present with headache, palpitations, sweating, etc.).

♦ PSYCHOTIC DISORDERS

SCHIZOPHRENIA (means "splitting of the mind")
**disorder with a minimum of 6-month duration that is characterized by an active psychotic phase* with two or more of the following symptoms present for at least one month:

- Delusions
- Hallucinations
- Disorganized speech
- Disorganized behavior

Etiology theories:

- Heredity;
- Abnormal neurotransmitter function;
- Free radical damage; environmental toxins;
- Possible childhood head injuries and/or birth trauma;
- Nutritional theories: high copper levels, which implies that a zinc deficiency may be underlying the problem;
- Hypoglycemia;
- "Cerebral allergy", due to increased histamine levels in a person with multiple allergies;
- Abnormal adrenal function, which allows cortisol release; in turn, in high quantities, cortisol affects the brain;
- EFA deficiency.

Nutrition and holistic approach:

- Identify the cause of the condition and take appropriate measures: food allergies, hypoglycemia, nutritional deficiencies, etc.;
- Ensure proper function of the liver, digestive tract and immune system;
- Increase flax seed oil intake, as it will turn into prostaglandins which help regulate neurocircuits;
- Increase intake of foods containing B vitamins, as they support the nervous system function;
- Carrots and cabbage are good sources of glutamine, which stimulates mental alertness and helps soothe abnormal behaviour;
- Avoid saturated fat, alcohol and smoking, which will make the condition worse.

Supplements:

- Vitamin B complex, 50-100mg /day;
- Vitamin C with bioflavonoids, 2 g/day;
- Flax seed oil, two tablespoons a day;
- Magnesium , 500 mg/day;
- Multivitamin and multimineral complex, as prescribed;
- Niacinamide 1-2 g/day; monitor liver enzymes.

Others:

- Gingko biloba and St. John's wort are helpful;
- Essential oils of chamomile, lavender and lemon balm are calming.

♦ MOOD DISTURBANCES

**mood means the emotional state in which ones lives for a period of time*

A. DEPRESSION

*when *five or more of the following present during the same two weeks period, different from previous levels of functioning;* the depressive episodes repeat, separated by two or more months;

- Depressed mood (irritability in children/adolescents);
- Decreased interest in most activities on a daily basis;
- Significant weight loss/gain when not on a diet;
- Sleep disturbances: insomnia or hypersomnia;
- Fatigue;
- Feelings of not being worthy or inappropriate guilt;
- Diminished ability to think, concentrate or make decisions;
- Recurrent thoughts of dying or suicide (beyond just fear of dying);
- Work, social or other areas of functioning significantly impaired.

Etiology:

- Psychological factors: when a person has to face loss, either of status, hope, self esteem, loss of somebody they loved; this sense of loss can be exacerbated by persistent pessimistic feelings;
- Neurotransmitters chemical imbalance (serotonin deficiency);
- Pre-existing medical condition: cancer, multiple sclerosis, chronic pain, diabetes, etc.;
- Hypothyroidism, defects in adrenal hormones regulation (increased cortisol will affect brain chemistry, by reducing the amount of tryptophan reaching the brain);
- Environmental toxins with nervous system affinity (heavy metals, solvents, pesticides);
- Smoking and alcohol abuse will affect the adrenal gland, the liver and the immune system;
- Hypoglycemia;
- Food allergies;
- Nutritional imbalances of folic acid and vitamin B_{12}, vitamin B_6 and EFA.

Nutrition and holistic approach:

- Very important: identify and manage appropriately: food allergies (in some cases it may result in depression, fatigue, muscle and joint pain, lack of concentration), liver toxic status, digestive system status;
- Avoid stressors: saturated fat (as it will displace the beneficial EFA molecules from the brain cell's membrane), refined carbohydrates, coffee, smoking, alcohol and stress itself;
- Increase intake of fruits and vegetables, grains and fish;
- Increase tryptophan rich foods.

<u>Supplements:</u>

- Good source multivitamin and mineral complex;
- Vitamin B complex, 100 mg/day;
- Folic acid and vitamin B_{12} , 800 mcg of each/day;
- Vitamin C and bioflavonoids, 2-3 g/day, or up to bowel tolerance;
- Flax seed oil one tablespoon/day.

Other measures:

- Lemon balm, vervain, limeflower, oats, borage and rosemary are helpful;
- St. John's wort is very useful; consult a herbalist before taking;
- Essential oils of jasmine, geranium, melissa, rose, lavender and sage are helpful;
- Meditation, hobbies, relaxation techniques, massages;
- Learn a positive attitude!

B. MANIA

**period lasting at least one week, with presence of abnormally elevated, expansive or irritable mood.*

Two or three of the following must be present:

- Exaggerated self esteem or grandiosity;
- Decreased need for sleep;
- Excessively loquacious/ talkative;
- Flight of ideas or feeling of thoughts racing;
- Easily distracted;
- Increase in goal-oriented activity;
- Work or social functioning significantly impaired;
- Difficulty assessing a situation correctly (excessive spending, wrong financial decisions).

C. BIPOLAR DISORDER (Manic Depression)

**mania alternating with depression* (the timing and cycling of the episodes varies)

The following aspects of **Etiology and **Nutritional and holistic approach** apply to mania aspect of the bipolar disorder only, as depression has been approached previously.

Etiology:

- Biochemical imbalances (tryptophan deficiency, phosphatidylcholine (the fat in our brain cell's membrane, that increases the brain activity for acetylcholine)deficiency;
- Nutritional imbalances: increased vanadium levels;
- Adrenal gland overexertion.

All bipolar disorder trends are much accentuated by stress exposure and /or exposure to coffee, smoking and alcohol.

Nutrition and holistic approach:

- Do employ all general measures outlined in *Depression*;
- Increased raw fruit and vegetables diet, as it seems to lower vanadium levels;
- Increase intake of tryptophan rich foods.

Supplements:

- Good source vitamin and mineral formula;
- Flax seed oil, one tablespoon/day;
- Vitamin C, 3-5 g/day, or up to bowel tolerance, in divided doses, as it seems to play a role in displacing vanadium;

- Vitamin B complex, 100 mg/day;
- Calcium and magnesium, 800 mg/day, respectively, 400 mg/day, as they have a calming effect and stabilize mood swings.

♦ COGNITIVE MENTAL DISORDERS

A. DEMENTIA

a mental syndrome characterized by a general loss of intellectual abilities (memory, judgment, personality), but not including depression or other functional disorder;

B. SENILE DEMENTIA

dementia appearing in old age

For A and B, the **classical symptoms** are:

- Memory impairment;
- In the beginning, insomnia, loss of interest, apathy;
- Cognitive disorder: not knowing where they are in terms of place and time;
- Deficits cause significant impaired social or work functioning;
- Gradual onset with continuing cognitive decline.

C. ALZHEIMER'S DISEASE

*a *degenerative brain disorder manifesting clinically as dementia, somehow characteristic EEG pattern (not yet proven) and distinctive brain tissue changes (definitive diagnosis is post mortem).*

*more prevalent in females than males.

Etiology theories:

- Genetic involvement (the presence of a " weak gene" on chromosome 21);
- Possible previous head trauma;
- Environmental toxicity (aluminum and/or mercury exposure) and free radical damage;
- Abnormal magnesium metabolism: magnesium competes with aluminum for absorption ;
- Nutritional deficiencies: EFA and/or nutrients that are responsible for producing neurotransmitters; also, low antioxidant status may contribute to the development of the disease;
- Arteriosclerosis: linked to decreased blood flow to the brain tissue.

Clinical aspect:

1. <u>Early stage:</u>

- The decline starts and progresses gradually, beginning with short term memory loss;
- Language problems, inability to perform normal, regular tasks, in the absence of a motor impairment;
- In time, confusion and disorientation appear; wandering away without knowing where they are and why are they there (cognitive impairment);
- Personality changes: anger, paranoia, depression.

2. Intermediate stage:
    - Personality changes accentuate: more aggressiveness, agitation, hostility;
    - Loss of sense of time and space;
    - Still ambulatory (able to move on their own), but signs of physical impairment start showing up: increased risk for falls and accidents.

3. Late stage:

- Physical deterioration present: inability to perform any activity necessary for their living; incontinence; inability to swallow and eat;
- Neurological signs start showing up (localized motor and/or sensory impairment);
- Complete memory loss; complete dependence on others;
- Coma and death, usually from infections.

Diagnosis:

- Clinical aspect; please, keep in mind that, at least in the first stages, Alzheimer's very much resembles Dementia, and a differential diagnosis between the above mentioned two is difficult;
- Usually, the diagnosis is by exclusion: all other causes of dementia (substance abuse, medications, toxic exposure, tumors, trauma, metabolic conditions, infections, vascular) are to be investigated by medical history, physical examination and laboratory testing;
- EEG seems to be somehow characteristic in Alzheimer;
- Abnormal fingerprints pattern;
- Post mortem: brain tissue modifications, like neurofibrillary tangles and senile plaques (agglomerations of devitalized tissue and proteins); also loss of neurons.

Nutrition and holistic approach:

- Sustained body support: mild liver detoxification; identification of possible allergies and/or nutritional abnormalities followed by correction;
- Digestive system and immune system status assessment; appropriate measures, if necessary;
- Avoid toxic and environmental additional exposure;
- Commence antioxidant rich diet;
- Increase intake of sulfur containing foods for detoxification purposes;
- Lecithin, as a building block for neurotransmitters (found in egg yolks, soy, cauliflower, cabbage, fish).

Supplements:

- Vitamin B complex , 50-100 mg/day;
- Vitamin B_{12}, 1000 mcg once or twice a day, as it is vital (along with folic acid) for the functioning of the nerves;
- Thiamin (vitamin B_1) seems to have a good effect in improving acetylcholine function;
- Vitamin C, 2-3 g/day associated with a good antioxidant complex;
- Zinc, 30-45 mg/day;
- Flax seed oil, one to two tablespoons/day.

Others:

- Gingko biloba, as it increases circulation to the brain;
- Ginseng powder, added to herbal teas, as it improves memory;
- Rosemary is a nervous tonic, especially for the elderly population;
- Orange blossoms are helpful in cases with confusion and depression;
- Geranium essential oil regulates the nervous system.

◆ANXIETY DISORDERS

**a feeling of fear and apprehension without an apparent clear cause;* associated with physiological changes (fast heart beat, sweating, etc);

Etiology:

- Stress overload; over stimulation;
- Increased toxic and/or environmental exposure;
- Physical illness (hyperthyroidism);
- Substance abuse (stimulants, drugs, etc.);
- Carbohydrate metabolism abnormalities: hypoglycemia, abnormal accumulation of lactic acid (some of the causes for this are: excessive coffee and alcohol intake, calcium, magnesium and vitamins B deficiency);
- EFA deficiency.

Types of anxiety disorders:

A. AGORAPHOBIA

**anxiety about being in open spaces, lack of boundaries;* fear of having a panic attack in such a situation. The place that initiates anxiety is avoided.

B. PANIC DISORDERS

**recurrent, unexpected panic attacks*

Panic attacks: brief periods of intense fear/discomfort, due to the fight or flight sympathetic response, including at least four of the following:

- Palpitations/tachycardia;
- Shaking, shortness of breath, choking feeling;
- Chest pain/discomfort; (frequently confused with heart attack);
- Nausea/abdominal upset;
- Dizziness, fear of losing control, fear of dying;
- Paresthesias, chills/hot flushes;

*at least one attack followed by one month or more of worry about getting into a similar situation

C. SOCIAL ANXIETY DISORDER

- Severe, persistent fear that one will act in a humiliating way in a social or performance situation; they know that fear does not have a clear supportive cause;
- Situation causing the fear is avoided at any length;
- This situation affects work/social life;
- Lasts for six or more months;

D. GENERALIZED ANXIETY DISORDER

- Excessive worry most days for six months or more about various aspects (money, job, health, love, etc.);
- Controlling the worry becomes a struggle;
- Three or more of the following anxiety-associated symptoms: restlessness, becomes tired easily, problems with concentration, irritability, muscle tension, insomnia;
- Worry causes significant work or social impairment;

E. POST-TRAUMATIC STRESS DISORDER

- Traumatic event occurred, which the person was part of;
- The event is persistently experienced in one or more of the following: recurrent images, thoughts, upsetting dreams;
- Intense distress when the person is exposed to a situation that reminds him/her of the traumatic event; they will avoid these situations at all costs;
- Increased symptoms of: insomnia, irritability, anger.

F. OBSESSIVE-COMPULSIVE DISORDER

- **Obsessions:** recurrent, persistent thoughts or images that can cause severe anxiety; for a while the person tries to ignore them somehow; the obsessions are the product of the person's own mind;
- **Compulsions:** overwhelming need to perform repeated actions/thoughts; are meant to avoid distress;
- At some point, the person recognizes the obsessions/compulsions as being unreasonable;
- O/C causes severe distress, consumes more than one hour daily and interferes with work/social life.

Nutrition and holistic approach for Anxiety Disorders:

Firstly keep in mind that the cause of the condition should be investigated and approached before implementing any specific remedies;

Secondly, but not less important, the invaluable contribution of good counseling for anxiety disorders must be emphasized; I have treated many cases of anxiety and panic attacks and whereas my combined nutrition and herbal approach has been extremely beneficial, the cases that benefited from serious counseling progressed undeniably, much better.

- Stress and toxic abuse greatly disturb the detoxification pathways and allow circulating toxins to harm us; therefore, employ a serious cause assessment and approach (liver, immune system, digestive system, carbohydrate metabolism);
- Avoid stimulants and excessive sugar and saturated fat intake;
- Employ a clean, healthy, supportive diet comprising of fresh fruits and vegetables, fish, grains and nuts;
- Increase the oats intake (rich in vitamins B_1 and B_5), as they are quite soothing and nourishing for the nervous system;
- Hazelnuts are a healing food for the nervous system.

Supplements:

- Vitamin B complex, 50 mg twice a day, as they support the health of the nervous system;
- Calcium and magnesium, 800 mg to 400 mg/day, as they have relaxant properties;
- Vitamin C and bioflavonoids, 2 g/day;
- Flax seed oil, one tablespoon a day;
- Good multivitamin and mineral complex.

Other measures are very helpful:

- Oats, hops, lavender, valerian, chamomile, lemon balm, passion flower or linden are excellent as teas or in a bath (ask a herbalist for advice on how to mix herbs);
- Essential oils of lavender, chamomile or lemon balm are very soothing;
- Relaxation, meditation, hobbies, support groups.

♦ EATING DISORDERS

**Disturbed (unusual, unhealthy) eating behaviours, generally accompanied by an excessive preoccupation with food and self body image;*

- high mortality rate (from suicide, metabolic problems or heart failure).

Etiology:

- Social pressure, peer pressure, fear of growing up, abuse;
- Psychological problems, self acceptance, children-parents' relationships, inter-partners relationships, tendency to a negative approach to situations and relationships (CNC: confirmed negativity condition);
- Nutritional deficiencies: zinc, serotonin.

BULIMIA * ***recurrent binge eating followed by inappropriate efforts to overcome the weight gain***	**ANOREXIA**** * ***disturbed sense of body image with abnormal fear of obesity***	**BINGE EATING DISORDER (COMPULSIVE OVEREATING)** * ***periods of binge eating or continuous overeating alternating with periods of fasting or dieting***
Recurrent binge eating more than two times per week for at least three months; Recurrent fasting, purging, excessive exercise; Excessive concern over body weight/shape; Addiction, remorse, guilt; Usually of normal weight; Metabolic disorders (electrolyte disturbance), Erosion of dental enamel, esophageal lesions, fatigue, muscle aches, chronic sore throat	Prevalent in adolescence and in females; Self starvation; extreme weight loss; Amenorrhea; Body weight less than 85% of expected body weight; Intense fear of weight gain; Inaccurate perception of body size; Addiction to control; obsession with food; Low heart beat, low BP (blood pressure), hypothermia, dehydration, malnutrition.	Continuous overeating, even when not hungry; not followed by purging; Sense of being unable to control eating; Periods of dieting or fasting; Occurs mostly in obese people.

Table 22.3 – Description of eating disorders

**rare in areas with food shortage; sometimes hospitalization for restoration of body weight

Treatment will vary depending on the individual circumstances. There is no one single treatment that has proven to be effective in all cases. Treatment aims to:

- Restore the person to a healthy weight;
- Restore healthy eating patterns;
- Treat any physical complications or associated mental health problems;
- Address thoughts, feelings and beliefs concerning food and body image;
- Enlist family support.

Nutrition and holistic approach:

- In the beginning, do not focus on diet diary or discussions about food and nutrition; work on building trust;
- If possible, avoid stimulants, excessive sugar;

- Focus on a diet as healthy as possible, with fruits, vegetables, grains, nuts;
- Increase intake of tryptophan containing foods;
- Bananas, walnuts and pineapple contain serotonin;
- Pumpkin and sunflower seeds contain zinc;
- Green drinks, if they are accepted.

<u>Supplements:</u> at this point, just do your best; they may refuse any supplement intake, but if they are receptive to your suggestions, here is a list:

- A good multivitamin and mineral complex, preferably in liquid form for absorption purposes;
- Zinc, 45-50 mg/day;
- Flax seed oil, one tablespoon/day.

<u>Others:</u>

- Definitely counseling;
- Teas of chamomile, gentian and mint may help increase the appetite;
- Stinging nettle is a good, nutrient rich herb;
- St. John's Wort may help in dealing with the feelings associated with these conditions;
- Ginseng will help energy levels; also, it is a rejuvenator;
- Take everything in small, but sure steps.

♦ PEDIATRIC DISORDERS

A. ATTENTION DEFICIT DISORDER

* *persistent patterns of inattention, and/or hyperactivity/impulsivity;*

* six or more of the following symptoms persisting for at least six months to a degree that is inconsistent with developmental level

1. <u>Inattention:</u>

- Difficulty sustaining attention in given tasks or play;
- Does not seem to listen when spoken to;
- Fails to finish chores, homework, duties;
- Difficulty organizing tasks and activities;

2. <u>Hyperactivity:</u>

- Fidgets with hands or feet and/or squirms in seat;
- Restlessness;
- Has difficulty playing or engaging in activities quietly;
- Talks excessively.

3. Impulsivity:

- Bursts out answers before questions have been completed;
- Has difficulty awaiting turn;
- Interrupts others.

TYPES:
1. ADD (Attention Deficit Disorder)
2. ADD with Hyperactivity

Etiology:

ADD	ADD with hyperactivity
• Chronic infections: especially otitis, which may result in hearing loss and impaired speech • Nutrient deficiency: any of the nutrients listed in the beginning of this chapter • Anemia: by impeding the cellular oxygenation with subsequent diminishing of the cellular functions • Heavy Metals: especially lead and mercury • Birth trauma, premature birth	• Food additives excess • Food sensitivities • Excessive sugar intake • Nutritional imbalances: magnesium and calcium • Possible imbalance of neurotransmitters (norepinephrine)

Table 22.4-ADD-etiology

Nutrition and holistic approach will apply to the cause of the condition
- Strongly avoid food additives, exposure to environmental toxins, excessive refined sugar intake or saturated fat;
- Employ, as much as possible a diet rich in fruits and vegetables, fish, nuts, grains;
- Aspartame is a neurotoxin; keep it out of the diet;
- Increase vitamin C and antioxidant rich foods; vitamin C is a weak chelator and it will bind and eliminate heavy metals; chlorella has the same effect;
- Coconut milk seems to help hyperactive children;
- Increase intake of zinc rich foods, as it helps with memory and learning problems; also, zinc deficiency can lead to hyperactivity

Supplements:
- A good multivitamin and mineral formula;
- Evening Primrose Oil (EPO), as prescribed, according to age;
- Calcium and magnesium, as prescribed, according to age.

Others:
- Counseling is very important and the whole family should try to get involved;
- Herbs like: oats, chamomile, lemon balm and passion flower are soothing and calming;
- Food allergy testing and heavy metals presence assessment are very important.

B. AUTISM

obvious abnormal or impaired development from a social and communication aspect; restricted level of activities and interests

*has a total of six or more items from the following categories:

1. Impairment in social interactions:

- Difficulty to look someone in the eyes;
- Failure to develop peer relationships according to age;
- Does not attempt to share enjoyment, interests, achievements;
- Lack of social or emotional reciprocity.

2. Impairment in communication:

- Delay or total lack of development in spoken language;
- Impairment in the ability to start or sustain a conversation ;
- Repetitive use of language;

3. Repetitive and stereotyped patterns of behavior, interests and activities:

- Always repeats the same activities and/or rituals;
- Repetitive movements.

Etiology theories
- Heavy metal and/or environmental toxicity;
- Weak immune system;
- Certain vaccinations;
- Malnutrition;
- Allergies;

Nutrition and holistic approach:
- Do try to identify a causative factor, and proceed accordingly;
- Approach digestive system status as nutritional deficiencies have been considered in the etiology of the condition;
- Employ a gluten*/casein free diet, as the literature suggests; improvements upon following it (it seems that children with very early autism have a problem with casein, whereas children with later development autism have difficulties with gluten; if the diet does not improve the situation within three months, we should look at factors other than nutrition);
- Wild lettuce is calming; so are oats.

*Gluten: protein in wheat, oats, barley, rye.

Supplements:

- Good multivitamin and mineral formula;
- Vitamin B complex, C, magnesium and EFA should be supplied according to age.

APPENDIX "A-1"

INFECTIOUS DISEASES

RESPIRATORY INFECTIONS

Disease	Pathogen	Transmission	Clinical aspect	Others
Viral respiratory infections	Rhinoviruses; (common cold) Influenza viruses;	Airborne	Varies: acute/chronic, sneezing, coughing, fever;	Can progress to bronchitis or pneumonia;
Bacterial respiratory infections	Many pathogens: pneumoccocus, haemophilus;	Airborne	Varies, pneumonia.	

GASTRO-INTESTINAL INFECTIONS

Disease	Pathogen	Transmission	Clinical aspect	Others
Viral enteritis	Rotavirus, Norwalk;	Fecal-oral	Diarrhea, nausea, vomiting;	
Bacterial enteritis	Shigella, Yersinia;	Fecal-oral	Bloody diarrhea with pus and mucus, abdominal cramps and tenesmus;	
Salmonellosis and Typhoid fever	Salmonella	Fecal-oral	Fever, nausea, watery diarrhea with pus;	
Amebiasis	Entamoeba histolytica;	Fecal-oral	Abdominal pain, fever, inflammation and abscesses;	"Traveler's diarrhea", commonly seen in AIDS.

PYOGENIC* BACTERIAL INFECTIONS

*pus forming

Disease	Pathogen	Transmission	Clinical aspect	Others
Staphylococcal infections	Staphylococcus aureus	Skin lesions; Respiratory droplets; Contaminated food;	Skin infections, food poisoning, Toxic Shock Syndrome, Endocarditis;	

APPENDIX "A-2"

INFECTIOUS DISEASES

SEXUALLY TRANSMITTED DISEASES

Disease	Pathogen	Transmission	Clinical aspect	Others
Genital herpes	Herpes virus	Sexually;Childbirth;	Outbreaks of vesicles, pruritus;	
Gonorrhea	Neisseria gonorrhea;	Sexually;	Male purulent urethritis, external genitalia abscesses in women;	Complications: PID, Salpingitis, urethral strictures and sterility;
Trichomoniasis	Trichomonas vaginalis;	Sexually	"strawberry mucosa";	Can be mildly symptomatic in men.

CHILDHOOD AND ADOLESCENCE DISEASES

Disease	Pathogen	Transmission	Clinical aspect	Others
Measles	Paramyxovirus;	Airborne	Fever, runny nose, sneezing, maculo-papular rash;	More serious than rubella;
Mumps (parotiditis)	Mumps virus	Airborne	Enlargement of parotid glands;	Complications: meningitis, orchitis, pancreatitis, encephalitis;
Mononucleosis	Epstein-Barr virus	Direct contact	Fever, sore throat lymphadenopathy, splenomegaly;	Young adults and adolescents;
Poliomyelitis	Polio virus	Fecal-oral	Necrosis of anterior horns of spinal cord: paralysis;	Rare
Chicken pox and Shingles	Varicella zoster virus;	Airborne Direct contact	**Chicken pox:** itchy peripheral rash **Shingles:** painful neuralgia	
Whooping Cough	Bordetella pertussis;	Airborne	Spasmodic cough, stridor in infants	
Diphteria	Corynebacterium diphteriae;	Airborne	Pseudo membrane formation, stridor, barking cough;	Can be fatal in infants

APPENDIX "A-3"

INFECTIOUS DISEASES

OPPORTUNISTIC AND AIDS-ASSOCIATED DISEASES

(infections that are normally dormant, appear with increased frequency in hosts with impaired immune system).

Disease	Pathogen	Transmission	Clinical aspect	Others
Pseudomonas infection	Pseudomonas aeruginosa;	Multiple	Pneumonia with necrosis; Swimmer's ear; osteomyelitis and endocarditis in drug users;	Involved in hospital infections;
Candidiasis	Candida albicans	Normal body flora; can be directly introduced in the body;	Thrush, vaginal candidiasis, diaper rash;	Frequent in immuno-compromised.

ZOONOTIC AND VECTOR-BORNE INFECTIONS

Disease	Pathogen	Transmission	Clinical aspect	Others
Rickettsial infections	Rickettsia	**Q fever**: tick **Thyphus**: direct contact (lice);	Typhus: rash, organ hemorrhages, enteritis; **Q fever**: interstitial pneumonitis;	
Lyme disease	Borrelia burgdoferi	Ticks	Disseminated annular rash, neurologic and cardiac symptoms;	Later, arthritic, MS and CNS involvement;
Malaria	Plasmodium	Mosquito bite	Periodic fever attacks	Liver, spleen and CNS involvement.

APPENDIX "B"

HEAVY METAL TOXICITY

Unfortunately and undeniably, since the Industrial revolution in late 19th century, we have all been exposed to a toxic and increasingly polluted world. Whereas not widely accepted as very harmful, environmental toxicity influences our lives more and more every day.
Some of these pollutants are heavy metals. The most widely abused and able to be tested are: **aluminum, antimony, arsenic, barium, beryllium, bismuth, cadmium, lead, mercury and silver.**

There is no metabolic function in a human body that may require the presence of these metals. They are considered to be toxic at any concentrations in the body and cause a vast array of psychological and physiological disturbances: headache, fatigue, muscle pain, indigestion, tremors, constipation, anemia, pallor, dizziness, poor coordination, short and long term memory loss, poor concentration, intellectual decline, irritability, fits of anger, depression, drowsiness, insomnia. Other signs and symptoms of heavy metal toxicity are: abdominal cramps, constipation or diarrhea, colitis, arrhythmia, alteration in blood pressure, dizziness, tinnitus, fine tremors, paresthesia ("pins and needles" sensation).

Heavy metal toxicity assessment:

1. Clinical appearance (as listed above);
2. Hair analysis (heavy metals may accumulate in the hair shaft);
3. Urine testing (heavy metals are eliminated via urine).

Heavy metal detoxification protocol:

1. High protein diet as the sulfur containing amino acids in the protein will facilitate detoxification;
2. Probiotics: it is vital to have a proper bowel flora for detoxification;
3. Increased fiber intake, because you should have two to three bowel movements per day (Freshly ground flax seed several teaspoons per day will help intestinal transit and also contribute beneficial essential fatty acids;.
4. Chlorella is an important part of the detoxification program, as a high amount of the heavy metals in our bodies is eliminated through the stool. Chlorella is an algae that has high levels of chlorophyll and other nutrients;
5. Ensure appropriate levels of stomach acid, as it will be very difficult to ionize mineral supplements to absorb them properly in the absence of hydrochloric acid;
6. Garlic, ideally fresh, but supplemental form is acceptable as well;
7. Cilantro will help mobilize mercury out of the tissue;
8. Mineral formula ; it seems that when you are deficient in magnesium, sodium, zinc and other minerals, the body, which has to work with something at least resembling a mineral, does not let go of the toxic metals very easily;
9. Essential fatty acids;
10. Antioxidant formula, containing vitamins E and C (vitamin C is a weak chelator itself) and Selenium;
11. Ensure liver and gall bladder health;
12. Chelation therapy (see Appendix H).

APPENDIX "C"

VITAMINS DEFICIENCIES, CONTRAINDICATIONS, INTERACTIONS

NUTRIENT	DEFICIENCY	CONTRAINDICATIONS/ TOXICITY	MISCELLANEOUS/ INTERACTIONS
VITAMIN C	Scurvy, delayed wound healing, reduced resistance to infections;	High doses can cause diarrhea and abdominal pain;	Caution when administered along with blood thinners Alcohol and smoking may decrease levels;
THIAMIN (B1)	Beriberi	Not significant	Not significant
RIBOFLAVIN (B2)	Associated with red and burning eyes, glossitis and decreased neurotransmitters function;	Not significant	Alcohol intake decreases absorption; use of antidepressants may increase riboflavin requirements;
NIACIN(B3)	Pellagra	Flushing, itching; not present with Niacinamide form; may increase liver enzymes;	May increase vasodilation;
VITAMIN B5	Not significant	Possible diarrhea in large doses;	Not significant
VITAMIN B6 (Pyridoxine)	Deficiency contributes to anemia;	Doses over 500mg/day can cause peripheral neuropathy!	Large doses will decrease effectiveness of Levodopa; oral contraceptives may increase the need for B_6;
VITAMIN B_{12}	Pernicious anemia	Not significant	Colchicines, alcohol, aspirin, may decrease absorption
FOLIC ACID	Megaloblastic anemia;	Large doses may promote seizures in epileptics;	Large doses impair Phenobarbital absorption; oral contraceptive may affect metabolism;
VITAMIN A	Immune impairment, dry skin and hair, eye disorders, impaired growth;	Liver damage, bone pain, fissures at mouth corners;	BCP may increase absorption;
VITAMIN D	Rickets; osteomalacia;	Very high doses: hypercalcemia, anorexia, nausea, H/A, depression, calcification of soft tissue, renal failure;	BCP may increase absorption; barbiturates may decrease effectiveness;
VITAMIN E	Muscle weakness	Nausea, diarrhea	Can potentiate action of blood thinners
VITAMIN K	Osteoporosis, coagulation problems	High doses may produce jaundice in infants	Antagonist of blood thinners

APPENDIX "D"

MINERAL DEFICIENCIES

NUTRIENT	DEFICIENCY	CONTRAINDICATIONS/ TOXICITY	MISCELLANEOUS/ INTERACTIONS
CALCIUM	Hypocalcemia, osteoporosis, muscle cramps, dental cavities;	Hypercalcemia;	Enhances effects of Digitalis; Decreases effects of tetracycline;
MAGNESIUM	Muscle spasms, poor growth, Tetany;	Arrhythmias, muscle weakness, diarrhea;	Depleted by some diuretics; Enhances CNS depressants;
SODIUM	Weight loss, electrolytes imbalance, nausea;	Hypernatremia, muscle weakness, CNS agitation, arrhythmias;	Very unlikely to have a deficiency state, as sodium is in every food;
POTASSIUM	Muscle weakness, arrhythmia, impaired growth, sterility;	Gastro-intestinal distress, heart block, nausea/vomiting;	Interactions with diuretics;
IRON	Iron deficiency anemia, fatigue;	Increased inflammatory status, may promote autoimmune diseases;	Increases vitamin C absorption; coffee and tea decrease absorption, antacids decrease absorption;
COPPER	Anemia, bone diseases;	Nausea and vomiting, malaise, hemolysis, retinal damage, renal tubular disorders;	Interacts with Zinc absorption;
ZINC	Dermatitis, diarrhea, immune deficiency, impaired functions of the male reproductive system;	Diarrhea, anemia, leucopenia, CNS depression, copper deficiency, increased cholesterol, muscle in coordination;	Impaired tetracycline absorption; absorption enhanced by glucose, lactose, soy, red wine.

APPENDIX "E"

SIGNS AND SYMPTOMS OF MALABSORPTION

	SIGNS AND SYMPTOMS	DEFICIENT NUTRIENT
GENERAL	Weight loss	Calories
	Muscle wasting	Proteins
SKIN	Psoriasis, eczema, scaling;	Zinc, vitamin A, EFA;
	Pallor (pale);	Folic acid, Iron, Vitamin B_{12};
	Bleeding;	Vitamin C;
	Flaking dermatitis;	Proteins, EFA, zinc;
	Bruising;	Vitamin K;
	Thickening and dryness of skin;	EFA;
HAIR	Sparse and thin, depigmentation, easy to pull out;	Proteins, vitamin A, zinc, EFA;
EYES	History of night blindness;	Vitamin A;
	Photophobia, blurring;	Vitamin A;
MOUTH	Bleeding gums;	Vitamin C, bioflavonoids;
	Cheilosis (fissures in the corners of the mouth);	Riboflavin;
BLOOD	Anemia	Iron, Vitamin B_{12}, Folic acid;

APPENDIX F

POST-SURGERY NUTRITIONAL PROTOCOL*

1. **High potency multivitamin and mineral formula**: for general support and maintenance; *this formula may be taken prior to surgery as well;*

2. **Vitamin C with bioflavonoids:** 1-2 g/day; to improve the strength of the blood vessels and also for new collagen formation, as many blood vessels and tissues have been affected by surgery;

3. **Vitamin A** 10000-15000 IU/day; antioxidant; skin and membranes repair and support; caution when liver pathologies present and also contraindicated in pregnancy; return to 5000 IU/day after 5-7 days;

4. **Zinc** 30-45 mg/day; very strong healing properties;

5. **Vitamin E** 400 IU/day; reduces scarring;

6. **EFA:** flax seed oil, one to two tablespoons/day; anti-inflammatory and protective effects; may increase the rate of tissue repair;

7. **Proteolytic enzymes**; to reduce inflammation and swelling of the surgery site and to promote resorption of tissue debris.

Notes: *applied after surgery

- This protocol may reduce the convalesce period;
- Attention to the fact that high vitamin C intake may thin the blood; do not suggest it prior to surgery.

APPENDIX "G"

THE IMPORTANCE OF B VITAMINS IN THE ENERGY PRODUCTION PATHWAY

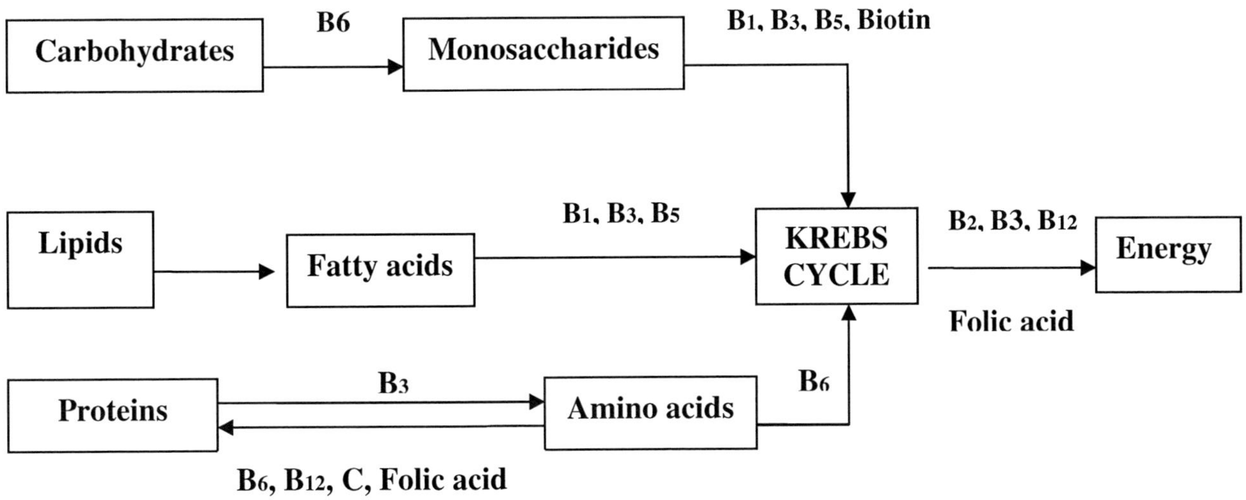

APPENDIX "H "

CHELATION THERAPY

Chelation is a therapeutic method utilizing chemical substances that attach to heavy metals in the body; as the chelating agent is eliminated (usually via urine), the heavy metal will be eliminated as well.

The word itself has its roots in the Greek word *(chela)* that describes the claw of a scorpion or crab. Historically speaking, chelating agents have been accepted since the time of the Second World War. Its beginnings employed a compound of sodium citrate that was used in 1941 to chelate lead from the bodies of people poisoned by this heavy metal. In time, research established that another compound, EDTA*, was able to remove heavy metals along with calcium (this is why chelation therapy is widely used (very controversially) in the treatment of cardio-vascular conditions).

Uses of chelation therapy

1. Cardio-vascular conditions (as it is eliminated from the body, EDTA will carry away calcium deposited in the arterial plaques, rendering the blood vessels much more elastic, therefore, improving the circulation and perfusion of the tissues);
    - Coronary Artery Disease;
    - High blood pressure (essential hypertension);
    - Peripheral circulation (Reynaud's disease);
    - Occlusion of blood flow to the extremities (intermittent claudication).
2. Heavy metal toxicity

Method:

This compound is introduced in the body intravenously, orally or as suppositories.
As it travels throughout the body, it "grabs" heavy metals from their hiding place and takes them with it via urine. Our bodies do not recognize or need EDTA, therefore it will be completely eliminated, along with its heavy load. Because it does not accumulate in our bodies, it will not elicit any side effects.

*EDTA stands for *ethyl diamine tetra acetic acid.*

GLOSSARY

Abscess: a collection of pus;
Acne: inflammation of skin;
Acute: severe symptoms and a short course;
Adipose: fatty;
Aerobic: requiring oxygen;
Anaerobic: in the absence of oxygen;
Angiography: radiography of the blood vessels;
Anorexia: loss of appetite;
Anoxia: oxygen deficiency;
Apoptosis: cell death;
Arrhythmia: abnormal heart rhythm
Arthritis: inflammation of the articular structures;
Astringent: reduces the size of tissues;
Asymptomatic: no symptoms;
Atria: upper heart chambers;
Atrophy: decrease in size of cells;
Auscultation: examination by listening.

BCP: birth control pills;
Benign: non malignant;
Bradypnea: low respiratory rate;
Bradycardia: low heart beat;
Buccal: pertaining to the cheek;

Calorie: unit of heat;
Cervical: refers to the neck;
CFS: chronic fatigue syndrome;
Cholecystitis: inflammation of the gall bladder;
Choryza: intense sneezing and runny nose;
Chronic: lasting for a long time (weeks, months);
Coagulation: clotting;
Colic: abdominal pain in children;
Conjunctivitis: inflammation of conjunctiva of the eye;
CTS: carpal tunnel syndrome;
Cutaneous: pertaining to skin
Cyanosis: bluish color of mucus membranes, due to lack of oxygen
Cystitis: inflammation of the urinary bladder

DVT: Deep Vein Thrombosis;
Deglutition: the act of swallowing;
Dehydration: condition arising because of excessive water loss;
Dermatitis: skin inflammation;
Dysbiosis: imbalance of gut flora
Dysmenorrhea: pain with menses;
Dyspareunia: pain with intercourse;
Dyspepsia: indigestion;
Dysphagia: difficulty swallowing;
Dysplasia: abnormal changes in the size and shape of cells;
Dyspnea: difficulty breathing;

Ectopic: not in the normal place;
Edema: accumulation of fluid;
Electrolyte: a substance that can conduct electricity;
Embolus: "traveling" obstacle which can lodge in a blood vessel;
Endocarditis: inflammation of the heart chambers lining;
Endocardium: the lining of the heart chambers;
Endometritis: inflammations of the uterus;
Enuresis: bed wetting;
Epistaxis: nose bleed;
EPO: evening primrose oil;
Eructation: belching;
Etiology: cause of disease;
Expiration: exhalation;

Fasciculation: small involuntary, local muscle contraction;
Flaccid: flabby, relaxed;

Flatulence: low gastro-intestinal tract gas;

Gangrene: death of tissue;
Gastralgia: stomach pain;
Geriatrics: specialty of medicine dealing with diseases of the aged;
Gerontology: the science that studies all aspects of aging;
Gestation: pertaining to pregnancy;
Gustation: pertaining to taste;
Gingivitis: inflammation of the gum;
Glossitis: inflammation of the tongue;
Goiter: benign enlargement of the thyroid gland;
Gynecology: specialty of medicine dealing with diseases of the genital tract.

H/A: headache;
Halitosis: bad breath;
Heart block: impaired transmission between the atria and the ventricles;
Hematemesis: upper gastro-intestinal bleeding;
Hematology: the science of blood elements'physiology and pathology;
Hematuria: passage of blood in urine;
Hemolysis: destruction of red blood cells;
Hemostasis: stoppage of blood flow;
HRT: hormone replacement therapy;
Hyperchlorhydria: high stomach acid;
Hyperglycemia: high blood sugar;
Hyperplasia: increase in cell number;
Hypertrophy: enlargement of an organ or part due to increase in size of its cells;
Hypochlorhydria: low stomach acid;
Hypoglycemia: low blood sugar;
Hypothermia: low body temperature;
Hypoxia: lack of Oxygen;
Hysterectomy: uterus removal.

IBD: Inflammatory Bowel Disease
IBS: Irritable Bowel Syndrome
Ileo-cecal valve: the valve that separates small from large intestine;
Infarct: localized area of ischemic necrosis;
Ingestion: taking a substance by mouth;
Inguinal: pertaining to the groin region;
Inspiration: inhalation;
Ischemic: lack of circulation.

Lacrimal: pertaining to tears;
LES: lupus erythematous disseminated;
Lesion: tissue injury or wound;
Leukocytosis: increased number of white blood cells
Lithotripsy: crushing of a urinary calculi
Lumen: the cavity within a tubular organ
Lymphadenopathy: swelling of the lymph nodes

Malabsorption: improper absorption
Malaise: a feeling of deep discomfort
Maldigestion: improper digestion
Malignant: cancerous
Melena: lower gastro-intestinal bleeding, black stools;
Menorrhagia: loss of blood with the menses;
Metabolism: all chemical reactions in the body;
Metastasis: spread of cancer;
Methrorrhagia: loss of blood between menses;
Micturition: urination;
Myocardium: the heart muscle;
Myometrium: the uterus muscle;
Myopia: nearsightedness;

Neuralgia: nerve pain;
Nocturia: urination in the nighttime;

Obstetrics: the branch of medicine dealing with pregnancy and labour;
Olfactory: pertains to smell;
Oncology: the study of tumors;
Onset: beginning, debut;
Ophthalmic: pertaining to the eye;
Oral: relating to the mouth;
Orchitis: inflammation of testis;
Osteopenia: reduced bone mass;
Osteoporosis: increased softening of bones;
Otic: pertaining to ear;

Palpation: examination by touch;
Palpitations: are perceived like "a *skipped beat";*
Paralysis: loss of muscle function;
Paraplegia: paralysis of the lower limbs;
Paresthesia: "pins and needles";
Parotiditis: inflammation of the parotid glands;
Pathogen: disease causing microorganism;
Pericarditis: inflammation of the pericardium;
Pericardium: outer layer of the heart;
Peritoneum: the lining of organs in the abdominal cavity;
Peritonitis: inflammation of the peritoneum;
Phlebitis: inflammation of the veins;
Phytoestrogens: estrogen like molecules from plants;
Plantar: pertaining to the sole of the foot;
Pleura: membrane covering the lungs;
Pleurisy: inflammation of pleura;
PMS: Premenstrual syndrome;
Pneumothorax: introducing of air in the pleural space;
Polycystic: containing many cysts;
Proctitis: inflammation of the rectal mucosa;
Prolapse: uterus or vagina slip forward
Prophylaxis: prevention;
Proteinuria: passage of proteins in the urine;
PUD: peptic ulcer disease
Pylorus: the final portion of the stomach;
Pyuria: pus in urine;

RA: rheumatoid arthritis;
RBC: red blood cells;

Salpingitis: inflammations the ovaries and/or the fallopian tubes;
Secretion: cellular product excreted to the exterior;
Septicemia: infection of blood;
Sign: objective, noticeable and /or measurable evidence pertaining to a person's status (rash, fever);
Sphincter: a muscular ring;
Stenosis: abnormal constriction or narrowing;
Stricture: narrowing;
Symptoms: subjective evidence, as perceived by a person (headache, abdominal pain);
Systemic: general, applied to the whole body;

Tachypnea: fast respiratory rate;
Tachycardia: fast heart beat;
Tendons: connective tissue that attaches the muscle to bone;
Thrombus: a stationary clot;
Tonus: muscle tone;

Ulcer: a loss of substance;
Urea: end product of protein metabolism;
Urethritis: inflammation of urethra;
Urinary calculi: kidney stones;

Vaginitis: inflammation of vaginal mucosa;
Varicocele: small varicose veins of the scrotum;
Vasoconstriction: narrowing of blood vessels;
Vasodilation: expansion of blood vessels;
Ventricles: lower heart chambers;
Vertigo: dizziness;
Vesicles: blisters;
Visceral: pertaining to the internal organs;

WBC: white blood cells;
Wheezing: a whistling respiratory sound;

Xenoestrogens: synthetic estrogen like molecules.

BIBLIOGRAPHY

Alternative Therapies, May-June 2004, vol.10 no 3;
Alternative Medicine Review, vol.9, no2, June 2004;
Alternative therapies in women's health, July 2004, vol.6 no7;
American Journal of Medicine, July 15, vol. 117, no2;
American Journal of Medicine, July 1, 2004, vol. 117 #1;
American Journal of Preventive Medicine, vol. 27(1), July 2004;
Annals of Allergy, Asthma and Immunology, June 2004, volume 92, no6. Published by American College of Allergy, Asthma and Immunology;
Austin, Steve, ND and Cathy Hitchcock, MSW. *"Breast Cancer, What You Should Know (but may not be told) about Prevention, Diagnosis and Treatment*, Prima Publishing, Rocklin, California, 1994;
Balch, James F. MD, and Phyllis A. Balch, C.N.C. "*Prescription for Nutritional Healing*", second edition, Avery, 1997;
Bateson-Koch, Carolee DC, ND. *"Allergies, Disease in Disguise"*. Alive Books, 1994;
Baumel, Syd. "*Dealing with Depression Naturally*". Keats publishing, 1995;
Bonnard, Marc, MD. *"The Viagra Alternative"*. Healing Arts Press, Rochester, Vermont, 1999;
Brecher, Harold and Arlene. *"Forty Something Forever, A Consumer's Guide to Chelation; Therapy and other Heart-Savers"*. Health Savers Press, Herndon, Virginia, 2000 ;
Brewer, Dr. Sarah and Michelle Berriedale-Johnson. "*Eat to Beat IBS*". Thorson Hammersmith, London 2004;
Cabot, Dr. Sandra, MD. "*The Liver Cleansing Diet*". SCB International Inc, 1996;
Canadian Journal of Dietetic Practice and Research, no 09797;
The Canadian Journal of Herbalism, 2004, vol. xxv, no2;
Cass, Hyla M.D. "*St. John's Wort, Nature's Blues Buster*". Avery Publishing Group, 1999;
Challem, Jack, Burton Berkson, M.D.Melissa Diane Smith. "*Syndrome X*"> Published by John Wiley & Sons, Inc.2000;
Clapp, Larry. *"Prostate Health in 90 Days"*. Hay House Inc., Carlsbad, California, 1997;
Clinical Nutrition Review, Oct 2001, vol. 21, 34;
Clinical Practice of Alternative Medicine, vol.3 no1, spring 2001;
Cotran, Ramzi S., M.D., Vinay Kumar, M.D., Stanley L. Robbins, M.D. "*Robbins-Pathologic Basis of Disease*". W.B. Saunders Company, 1994;
Curry, Katharine R., Any Jaffe. "*Nutrition Counseling and Communications skills*". W.B. Saunders Company, 1998;
Cutler, Ellen W., DC. "*Winning the War against Immune Disorders and Allergies*". Delmar Publishers, 1998;
Davies, Brenda, RD & Tom Barnard, MD. "*Defeating Diabetes*", Healthy Living Publications, Summertown Tennessee, 2003;
Davies, Jill Rosemary. "*Saw Palmetto*". Element Books Limited, 2000;
Erasmus, Udo. "*Fats and oils*". Alive Books, Vancouver, BC, 1986;
European Journal of Clinical Nutrition, vol. 58, no1, January 2004;
European Journal of Clinical Nutrition, vol. 58, no7, July 2004;
European Journal of Herbal Medicine, vol.5, no2, Summer 2000;
Evidence based Preventive Medicine, vol. 1, #2, 2004;
Evidence based Preventive Medicine, vol. 1 #1, 2003;

Evidence based Integrative Medicine, vol. 1, #2, 2004;
Fetrow, C.W., PharmD, Juan R. Avila, PharmD, "*Professional's handbook of Complementary and Alternative Medicines*", second edition, Springhouse, Pennsylvania, 2001;
Frahm, Anne E with David J. Frahm. "*A Cancer Battle Plan*". Jeremy P. Tarcher, Putnam, NY 1992;
Frahm, Dave, "*Cancer Battle Plan Source Book*". Jeremy Tarcher, Putnam NY 2000;
Grossman, Marc, & Glen Swartwout. "*Natural Eye Care*". Keats Publishing, 1999;
Gursche, Siegfried MH, Zoltan Rona, M.D., MSc. "*Encyclopedia of Natural Healing*", Alive Books, 1997;
Haas, Elson M., M.D., "*Staying Healthy with Nutrition*". Celestial Arts, Berkeley, California, 1992;
Heineman, John. "*Heinemann's Encyclopedia of Nuts, Berries and Seeds*". Parker Publishing Company, New York, 1995;
Herbs for Health, august 2004;
Herbs foe Health, Nov/Dec 2003;
Hudson, Tori, ND. "*Women's Encyclopedia of Natural Medicine*". Keats Publishing, Los Angeles, 1999;
Ingham, Christine. "*Panic Attacks*". Thorsons, 2000;
Integrative Cancer Therapies, vol.3 no2, June 2004;
Integrative Cancer Therapies, vol.3 no1, March 2004
Journal of Medicinal Food, vol.7 no1, spring 2004;
Journal of Medicinal Food, vol. 7 no2, summer 2004;
Journal of Nutrition, Education and behavior, vol 36, no3, May-June 2004;
Journal of Nutritional sciences and Vitaminology, vol.50, #2, 2004;
Kaur, Sat Dharam. "*A call to Women*". Quarry Health Books, Kingston, Ontario, 2000;
Legato, Marianne J., MD, and Carol Colman. "*The female heart*". Quill Harper Collins Books, 2000;
L'esperance, Carrie. "*The Seasonal Detoxification Diet*". Healing Arts Press, Rochester, Vermont, 2002;
Levin, Buck, PhD, RD. "*Environmental Nutrition, Understanding the link between Environment, Food Quality and Disease*", Hinge Pin, Washington, 1990;
Marieb, Elaine N. "*Essentials of Human Anatomy and Physiology*". Seventh Edition, Benjamin Cummings, 2003;
Matsen, Dr. Jonn ND, "*Eating Alive, Prevention Thru Good Digestion*". Crompton Books, North Vancouver, 2002;
McCance, Kathryn L., Sue E. Huether. "*Pathophysiology, The Biologic Basis for Disease in Adults and Children*", Third edition. Mosby, 1998;
Meara, Dr. Jolyon and Professor William C. Koller. "*Parkinson Disease and Parkinsonism in the Elderly*". Cambridge University Press, 2000;
Mendelsohn, Robert S., MD. "*Confessions of a Medical Heretic*". Contemporary Books, 1979;
Mindell, Earl, R.Ph., Ph.D "*Earl Mindell's antiaging bible*". A Fireside Book, New York, 1996;
Moore, Richard D. "*The High Blood Pressure Solution*". Healing Arts Press, Rochester, Vermont, 2001;
Moss, Ralph W. PhD. "*Herbs Against Cancer-History and Controversy*". Equinox Press Inc. New York, 1998;
Murray, "Michael T. "*Diabetes and Hypoglycemia*". Prima Publishing, Roseville, California, 1994;
Murray, Michael, ND and Joseph Pizzorno, ND. "*Encyclopedia of Natural Medicine*". Prima Health, a division of Prima Publishing, 1998;

Nelson, Miriam E. "*Strong Women and Men Beat Arthritis*". A Perigree Book, published by The Berkeley Publishing Group, NY 2002;
Northrup, Christiane. "*Women's Bodies, Women's Wisdom*". Bantam Books, 1998;
Nutrition Research Newsletter, vol. XXIII, #7, July 2004;
Olivier, Suzannah, "*The Detox Manual*". Pocket Books, an imprint of Simon and Shuster, UK, Ltd.;
Pagana, Kathleen D., Timothy J Pagana. "*Mosby's Manual of Diagnostic and Laboratory Tests*". Mosby 1998;
Pepe, Celeste, DC, ND, and Lisa Hammond, "*Reversing MS-9 effective steps to recover your health*". Hampton Roads Publishing Company Inc 2001;
Pizzorno, Joseph E. Jr., Michael T. Murray. "*Textbook of Natural Medicine*", second edition, Churchill Livingstone, 1999;
Premkumar, Dr.Kalyani, "*Pathology A to Z-a Handbook for Massage Therapists*". Van Pub Books, Calgary, 1999;
Redmon, George L, PhD, ND. "*Energy for Life*". Vital Health Publishing, 2000;
Sharon, Dr. Michael. "*Complete Nutrition-how to live in total health*". Imago, 1989,
Swank, Roy Laver, MD, PhD, and Barbara Brewer Dugan. "*The Multiple Sclerosis Diet Book*", Doubleday, 1987;
The American Journal of Cardiology, Nov 6, 2003;
The Journal of Nutrition, vol.134 no7, July 2004;
The Lancet, vol.364, no 9429, July 10-16, 2004;
The Merck Manual, Seventeenth Edition, Published by Merck Research Laboratories, 1999;
The New England Journal of Medicine, vol 351 no 3, July 15, 2004;
The New England Journal of Medicine, vol 351 no 6, august 5, 2004;
The New England Journal of Medicine, vol 351 no 5, July 29, 2004;
Townsend Letter for Doctors and Patients, no 252, July 2004;
Townsend Letter for Doctors and Patients, 3238, May 2003;
Townsend Letter for Doctors and Patients, no 239, June 2003;
Townsend Letter for Doctors and Patients, no 240, July 2003;
Townsend Letter for Doctors and Patients, no. 241/242, august Sept. 2003;
Whillier, Stephney. "*Nutritional Pathology and the Health Care of the Future*". CSNN Publishing, 1999.

INDEX

A

B

C

INDEX OF TABLES

Chapter 11: Nervous system disorders

Chapter 12: Ophthalmologic, ear, nose and throat disorders

Chapter 13: Endocrine and metabolic disorders

Chapter 14: Integumentary system diseases

Chapter 15: Pulmonary disorders

Chapter 16: Cardiovascular disorders

Chapter 17: Hematology and oncology

INDEX OF DIAGRAMS

Chapter 13: Endocrine and metabolic disorders

Chapter 16: Cardiovascular disorders

Chapter 17: Hematology and oncology